Nutrition, Exercise, and End-of-Life Discussion in the Cardiovascular Field

Nutrition, Exercise, and End-of-Life Discussion in the Cardiovascular Field

Editor

Yoshihiro Fukumoto

MDPI • Basel • Beijing • Wuhan • Barcelona • Belgrade • Manchester • Tokyo • Cluj • Tianjin

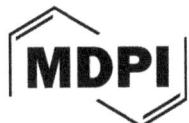

Editor
Yoshihiro Fukumoto
Kurume University School of
Medicine
Japan

Editorial Office
MDPI
St. Alban-Anlage 66
4052 Basel, Switzerland

This is a reprint of articles from the Special Issue published online in the open access journal *Nutrients* (ISSN 2072-6643) (available at: https://www.mdpi.com/journal/nutrients/special_issues/ Nutrition_Exercise_and_End_of_Life_Discussion_in_the_Cardiovascular_Field).

For citation purposes, cite each article independently as indicated on the article page online and as indicated below:

LastName, A.A.; LastName, B.B.; LastName, C.C. Article Title. *Journal Name* **Year**, *Volume Number*, Page Range.

ISBN 978-3-0365-3891-4 (Hbk)
ISBN 978-3-0365-3892-1 (PDF)

© 2022 by the authors. Articles in this book are Open Access and distributed under the Creative Commons Attribution (CC BY) license, which allows users to download, copy and build upon published articles, as long as the author and publisher are properly credited, which ensures maximum dissemination and a wider impact of our publications.

The book as a whole is distributed by MDPI under the terms and conditions of the Creative Commons license CC BY-NC-ND.

Contents

About the Editor ix

Yoshihiro Fukumoto
Nutrition and Cardiovascular Diseases
Reprinted from: *Nutrients* **2022**, *14*, 94, doi:10.3390/nu14010094 1

Yuki Ishida, Daigo Yoshida, Takanori Honda, Yoichiro Hirakawa, Mao Shibata, Satoko Sakata, Yoshihiko Furuta, Emi Oishi, Jun Hata, Takanari Kitazono and Toshiharu Ninomiya
Influence of the Accumulation of Unhealthy Eating Habits on Obesity in a General Japanese Population: The Hisayama Study
Reprinted from: *Nutrients* **2020**, *12*, 3160, doi:10.3390/nu13113916 5

Ruixin Zhu, Mikael Fogelholm, Sally D. Poppitt, Marta P. Silvestre, Grith Møller, Maija Huttunen-Lenz, Gareth Stratton, Jouko Sundvall, Laura Råman, Elli Jalo, Moira A. Taylor, Ian A. Macdonald, Svetoslav Handjiev, Teodora Handjieva-Darlenska, J. Alfredo Martinez, Roslyn Muirhead, Jennie Brand-Miller and Anne Raben
Adherence to a Plant-Based Diet and Consumption of Specific Plant Foods—Associations with 3-Year Weight-Loss Maintenance and Cardiometabolic Risk Factors: A Secondary Analysis of the PREVIEW Intervention Study
Reprinted from: *Nutrients* **2021**, *13*, 3916, doi:10.3390/nu13113916 15

Chaochen Wang, Hiroshi Yatsuya, Yingsong Lin, TaeSasakabe, Sayo Kawai, Shogo Kikuchi, Hiroyasu Iso and Akiko Tamakoshi
Milk Intake and Stroke Mortality in the Japan Collaborative Cohort Study—A Bayesian Survival Analysis
Reprinted from: *Nutrients* **2020**, *12*, 2743, doi:10.3390/nu12092743 31

Urban Alehagen, Jan Aaseth, Tomas L. Lindahl, Anders Larsson and Jan Alexander
Dietary Supplementation with Selenium and Coenzyme Q_{10} Prevents Increase in Plasma D-Dimer While Lowering Cardiovascular Mortality in an Elderly Swedish Population
Reprinted from: *Nutrients* **2021**, *13*, 1344, doi:10.3390/nu13041344 43

Futoshi Eto, Kazuo Washida, Masaki Matsubara, Hisashi Makino, Akio Takahashi, Kotaro Noda, Yorito Hattori, Yuriko Nakaoku, Kunihiro Nishimura, Kiminori Hosoda and Masafumi Ihara
Glucose Fluctuation and Severe Internal Carotid Artery Siphon Stenosis in Type 2 Diabetes Patients
Reprinted from: *Nutrients* **2021**, *13*, 2379, doi:10.3390/nu13072379 57

Miki Sugiyama, Takuma Hazama, Kaoru Nakano, Kengo Urae, Tomofumi Moriyama, Takuya Ariyoshi, Yuka Kurokawa, Goh Kodama, Yoshifumi Wada, Junko Yano, Yoshihiko Otsubo, Ryuji Iwatani, Yukie Kinoshita, Yusuke Kaida, Makoto Nasu, Ryo Shibata, Kyoko Tashiro and Kei Fukami
Effects of Reducing L-Carnitine Supplementation on Carnitine Kinetics and Cardiac Function in Hemodialysis Patients: A Multicenter, Single-Blind, Placebo-Controlled, Randomized Clinical Trial
Reprinted from: *Nutrients* **2021**, *13*, 1900, doi:10.3390/nu13061900 69

Keiko Matsuzaki, Nobuko Fukushima, Yutaka Saito, Naoya Matsumoto, Mayu Nagaoka, Yousuke Katsuda and Shin-ichiro Miura
The Effects of Long-Term Nutrition Counseling According to the Behavioral Modification Stages in Patients with Cardiovascular Disease
Reprinted from: *Nutrients* 2021, *13*, 414, doi:10.3390/nu13020414 81

Tomoaki Okada, Toru Miyoshi, Masayuki Doi, Kosuke Seiyama, Wataru Takagi, Masahiro Sogo, Kazumasa Nosaka, Masahiko Takahashi, Keisuke Okawa and Hiroshi Ito
Secular Decreasing Trend in Plasma Eicosapentaenoic and Docosahexaenoic Acids among Patients with Acute Coronary Syndrome from 2011 to 2019: A Single Center Descriptive Study
Reprinted from: *Nutrients* 2021, *13*, 253, doi:10.3390/nu13010253 95

Andrea Greco, Agostino Brugnera, Roberta Adorni, Marco D'Addario, Francesco Fattirolli, Cristina Franzelli, Cristina Giannattasio, Alessandro Maloberti, Francesco Zanatta and Patrizia Steca
Protein Intake and Physical Activity in Newly Diagnosed Patients with Acute Coronary Syndrome: A 5-Year Longitudinal Study
Reprinted from: *Nutrients* 2021, *13*, 634, doi:10.3390/nu13020634 107

Naoki Itaya, Ako Fukami, Tatsuyuki Kakuma and Yoshihiro Fukumoto
Nutrition Status and Renal Function as Predictors in Acute Myocardial Infarction with and without Cancer: A Single Center Retrospective Study
Reprinted from: *Nutrients* 2021, *13*, 2663, doi:10.3390/nu13082663 123

Naoaki Matsuo, Toru Miyoshi, Atsushi Takaishi, Takao Kishinoue, Kentaro Yasuhara, Masafumi Tanimoto, Yukari Nakano, Nobuhiko Onishi, Masayuki Ueeda and Hiroshi Ito
High Plasma Docosahexaenoic Acid Associated to Better Prognoses of Patients with Acute Decompensated Heart Failure with Preserved Ejection Fraction
Reprinted from: *Nutrients* 2021, *13*, 371, doi:10.3390/nu13020371 137

Yoshikuni Obata, Naoya Kakutani, Shintaro Kinugawa, Arata Fukushima, Takashi Yokota, Shingo Takada, Taisuke Ono, Takeshi Sota, Yoshiharu Kinugasa, Masashige Takahashi, Hisashi Matsuo, Ryuichi Matsukawa, Ichiro Yoshida, Isao Yokota, Kazuhiro Yamamoto and Miyuki Tsuchihashi-Makaya
Impact of Inadequate Calorie Intake on Mortality and Hospitalization in Stable Patients with Chronic Heart Failure
Reprinted from: *Nutrients* 2021, *13*, 874, doi:10.3390/nu13030874 151

Kenya Kusunose, Yuichiro Okushi, Yoshihiro Okayama, Robert Zheng, Miho Abe, Michikazu Nakai, Yoko Sumita, Takayuki Ise, Takeshi Tobiume, Koji Yamaguchi, Shusuke Yagi, Daiju Fukuda, Hirotsugu Yamada, Takeshi Soeki, Tetsuzo Wakatsuki and Masataka Sata
Association between Vitamin D and Heart Failure Mortality in 10,974 Hospitalized Individuals
Reprinted from: *Nutrients* 2021, *13*, 335, doi:10.3390/nu13020335 161

Tatsuhiro Shibata, Kazutoshi Mawatari, Naoko Nakashima, Koutatsu Shimozono, Kouko Ushijima, Yumiko Yamaji, Kumi Tetsuka, Miki Murakami, Kouta Okabe, Toshiyuki Yanai, Shoichiro Nohara, Jinya Takahashi, Hiroki Aoki, Hideo Yasukawa and Yoshihiro Fukumoto
Multidisciplinary Team-Based Palliative Care for Heart Failure and Food Intake at the End of Life
Reprinted from: *Nutrients* 2021, *13*, 2387, doi:10.3390/nu13072387 173

About the Editor

Yoshihiro Fukumoto: MD, PhD, FJCC, FESC, FAHA, FJCS. Professor and Chairman, Division of Cardiovascular Medicine, Department of Internal Medicine, Kurume University School of Medicine. Deputy Director of Kurume University Hospital. He works in the cardiology field, especially on atherosclerosis, heart failure, pulmonary hypertension, and onco-cardiology.

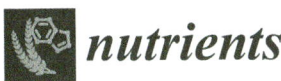

Editorial

Nutrition and Cardiovascular Diseases

Yoshihiro Fukumoto

Division of Cardiovascular Medicine, Department of Internal Medicine, Kurume University School of Medicine, Kurume 830-0011, Japan; fukumoto_yoshihiro@med.kurume-u.ac.jp; Tel.: +81-942-31-7562; Fax: +81-942-33-6509

Citation: Fukumoto, Y. Nutrition and Cardiovascular Diseases. *Nutrients* 2022, 14, 94. https://doi.org/10.3390/nu14010094

Received: 30 November 2021
Accepted: 16 December 2021
Published: 27 December 2021

Publisher's Note: MDPI stays neutral with regard to jurisdictional claims in published maps and institutional affiliations.

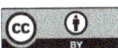

Copyright: © 2021 by the author. Licensee MDPI, Basel, Switzerland. This article is an open access article distributed under the terms and conditions of the Creative Commons Attribution (CC BY) license (https://creativecommons.org/licenses/by/4.0/).

Unhealthy food intake and insufficient physical activities are related with obesity or life-style diseases, which can cause cardiovascular diseases, finally leading to death [1,2]. First, to prevent the progression of obesity or life-style diseases, nutrition and exercise are the most important issues. However, many people are not aware of their importance. Second, after the development of obesity or life-style diseases, nutrition and exercise control with appropriate medical therapies are required. Still, many patients do not recognize this. Third, after the cardiovascular diseases, nutrition and exercise with optimal medical and/or interventional therapies are required. However, some patients are not able to control their food intake and physical activities. Finally, patients with end-stage cardiovascular diseases need their end-of-life discussion. In the current Special Issue of Nutrients, the importance of nutrition was reported before and after cardiovascular diseases development.

Regarding BEFORE cardiovascular diseases development, Wang et al. [3] have shown the strong evidence that daily milk intake among Japanese men was associated with delayed and lower risk of mortality from stroke (especially cerebral infarction, using data from the JACC study) as a good eating habit. The time before an event of stroke mortality occurred was slowed down among men who drank milk regularly. [3] Also in the aspect of healthy food, Zhu et al. [4] have demonstrated that their secondary analysis showed that long-term consumption of specific healthy plant foods including nuts, fruits, and vegetables improved weight management and cardiometabolic health, whereas adherence to an overall plant-based diets benefited weight management only, supporting the hypothesis that specific components in plant-based diets are important as well. As a good habit in a high-risk group, Alehagen et al. [5] have reported the relationship between D-dimer and a dietary supplement consisting of selenium and coenzyme Q10 in an elderly community-living population. They observed a significantly reduced cardiovascular mortality in the population with a high D-dimer level when given selenium and coenzyme Q10, as compared to those on placebo [5].

Conversely, unhealthy food issues were also reported. Ishida et al. [6] have revealed dose-response-positive associations between the number of accumulated unhealthy eating habits and the likelihood of obesity and central obesity in a general Japanese population, suggesting that modifying individual unhealthy eating habits and avoiding their accumulation might reduce the burden of obesity and central obesity [6]. As indicated in this article, healthcare professionals need to encourage those who have unhealthy eating habits to modify each of their habits individually, including avoidance of accumulating multiple unhealthy habits, in order to prevent cardiovascular diseases [6]. Further longitudinal studies should be performed to examine whether a causal relationship exists between the accumulation of unhealthy eating habits and the incidence of obesity or central obesity [6].

Regarding AFTER cardiovascular diseases development, the importance of nutrition in various types of cardiovascular diseases was reported. Matsuzaki et al. [7] have demonstrated that acquisition of effective behaviour modifications by long-term nutrition counselling, according to behavioural modification stages, was important for patients with cardiovascular diseases.

In acute coronary syndrome (ACS), Okada et al. [8] have found a decreasing trend in eicosapentaenoic acid (EPA) and docosahexaenoic acid (DHA) levels, and EPA to arachidonic acid ratio in men from 2011 to 2019 without significant changes in low-density lipoprotein and high-density lipoprotein cholesterol levels, in which decreasing trend in EPA and DHA levels did not depend on age and was significant only in men in patients with ACS. Administration of a sufficient dose of n-3 polyunsaturated fatty acids may be effective in the secondary prevention of ACS, but further studies are needed to obtain robust evidence. Next, Creco A, et al. [9] have indicated that patients with ACS experience difficulties in achieving and mostly maintaining adequate levels of a healthy diet and physical activity over time, of which difficulties were modulated by environmental conditions, and most importantly, by psychological characteristics, suggesting how to perform tailor diet and physical activity interventions. They considered that tailoring should be aimed at promoting cognitive awareness of the risks associated with cardiovascular diseases recurrence. In fact, they showed that patients, who were more anxious, and therefore more concerned and somehow aware of their health, were more able to maintain healthy behaviour over time [9]. Cognitive awareness of the risks associated with cardiovascular diseases recurrence may be a useful tool to sustain patients' capabilities to self-regulate their behaviours and to ameliorate lifestyle behaviour [9]. In atherosclerosis, blood glucose fluctuations are also important. Eto et al. [10] have indicated that patients with severe internal carotid artery siphon stenosis had higher blood glucose fluctuations as assessed with standard deviation, coefficient of variation, and mean amplitude of glycaemic excursions. Meanwhile, there were no significant differences in other vascular risk factors, such as hypertension, dyslipidaemia, mean blood glucose levels, haemoglobin A1c, and duration in years of type 2 diabetes mellitus, suggesting that glucose fluctuation can be a target of preventive therapies for intracranial artery stenosis and ischemic stroke [10].

In advanced cardiovascular diseases, low nutrition status is another problem. In this special issue, the correlation between nutrition status and acute myocardial infarction (AMI) with cancer was also reported. Itaya et al. [11] have indicated that the prevalence of cancer in AMI was 13%, and that worse nutrition status and renal dysfunction were associated with AMI with cancer, in which nutrition status was a major different characteristic from non-cancer. Further, they have developed formulas to predict the presence of cancer in AMI [11].

Next, in heart failure (HF), Kurunose et al. [12] have shown that patients with vitamin D supplementation had a lower in-hospital mortality for HF than patients without vitamin D supplementation in the propensity matched cohort. The causality should be tested in the future RCTs in specific population based on their study [12]. As also reported in ACS, Matsuo et al. [13] have found that low plasma DHA levels were significantly associated with an increase in all-cause death in patients with acute decompensated heart failure with preserved ejection fraction (HFpEF), independent of nutritional status, in which measurement of plasma DHA levels may be useful in identifying high-risk patients with HFpEF, and supplementation with DHA may be a potential therapeutic target in these patients.

After HF development, adequate nutrition intake is important. Obata et al. [14] indicated that inadequate dietary calorie intake was independently associated with an increased risk of adverse clinical events including all-cause death and hospitalization due to worsening HF in stable patients with chronic HF. To meet the humanly end of HF life, nutritional care is quite important. Shibata et al. [15] have demonstrated that HF palliative care team activities were able to provide an opportunity to discuss end-of-life care with patients, reduce the burden of physical and mental symptoms, and shift the goals of end-of-life nutritional care to ensuring comfort and quality of life.

In patients with end-stage kidney disease, HF is a serious condition characterized by decreased myocardial contractility and abnormal hemodynamic state [16]. It has been demonstrated that L-carnitine supplementation could improve clinical symptoms and cardiac function and decrease serum levels of B-type natriuretic peptide (BNP) and NT-proBNP in patients with chronic HF, [17] which might also improve cardiac function in hemodialysis patients [18], suggesting that L-carnitine treatment may have protective effects on HF in hemodialysis patients with carnitine deficiency. In the current issue,

Sugiyama et al. [16] have reported that reducing L-carnitine administration for six months significantly decreased both plasma and red blood cell carnitine levels. Moreover, stopping L-carnitine increased plasma BNP levels. However, this stoppage did not influence cardiac function in hemodialysis patients [16].

Nutrition should be considered before and after cardiovascular development. According to these findings, we should pay more attention to preventive and therapeutic strategies for cardiovascular diseases.

Conflicts of Interest: The authors declare no conflict of interest.

References

1. Adachi, H.; Enomoto, M.; Fukami, A.; Nakamura, S.; Nohara, Y.; Kono, S.; Sakaue, A.; Hamamura, H.; Toyomasu, K.; Yamamoto, M.; et al. Trends in nutritional intake and coronary risk factors over 60 years among Japanese men in Tanushimaru. *Heart Vessel.* **2020**, *35*, 901–908. [CrossRef] [PubMed]
2. Sakaue, A.; Adachi, H.; Enomoto, M.; Fukami, A.; Kumagai, E.; Nakamura, S.; Nohara, Y.; Kono, S.; Nakao, E.; Morikawa, N.; et al. Association between physical activity, occupational sitting time and mortality in a general population: An 18-year prospective survey in Tanushimaru, Japan. *Eur. J. Prev. Cardiol.* **2020**, *27*, 758–766. [CrossRef] [PubMed]
3. Wang, C.; Yatsuya, H.; Lin, Y.; Sasakabe, T.; Kawai, S.; Kikuchi, S.; Iso, H.; Tamakoshi, A. Milk Intake and Stroke Mortality in the Japan Collaborative Cohort Study—A Bayesian Survival Analysis. *Nutrients* **2020**, *12*, 2743. [CrossRef] [PubMed]
4. Zhu, R.; Robertson, K.; Protudjer, J.L.; Macikunas, A.; Kim, R.; Jeimy, S.; Kim, H. Impact of age on adherence and efficacy of peanut oral-immunotherapy using a standardized protocol. *Pediatr. Allergy Immunol.* **2021**, *32*, 783–786. [CrossRef] [PubMed]
5. Alehagen, U.; Aaseth, J.; Lindahl, T.; Larsson, A.; Alexander, J. Dietary Supplementation with Selenium and Coenzyme Q_{10} Prevents Increase in Plasma D-Dimer While Lowering Cardiovascular Mortality in an Elderly Swedish Population. *Nutrients* **2021**, *13*, 1344. [CrossRef] [PubMed]
6. Ishida, Y.; Yoshida, D.; Honda, T.; Hirakawa, Y.; Shibata, M.; Sakata, S.; Furuta, Y.; Oishi, E.; Hata, J.; Kitazono, T.; et al. Influence of the Accumulation of Unhealthy Eating Habits on Obesity in a General Japanese Population: The Hisayama Study. *Nutrients* **2020**, *12*, 3160. [CrossRef] [PubMed]
7. Matsuzaki, K.; Fukushima, N.; Saito, Y.; Matsumoto, N.; Nagaoka, M.; Katsuda, Y.; Miura, S.-I. The Effects of Long-Term Nutrition Counseling According to the Behavioral Modification Stages in Patients with Cardiovascular Disease. *Nutrients* **2021**, *13*, 414. [CrossRef] [PubMed]
8. Okada, T.; Miyoshi, T.; Doi, M.; Seiyama, K.; Takagi, W.; Sogo, M.; Nosaka, K.; Takahashi, M.; Okawa, K.; Ito, H. Secular Decreasing Trend in Plasma Eicosapentaenoic and Docosahexaenoic Acids among Patients with Acute Coronary Syndrome from 2011 to 2019: A Single Center Descriptive Study. *Nutrients* **2021**, *13*, 253. [CrossRef] [PubMed]
9. Greco, A.; Brugnera, A.; Adorni, R.; D'Addario, M.; Fattirolli, F.; Franzelli, C.; Giannattasio, C.; Maloberti, A.; Zanatta, F.; Steca, P. Protein Intake and Physical Activity in Newly Diagnosed Patients with Acute Coronary Syndrome: A 5-Year Longitudinal Study. *Nutrients* **2021**, *13*, 634. [CrossRef]
10. Eto, F.; Washida, K.; Matsubara, M.; Makino, H.; Takahashi, A.; Noda, K.; Hattori, Y.; Nakaoku, Y.; Nishimura, K.; Hosoda, K.; et al. Glucose Fluctuation and Severe Internal Carotid Artery Siphon Stenosis in Type 2 Diabetes Patients. *Nutrients* **2021**, *13*, 2379. [CrossRef]
11. Itaya, N.; Fukami, A.; Kakuma, T.; Fukumoto, Y. Nutrition Status and Renal Function as Predictors in Acute Myocardial Infarction with and without Cancer: A Single Center Retrospective Study. *Nutrients* **2021**, *13*, 2663. [CrossRef]
12. Kusunose, K.; Okushi, Y.; Okayama, Y.; Zheng, R.; Abe, M.; Nakai, M.; Sumita, Y.; Ise, T.; Tobiume, T.; Yamaguchi, K.; et al. Association between Vitamin D and Heart Failure Mortality in 10,974 Hospitalized Individuals. *Nutrients* **2021**, *13*, 335. [CrossRef]
13. Matsuo, N.; Miyoshi, T.; Takaishi, A.; Kishinoue, T.; Yasuhara, K.; Tanimoto, M.; Nakano, Y.; Onishi, N.; Ueeda, M.; Ito, H. High Plasma Docosahexaenoic Acid Associated to Better Prognoses of Patients with Acute Decompensated Heart Failure with Preserved Ejection Fraction. *Nutrients* **2021**, *13*, 371. [CrossRef]
14. Obata, Y.; Kakutani, N.; Kinugawa, S.; Fukushima, A.; Yokota, T.; Takada, S.; Ono, T.; Sota, T.; Kinugasa, Y.; Takahashi, M.; et al. Impact of Inadequate Calorie Intake on Mortality and Hospitalization in Stable Patients with Chronic Heart Failure. *Nutrients* **2021**, *13*, 874. [CrossRef] [PubMed]
15. Shibata, T.; Mawatari, K.; Nakashima, N.; Shimozono, K.; Ushijima, K.; Yamaji, Y.; Tetsuka, K.; Murakami, M.; Okabe, K.; Yanai, T.; et al. Multidisciplinary Team-Based Palliative Care for Heart Failure and Food Intake at the End of Life. *Nutrients* **2021**, *13*, 2387. [CrossRef]
16. Sugiyama, M.; Hazama, T.; Nakano, K.; Urae, K.; Moriyama, T.; Ariyoshi, T.; Kurokawa, Y.; Kodama, G.; Wada, Y.; Yano, J.; et al. Effects of Reducing L-Carnitine Supplementation on Carnitine Kinetics and Cardiac Function in Hemodialysis Patients: A Multicenter, Single-Blind, Placebo-Controlled, Randomized Clinical Trial. *Nutrients* **2021**, *13*, 1900. [CrossRef]

17. Song, X.; Qu, H.; Yang, Z.; Rong, J.; Cai, W.; Zhou, H. Efficacy and Safety of L-Carnitine Treatment for Chronic Heart Failure: A Meta-Analysis of Randomized Controlled Trials. *BioMed Res. Int.* **2017**, *2017*, 6274854. [CrossRef]
18. Higuchi, T.; Abe, M.; Yamazaki, T.; Okawa, E.; Ando, H.; Hotta, S.; Oikawa, O.; Kikuchi, F.; Okada, K.; Soma, M. Levocarnitine Improves Cardiac Function in Hemodialysis Patients With Left Ventricular Hypertrophy: A Randomized Controlled Trial. *Am. J. Kidney Dis.* **2016**, *67*, 260–270. [CrossRef] [PubMed]

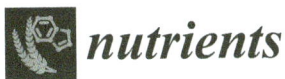

Article

Influence of the Accumulation of Unhealthy Eating Habits on Obesity in a General Japanese Population: The Hisayama Study

Yuki Ishida [1], Daigo Yoshida [1,*], Takanori Honda [1], Yoichiro Hirakawa [1,2], Mao Shibata [1,3], Satoko Sakata [1,2,3], Yoshihiko Furuta [1,2], Emi Oishi [1,2], Jun Hata [1,2,3], Takanari Kitazono [2,3] and Toshiharu Ninomiya [1,3]

[1] Department of Epidemiology and Public Health, Graduate School of Medical Sciences, Kyushu University, Fukuoka 812-8582, Japan; ishida-y@eph.med.kyushu-u.ac.jp (Y.I.); honda-t@eph.med.kyushu-u.ac.jp (T.H.); you1@eph.med.kyushu-u.ac.jp (Y.H.); shibata.mao.276@m.kyushu-u.ac.jp (M.S.); ssakata@eph.med.kyushu-u.ac.jp (S.S.); furuta.yoshihiko.496@m.kyushu-u.ac.jp (Y.F.); oishiemi@eph.med.kyushu-u.ac.jp (E.O.); junhata@eph.med.kyushu-u.ac.jp (J.H.); nino@eph.med.kyushu-u.ac.jp (T.N.)
[2] Department of Medicine and Clinical Science, Graduate School of Medical Sciences, Kyushu University, Fukuoka 812-8582, Japan; kitazono@intmed2.med.kyushu-u.ac.jp
[3] Center for Cohort Studies, Graduate School of Medical Sciences, Kyushu University, Fukuoka 812-8582, Japan
* Correspondence: dyoshida@eph.med.kyushu-u.ac.jp

Received: 24 September 2020; Accepted: 14 October 2020; Published: 16 October 2020

Abstract: Few studies have examined the association between the accumulation of unhealthy eating habits and the likelihood of obesity or central obesity in a general Japanese population. We examined this association in a sample of 1906 community-dwelling Japanese subjects (age: 40–74 years) who participated in a health check-up in 2014. A face-to-face questionnaire interview was conducted to collect information about three unhealthy eating habits, i.e., snacking, eating quickly, and eating late-evening meals. Obesity was defined as body mass index ≥ 25 kg/m^2 and central obesity was defined as waist circumference ≥ 90 cm in men and ≥ 80 cm in women. The odds ratios (OR) were estimated by using a logistic regression analysis. Subjects with any one of the three eating habits had a significantly higher likelihood of obesity than those without that habit after adjusting for confounding factors. The multivariable-adjusted OR for obesity increased linearly with an increase in the number of accumulated unhealthy eating habits (p for trend <0.001). Similar associations were observed for central obesity. Our findings suggest that modifying each unhealthy eating habit and avoiding an accumulation of multiple unhealthy eating habits might be important to reduce the likelihood of obesity.

Keywords: unhealthy eating habits; accumulation; obesity; central obesity; general Japanese population

1. Introduction

The number of people with obesity is increasing globally [1]. Obesity is a major risk factor for chronic diseases, such as hypertension, diabetes, hyperlipidemia, cardiovascular disease, and cancer [2]. Central obesity, defined by an increased waist circumference, has also been reported to increase the risk of cardiovascular disease and death [3,4]. In order to reduce the burden of obesity-related diseases, the prevention of obesity must be a public health priority.

Among the various strategies for health promotion, one commonality is the importance of healthy eating habits to prevent obesity [2]. Several epidemiologic studies have indicated that unhealthy eating habits, such as snacking [5–8], eating quickly [7,9,10], and eating late-evening meals [11,12], are significantly associated with an increased risk of obesity or central obesity. These previous studies investigated the influence of each eating habit separately, but it is also important to consider the influence of the accumulation of unhealthy eating habits on obesity and central obesity, since unhealthy eating habits tend to overlap. However, there have been few population-based studies evaluating the influence of the accumulation of multiple unhealthy eating habits on having obesity and central obesity in Japanese.

Therefore, the aim of the present study was to examine the associations of both individual and accumulated unhealthy eating habits with the likelihood of having obesity and central obesity in a general Japanese population.

2. Materials and Methods

2.1. Study Population

The Hisayama Study is a population-based prospective cohort study of cardiovascular disease and its risk factors, which was begun in 1961 in the town of Hisayama, a suburb of the Fukuoka metropolitan area on Kyushu Island, Japan. According to the national census, the age and occupational distributions in Hisayama have been almost identical to those of all of Japan since the 1960s [13,14]. The present cross-sectional study was based on a screening survey conducted in 2014. A total of 1930 residents aged 40–74 years (51.7% of the total population of this age group) underwent a health check-up and completed an interviewer-administered questionnaire about eating habits. After excluding 4 individuals who did not provide consent to participate in the study and 20 without available data of eating habits, the remaining 1906 subjects (835 men and 1071 women) were enrolled in this study.

2.2. Definition of Obesity and Central Obesity

Body height and weight were measured using an automated digital scale (DC-250, Tanita, Tokyo, Japan) in light clothing without shoes, and body mass index (BMI) was calculated as weight (kg) divided by height squared (m^2). Obesity was defined as a BMI $\geq$25 kg/m^2. Waist circumference at the umbilical level was measured by trained nurses using a non-stretchable tape measure with the participant in the standing position, and central obesity was defined as a waist circumference $\geq$90 cm in men and $\geq$80 cm in women according to International Obesity Task Force central obesity criteria for Asia [15].

2.3. Definition of Unhealthy Eating Habits

A face-to-face interview by registered dietitians was conducted to collect the information on eating habits using a questionnaire, which was modified from the questionnaire for the Standard Health Check-up and Counseling Guidance to prevent metabolic syndrome proposed by the Japanese Ministry of Health, Labour and Welfare [16]. The original questionnaire is widely used in the nationwide health check-ups for residents aged 40 to 74 years in Japan.

Eating habits were determined by the following questions: "Do you eat snacks?" (snacking); "Does your eating speed more quickly than other people?" (eating quickly); "Do you have late-evening meals within two hours before bedtime?" (eating late-evening meals). The answer options were "yes" or "no". Those who answered yes to a question were defined as having that particular unhealthy eating habit. The number of accumulated unhealthy eating habits was determined by summing up the positive responses, ranging from 0 to 3.

2.4. Measurement of Other Risk Factors

Each participant completed a self-administered questionnaire including smoking habits, drinking habits, regular exercise, marital status, living status, and employment status. Smoking habits and drinking habits were classified into currently habitual or not. The subjects who reported engaging in sports or other forms of exertion $\geq$3 times a week during their leisure time made up the regular exercise group. Marital status was classified as currently "married" or "unmarried, divorced, or widowed".

Living status was categorized as "living alone" or "living with others". Employment status was categorized as currently "employed" or "unemployed"; housewives were classified as "unemployed" in the present study. The questionnaire was checked by trained interviewers at the screening.

2.5. Statistical Analysis

Descriptive statistics according to the response to each unhealthy eating habit and the number of accumulated eating habits were presented as age- and sex-adjusted means or frequencies. The group differences were tested by analysis of covariance and a logistic regression model. The age- and sex-adjusted mean values of BMI and waist circumference according to the status of each unhealthy eating habit and the numbers of accumulated eating habits were estimated by using the analysis of covariance. The means of BMI and waist circumference across the numbers of accumulated unhealthy eating habits were tested by a linear regression model. The odds ratios (OR) and their 95% confidence intervals (CIs) for the presence of obesity and central obesity according to each unhealthy eating habit and the number of accumulated eating habits were computed with the use of the logistic regression model. The trends in the estimates across the number of accumulated unhealthy eating habits were tested by including the ordinal number (0, 1, 2, or 3) representing the number of the accumulated eating habits in the relevant model. The heterogeneities in the association between subgroup covariates were tested by adding the multiplicative interaction term to the relevant model. All statistical analyses were performed using the SAS program package version 9.4 (SAS Institute Inc., Cary, NC, USA). Two-tailed p-values of < 0.05 were considered significant.

2.6. Ethical Considerations

The study protocol was approved by the Kyushu University Institutional Review Board for Clinical Research, and the procedures followed were in accordance with national guidelines. All participants provided written informed consent.

3. Results

Table 1 shows the age- and sex-adjusted mean values or frequencies of covariates according to the status of each of the unhealthy eating habits. Subjects who snacked were more likely to be women, and less likely to be current smokers, current drinkers, living alone, and employed than those without. Subjects who ate quickly were younger than those who were not. Subjects who ate late-evening meals were younger, and more likely to be men, current smokers, current drinkers, living alone, and employed than those who did not.

Table 1. Age- and sex-adjusted participant characteristics according to the status of each unhealthy eating habit.

	Snacking			Eating Quickly			Eating Late-Evening Meals		
	No ($n = 832$)	Yes ($n = 1074$)	p Value	No ($n = 1037$)	Yes ($n = 869$)	p Value	No ($n = 1399$)	Yes ($n = 507$)	p Value
Age, year	60.8 (0.3)	60.0 (0.3)	0.11	61.3 (0.3)	59.1 (0.3)	<0.001	61.8 (0.3)	56.4 (0.4)	<0.001
Women, %	40.5	68.3	<0.001	57.8	54.3	0.13	63.1	37.3	<0.001
Current smoking, %	15.9	11.5	0.005	14.3	12.2	0.16	12.2	16.9	0.006
Current drinking, %	64.6	50.0	<0.001	57.6	54.8	0.27	53.2	65.1	<0.001
Regular exercise, %	16.0	15.5	0.77	15.1	16.4	0.42	16.3	14.1	0.27
Married, %	80.2	83.7	0.06	80.9	83.7	0.11	82.7	80.8	0.38
Living alone, %	7.1	4.9	0.04	6.2	5.4	0.44	5.0	8.2	0.02
Current employment, %	52.2	45.9	0.03	47.3	50.2	0.29	44.8	60.0	<0.001

Values are expressed as adjusted mean (standard error), or frequency. Mean values of age were adjusted for sex. Frequencies of women were adjusted for age.

Among the 1906 subjects, 504 (26.4%) had obesity and 860 (45.1%) had central obesity. As shown in Table 2, the age- and sex-adjusted mean values of BMI and waist circumference were higher in the subjects with any one of the unhealthy eating habits than in those without that habit (all p values < 0.05; except for BMI in subjects who ate late-evening meals). Subjects with any one of the unhealthy eating habits had a significantly greater likelihood of the presence of obesity (snacking:

OR 1.49 [95% CI 1.19–1.86]; eating quickly: 2.11 [1.71–2.61]; eating late-evening meals: 1.39 [1.09–1.77]) and central obesity (snacking: 1.29 [1.05–1.58]; eating quickly: 1.89 [1.55–2.30]; eating late-evening meals: 1.36 [1.08–1.72]) after adjusting for age, sex, current smoking, current drinking, regular exercise, marital status, living status, and employment status.

Table 2. Multivariable-adjusted likelihood of the presence of obesity and central obesity according to the status of each unhealthy eating habit.

Outcomes Unhealthy Eating Habits	Age- and Sex-Adjusted Mean (95% CI) of BMI or WC	No. of Obese or Central Obese Subjects/Total Subjects	Model 1 [a]		Model 2 [b]	
			OR (95% CI)	p Value	OR (95% CI)	p Value
Obesity	BMI (kg/m^2)					
Snacking						
No	22.8 (22.5–23.0) [c]	200/832	1.00 (reference)		1.00 (reference)	
Yes	23.5 (23.2–23.7) [c],**	304/1074	1.50 (1.20–1.86)	<0.001	1.49 (1.19–1.86)	<0.001
Eating quickly						
No	22.6 (22.3–22.8) [c]	207/1037	1.00 (reference)		1.00 (reference)	
Yes	23.9 (23.7–24.1) [c],**	297/869	2.12 (1.72–2.61)	<0.001	2.11 (1.71–2.61)	<0.001
Eating late-evening meals						
No	23.1 (22.9–23.3) [c]	342/1399	1.00 (reference)		1.00 (reference)	
Yes	23.4 (23.1–23.7) [c]	162/507	1.38 (1.09–1.74)	0.008	1.39 (1.09–1.77)	0.007
Central obesity	WC (cm)					
Snacking						
No	82.9 (82.2–83.5) [d]	315/832	1.00 (reference)		1.00 (reference)	
Yes	84.7 (84.1–85.3) [d],**	545/1074	1.30 (1.06–1.58)	0.01	1.29 (1.05–1.58)	0.01
Eating quickly						
No	82.4 (81.9–83.0) [d]	413/1037	1.00 (reference)		1.00 (reference)	
Yes	85.7 (85.1–86.3) [d],**	447/869	1.88 (1.55–2.29)	<0.001	1.89 (1.55–2.30)	<0.001
Eating late-evening meals						
No	83.6 (83.1–84.1) [d]	645/1399	1.00 (reference)		1.00 (reference)	
Yes	84.7 (83.9–85.6) [d],*	215/507	1.35 (1.07–1.70)	0.01	1.36 (1.08–1.72)	0.009

Abbreviations: BMI, body mass index; OR, odds ratio; CI, confidence interval; WC, waist circumference. [a] Adjusted for age and sex. [b] Adjusted for age, sex, current smoking, current drinking, regular exercise, marital status, living status, and employment status. [c] The values are shown as the age- and sex-adjusted mean values (95% CI) of BMI (unit: kg/m^2). [d] The values are shown as the age- and sex-adjusted mean values (95% CI) of WC (unit: cm). * $p < 0.05$, ** $p < 0.01$ vs. "No".

Next, we investigated the association between the number of accumulated unhealthy eating habits and the likelihood of obesity and central obesity. Descriptive statistics according to the number of accumulated unhealthy eating habits are shown in Table 3. Subjects with a higher number of accumulated unhealthy eating habits were more likely to be younger. A higher number of accumulated unhealthy eating habits were significantly associated with the age- and sex-adjusted mean values of BMI and waist circumference (both p for trend <0.001; Figure 1). The multivariable-adjusted OR for having obesity or central obesity increased linearly with a higher number of accumulated unhealthy eating habits (obesity: OR 1.53 [95% CI 1.11–2.12], 2.62 [1.89–3.63], and 3.65 [2.36–5.63] for one, two, and three unhealthy eating habits, respectively, p for trend <0.001; central obesity: 1.53 [1.16–2.01], 2.28 [1.71–3.05], and 2.87 [1.89–4.36], p for trend <0.001; Figure 2).

Table 3. Age- and sex-adjusted characteristics of the study participants according to the number of accumulated unhealthy eating habits.

	Number of Unhealthy Eating Habits				
	0 ($n = 367$)	1 ($n = 779$)	2 ($n = 609$)	3 ($n = 151$)	p for Trend
Age, year	63.3 (0.5)	61.0 (0.3)	58.7 (0.4)	56.2 (0.8)	<0.001
Women, %	45.6	61.7	57.2	49.5	0.20
Current smoking, %	14.1	14.3	11.5	13.9	0.36
Current drinking, %	60.6	57.2	52.6	56.0	0.06
Regular exercise, %	15.5	16.4	14.8	16.2	0.81
Married, %	76.9	83.0	85.6	76.9	0.12
Living alone, %	6.2	6.3	4.8	7.2	0.64
Current employment, %	46.4	46.7	51.1	54.4	0.08

Values are expressed as adjusted mean (standard error), or frequency. Mean values of age were adjusted for sex. Frequencies of women were adjusted for age.

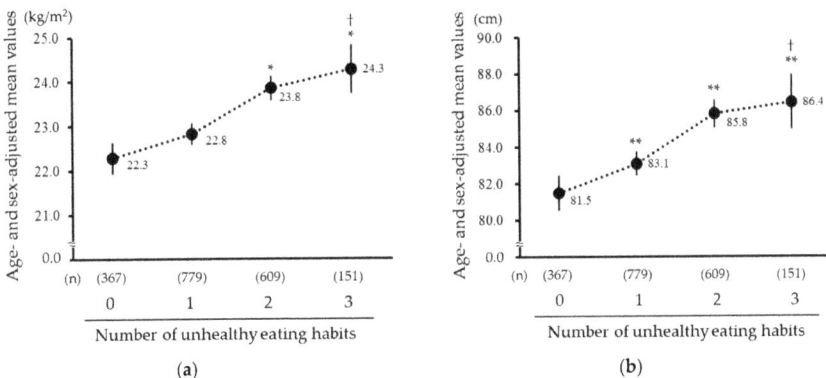

Figure 1. Age- and sex-adjusted mean values of body mass index and waist circumference according to the number of accumulated unhealthy eating habits: (**a**) Body mass index; (**b**) Waist circumference. Solid circles and vertical bars represent the mean values and 95% confidence intervals of each parameter, respectively. * $p < 0.05$, ** $p < 0.01$ vs. "0", † p for trend <0.001.

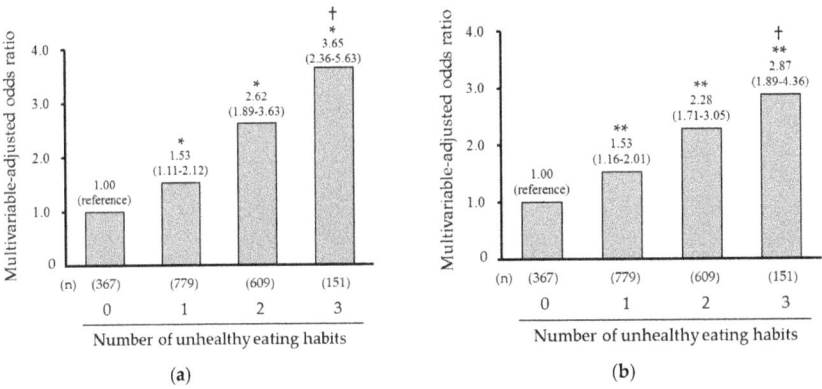

Figure 2. Multivariable-adjusted odds ratio of obesity and central obesity according to the number of accumulated unhealthy eating habits: (**a**) Obesity; (**b**) Central obesity. The values on the bars show the odds ratios (95% confidence intervals), which were adjusted for age, sex, current smoking, current drinking, regular exercise, marital status, living status, and employment status. * $p < 0.05$, ** $p < 0.01$ vs. "0", † p for trend <0.001.

Finally, we compared the age- and sex-adjusted ORs of the presence of obesity and central obesity per every one increment in the number of accumulated unhealthy eating habits between the subgroups of covariates (Table 4). The magnitudes of the association between the number of accumulated unhealthy eating habits and the likelihood of obesity and central obesity were stronger in the subgroups of subjects aged 40–59 years, male subjects, and employed subjects than in subjects aged 60–74 years, female subjects, and unemployed subjects (all p for heterogeneity <0.05). In addition, the likelihood of obesity per the number of accumulated unhealthy eating habits was greater in subjects with regular exercise than in those without it. Meanwhile, the association with central obesity tended to be heterogeneous between the drinking habit subgroups (p for heterogeneity =0.09). No clear heterogeneity was detected between the subgroups of smoking habits, marital status, and living status (all p for heterogeneity >0.3).

Table 4. Age- and sex-adjusted odds ratios and 95% confidence intervals of the presence of obesity and central obesity per every one increment in the number of accumulated unhealthy eating habits in the subgroups of covariates.

Subgroups	Obesity				Central Obesity			
	No. of Events	No. of Subjects	OR (95% CI) per 1 Increment in the Number of Unhealthy Eating Habits	p for Hetero.	No. of Events	No. of Subjects	OR (95% CI) per 1 Increment in the Number of Unhealthy Eating Habits	p for Hetero.
Age								
40–59 years	186	757	1.98 (1.60–2.45)		298	757	1.71 (1.42–2.05)	
60–74 years	318	1149	1.40 (1.20–1.63)	0.01	562	1149	1.27 (1.10–1.47)	0.01
Sex								
Men	267	835	1.75 (1.48–2.08)		243	835	1.63 (1.37–1.93)	
Women	237	1071	1.41 (1.17–1.69)	0.02	617	1071	1.32 (1.13–1.54)	0.007
Current smoking								
No	413	1576	1.55 (1.35–1.78)		760	1576	1.44 (1.27–1.64)	
Yes	91	330	1.77 (1.33–2.35)	0.38	100	330	1.53 (1.16–2.01)	0.47
Current drinking								
No	214	855	1.55 (1.27–1.88)		439	855	1.31 (1.11–1.56)	
Yes	290	1051	1.62 (1.38–1.91)	0.66	421	1051	1.58 (1.36–1.85)	0.09
Regular exercise								
No	422	1595	1.69 (1.47–1.93)		741	1595	1.51 (1.33–1.72)	
Yes	82	309	1.20 (0.90–1.62)	0.046	119	309	1.21 (0.90–1.61)	0.22
Marital status								
Unmarried, divorced, and widowed	77	346	1.45 (1.94–1.92)		150	346	1.35 (1.05–1.74)	
Married	427	1560	1.63 (1.42–1.87)	0.49	710	1560	1.48 (1.30–1.69)	0.47
Living status								
Living with others	477	1790	1.62 (1.43–1.84)		807	1790	1.47 (1.30–1.65)	
Living alone	27	116	1.23 (0.75–2.03)	0.34	53	116	1.35 (0.85–2.14)	0.66
Employment status								
Unemployed	239	983	1.39 (1.16–1.66)		513	983	1.25 (1.07–1.47)	
Employed	265	923	1.82 (1.53–2.17)	0.048	347	923	1.71 (1.45–2.02)	0.006

Abbreviations: OR, odds ratio; CI, confidence intervals; hetero., heterogeneity.

4. Discussion

In the present study, we clearly demonstrated that subjects with unhealthy eating habits—namely, snacking, eating quickly, and eating late-evening meals—had a significantly greater likelihood of the presence of obesity and central obesity. Notably, the accumulation of these unhealthy eating habits was linearly associated with a higher likelihood of obesity and central obesity after adjusting for demographic, socioeconomic, and lifestyle factors in a general Japanese adult population. These findings highlight that unhealthy eating habits, and especially their accumulation, have a major influence on obesity and central obesity, and may suggest that an improvement in these unhealthy eating habits would help to prevent obesity or central obesity.

Epidemiological evidence from cross-sectional and longitudinal studies has shown that individual unhealthy eating habits play a significant role in the development of obesity [5–12]. However, there have been few studies addressing the influence of the accumulation of unhealthy eating habits on obesity or central obesity. Three cross-sectional studies have shown that an accumulation of unhealthy eating habits was positively associated with the prevalence of obesity or metabolic syndrome in adult Japanese populations [12,17,18]. A community-based study conducted in northeast Japan showed that the multivariate-adjusted OR for obesity increased with an increase in the number of unhealthy eating habits, which in this case were skipping breakfast, eating quickly, and eating late-evening meals [18]. These findings were similar to our findings. In addition, one longitudinal study of working adults revealed that individuals who had both of two unhealthy eating habits—namely, snacking after dinner and eating late-evening meals—had an approximately twofold greater likelihood of having obesity than those with only one or neither of these habits [11]. Therefore, it seems reasonable to speculate that the accumulation of multiple unhealthy eating habits might increase the likelihood of obesity and central obesity in Japanese adults.

There are several possible mechanisms underlying the significant association between individual unhealthy eating habits and the greater likelihood of having obesity or central obesity. Subjects with a snacking habit were shown to have a higher total energy intake than those without a snacking habit [19,20]. In general, snacks tend to be high in calories, carbohydrates, and fats [21]. In the US population, the number of individuals with a snacking habit has increased over the last 30 years, and the energy intake from snacking has been estimated to be approximately 280 kcal/day, which is equivalent to 15.4% of the average energy intake of US adults [22,23]. In addition, eating speed is likely to influence the blood concentrations of appetite suppressant hormones. Subjects who eat quickly have been reported to have lower blood concentrations of pancreatic or gut hormones that are expected to suppress appetite (e.g., insulin, glucagon-like peptide 1, and peptide YY) than those who do not [24]. A systematic review revealed that subjects who ate quickly had a higher energy intake than those who ate slowly [25]. These results suggest that subjects with the unhealthy eating habit of eating quickly are more likely to have a higher energy intake due to an increased appetite than those without this habit. Meanwhile, eating late-evening meals has been considered to lead to an energy surplus, because diet-induced thermogenesis is lower at night than in the daytime [26,27]. Moreover, the sympathetic nerve activation and subsequent sleep disturbance caused by increased leptin secretion after a meal may be involved in the excess risk of obesity from eating late-evening meals [28,29]. Insufficient sleep leads to elevated ghrelin, which is an orexigenic peptide that may increase appetite [30]. As we noted above, several independent mechanisms, including behavioral, endocrine, and energy metabolic mechanisms, may be at play in the relation between unhealthy eating habits and obesity, and therefore the accumulation of unhealthy eating habits might additively increase the likelihood of having obesity or central obesity.

In the present study, the subgroup analysis showed that the magnitude of the influence of the accumulation of unhealthy eating habits on the excess likelihood of having obesity or central obesity were stronger in the groups of middle-aged subjects, male subjects, current drinkers, subjects who did not perform regular exercise, and subjects who currently engaged in work than in their counterpart groups (non-middle-aged subjects, female subject, etc.). In general, middle-aged male subjects tend to have a greater energy intake than older subjects and/or women [31,32]. The significant heterogeneity in obesity and central obesity observed between subjects in the current drinking and non-current drinking subgroups and subjects in the employed and unemployed subgroups may also reflect the high energy consumption: Middle-aged men are more likely to have a drinking habit and to be employed. In addition, the absence of a regular exercise habit could contribute to decreased energy expenditure, resulting in a further energy surplus. Our findings suggest that middle-aged male subjects and subjects who do not perform exercise regularly are more likely to be affected by the adverse effects of accumulated unhealthy eating habits on obesity.

The present study has several limitations. First, because of the cross-sectional nature of this study, we were not able to determine whether there was a causal association between unhealthy eating habits and either obesity or central obesity. Second, the information about the unhealthy eating habits was derived from questioning the participants rather than observing their actual behaviors. However, a moderate-to-high level of concordance between the self-reported and friend-reported rate of eating was shown in a previous study [33]. Finally, we did not have information on the energy intake and nutrients. Further studies will be needed to assess these parameters carefully in order to clarify whether unhealthy eating habits increase the likelihood of obesity and central obesity through excessive intake of energy, fat, and carbohydrates.

5. Conclusions

The present study revealed dose–response-positive associations between the number of accumulated unhealthy eating habits and the likelihood of obesity and central obesity in a general Japanese population. Our findings suggest that modifying individual unhealthy eating habits and avoiding their accumulation might reduce the burden of obesity and central obesity. Healthcare professionals need to encourage those who have unhealthy eating habits to modify each of their habits individually as well as to avoid accumulating multiple unhealthy habits. Further longitudinal studies will be needed to elucidate whether a causal relationship exists between the accumulation of unhealthy eating habits and the incidence of obesity or central obesity.

Author Contributions: Study concept and design, Y.I. and D.Y.; data collection, D.Y., T.H., Y.H., M.S., S.S., Y.F., E.O., J.H., and T.N.; interpretation of data, Y.I., D.Y., T.H., Y.H., M.S., S.S., Y.F., E.O., J.H., T.K., and T.N.; statistical analysis, Y.I. and D.Y.; study coordinator, T.N.; funding acquisition, T.N.; writing—original manuscript, Y.I. and D.Y.; writing—review and editing, Y.I., D.Y., T.H., Y.H., M.S., S.S., Y.F., E.O., J.H., T.K., and T.N. All authors have read and agreed to the published version of the manuscript.

Funding: This study was supported in part by Grants-in-Aid for Scientific Research A (JP16H02692), B (JP17H04126, JP18H02737, and JP19H03863), C (JP18K07565, JP18K09412, JP19K07890, JP20K10503, and JP20K11020), Grants-in-Aid for Early-Career Scientists (JP18K17925), and Grants-in-Aid for Research Activity Start-up (JP19K23971) from the Ministry of Education, Culture, Sports, Science and Technology of Japan; by Health and Labour Sciences Research Grants of the Ministry of Health, Labour and Welfare of Japan (20FA1002); and by the Japan Agency for Medical Research and Development (JP20dk0207025, JP20km0405202, and JP20fk0108075).

Acknowledgments: The authors thank the residents of the town of Hisayama for their participation in the survey and the staff of the Division of Health and Welfare of Hisayama for their cooperation with this study. The statistical analyses were carried out using the computer resources offered under the category of General Projects by Research Institute for Information Technology, Kyushu University.

Conflicts of Interest: The authors have no conflict of interest to declare.

References

1. NCD Risk Factor Collaboration. Trends in adult body-mass index in 200 countries from 1975 to 2014: A pooled analysis of 1698 population-based measurement studies with 19.2 million participants. *Lancet* **2016**, *387*, 1377–1396. [CrossRef]
2. WHO; FEC. *Diet, Nutrition and the Prevention of Chronic Diseases, WHO Technical Report Series 916*; WHO: Geneva, Switzerland, 2003.
3. Saito, I.; Kokubo, Y.; Kiyohara, Y.; Doi, Y.; Saitoh, S.; Ohnishi, H.; Miyamoto, Y. Prospective study on waist circumference and risk of all-cause and cardiovascular mortality. *Circ. J.* **2012**, *76*, 2867–2874. [CrossRef]
4. Schneider, H.J.; Friedrich, N.; Klotsche, J.; Pieper, L.; Nauck, M.; John, U.; Dörr, M.; Felix, S.; Lehnert, H.; Pittrow, D.; et al. The predictive value of different measures of obesity for incident cardiovascular events and mortality. *J. Clin. Endocrinol. Metab.* **2010**, *95*, 1777–1785. [CrossRef]
5. Liu, X.; Zheng, C.; Xu, C.; Liu, Q.; Wang, J.; Hong, Y.; Zhao, P. Nighttime snacking is associated with risk of obesity and hyperglycemia in adults: A cross-sectional survey from Chinese adult teachers. *J. Biomed. Res.* **2017**, *31*, 541–547.
6. Murakami, K.; Livingstone, M.B.E. Eating Frequency is positively associated with overweight and central obesity in US adults. *J. Nutr.* **2015**, *145*, 2715–2724. [CrossRef]
7. Mesas, A.E.; Muñoz-Pareja, M.; López-Garcia, E.; Rodríguez-Artalejo, F. Selected eating behaviours and excess body weight: A systematic review. *Obes. Rev.* **2012**, *13*, 106–135. [CrossRef]
8. Bes-Rastrollo, M.; Sanchez-Villegas, A.; Basterra-Gortari, F.J.; Nunez-Cordoba, J.M.; Toledo, E.; Serrano-Martinez, M. Prospective study of self-reported usual snacking and weight gain in a Mediterranean cohort: The SUN project. *Clin. Nutr.* **2010**, *29*, 323–330. [CrossRef]
9. Ohkuma, T.; Hirakawa, Y.; Nakamura, U.; Kiyohara, Y.; Kitazono, T.; Ninomiya, T. Association between eating rate and obesity: A systematic review and meta-analysis. *Int. J. Obes.* **2015**, *39*, 1589–1596. [CrossRef]
10. Ohkuma, T.; Fujii, H.; Iwase, M.; Kikuchi, Y.; Ogata, S.; Idewaki, Y.; Ide, H.; Doi, Y.; Hirakawa, Y.; Mukai, N.; et al. Impact of eating rate on obesity and cardiovascular risk factors according to glucose tolerance status: The Fukuoka Diabetes Registry and the Hisayama Study. *Diabetologia* **2013**, *56*, 70–77. [CrossRef]
11. Yoshida, J.; Eguchi, E.; Nagaoka, K.; Ito, T.; Ogino, K. Association of night eating habits with metabolic syndrome and its components: A longitudinal study. *BMC Public Health* **2018**, *18*, 1366. [CrossRef]
12. Kutsuma, A.; Nakajima, K.; Suwa, K. Potential association between breakfast skipping and concomitant late-night-dinner eating with metabolic syndrome and proteinuria in the Japanese population. *Scientifica* **2014**, *2014*, 253581. [CrossRef] [PubMed]

13. Hata, J.; Ninomiya, T.; Hirakawa, Y.; Nagata, M.; Mukai, N.; Gotoh, S.; Fukuhara, M.; Ikeda, F.; Shikata, K.; Yoshida, D.; et al. Secular trends in cardiovascular disease and its risk factors in Japanese: Half-century data from the Hisayama Study (1961–2009). *Circulation* **2013**, *128*, 1198–1205. [CrossRef] [PubMed]
14. Ninomiya, T. Japanese legacy cohort studies: The Hisayama Study. *J. Epidemiol.* **2018**, *28*, 444–451. [CrossRef] [PubMed]
15. Alberti, K.G.M.M.; Eckel, R.H.; Grundy, S.M.; Zimmet, P.Z.; Cleeman, J.I.; Donato, K.A.; Fruchart, J.; James, W.P.T.; Loria, C.M.; Smith, S.C., Jr. Harmonizing the metabolic syndrome: A joint interim statement of the International Diabetes Federation Task Force on Epidemiology and Prevention; National Heart, Lung, and Blood Institute; American Heart Association; World Heart Federation; International Atherosclerosis Society; and International Association for the Study of Obesity. *Circulation* **2009**, *120*, 1640–1645. [PubMed]
16. Ministry of Health, Labour and Welfare, Japan. Standardized Health Check-Up and Intervention Program. 2007. Available online: http://tokutei-kensyu.tsushitahan.jp/manage/wp-content/uploads/2014/05/36ec0bcdf91b61a94a1223627abffe8d.pdf (accessed on 3 September 2020).
17. Kimura, Y.; Nanri, A.; Matsushita, Y.; Sasaki, S.; Mizoue, T. Eating behavior in relation to prevalence of overweight among Japanese men. *Asia Pac. J. Clin. Nutr.* **2011**, *20*, 29–34.
18. Lee, J.S.; Mishra, G.; Hayashi, K.; Watanabe, E.; Mori, K.; Kawakubo, K. Combined eating behaviors and overweight: Eating quickly, late evening meals, and skipping breakfast. *Eat. Behav.* **2016**, *21*, 84–88. [CrossRef] [PubMed]
19. Larson, N.I.; Miller, J.M.; Watts, A.W.; Story, M.T.; Neumark-Sztainer, D.R. Adolescent snacking behaviors are associated with dietary intake and weight status. *J. Nutr.* **2016**, *146*, 1348–1355. [CrossRef] [PubMed]
20. de Graaf, C. Effects of snacks on energy intake: An evolutionary perspective. *Appetite* **2006**, *47*, 18–23. [CrossRef] [PubMed]
21. Ministry of Education, Culture, Sports, Science and Technology-JAPAN. Standard Tables of Food Composition in Japan. 2015. Available online: https://www.mext.go.jp/en/policy/science_technology/policy/title01/detail01/1374030.htm (accessed on 3 September 2020).
22. Duffey, K.J.; Popkin, B.M. Energy density, portion size, and eating occasions: Contributions to increased energy intake in the United States, 1977–2006. *PLoS Med.* **2011**, *8*, e1001050. [CrossRef]
23. Nielsen, S.J.; Siega-Riz, A.M.; Popkin, B.M. Trends in energy intake in U.S. between 1977 and 1996: Similar shifts seen across age groups. *Obes. Res.* **2002**, *10*, 370–378. [CrossRef]
24. Karl, J.P.; Young, A.J.; Rood, J.C.; Montain, S.J. Independent and combined effects of eating rate and energy density on energy intake, appetite, and gut hormones. *Obesity* **2013**, *21*, E244–E252. [CrossRef]
25. Robinson, E.; Almiron-Roig, E.; Rutters, F.; de Graaf, C.; Forde, C.G.; Smith, C.T.; Nolan, S.J.; Jebb, S.A. A systematic review and meta-analysis examining the effect of eating rate on energy intake and hunger. *Am. J. Clin. Nutr.* **2014**, *100*, 123–151. [CrossRef]
26. Bo, S.; Fadda, M.; Castiglione, A.; Ciccone, G.; de Francesco, A.; Fedele, D.; Guggino, A.; Caprino, M.P.; Ferrara, S.; Boggio, M.V.; et al. Is the timing of caloric intake associated with variation in diet-induced thermogenesis and in the metabolic pattern? a randomized cross-over study. *Int. J. Obes.* **2015**, *39*, 1689–1695. [CrossRef] [PubMed]
27. Romon, M.; Edme, J.L.; Boulenguez, C.; Lescroart, J.L.; Frimat, P. Circadian variation of diet-induced thermogenesis. *Am. J. Clin. Nutr.* **1993**, *57*, 476–480. [CrossRef] [PubMed]
28. Imayama, I.; Prasad, B. Role of leptin in obstructive sleep apnea. *Ann. Am. Thorac. Soc.* **2017**, *14*, 1607–1621. [CrossRef]
29. Yasumoto, Y.; Hashimoto, C.; Nakao, R.; Yamazaki, H.; Hiroyama, H.; Nemoto, T.; Yamamoto, S.; Sakurai, M.; Oike, H.; Wada, N.; et al. Short-term feeding at the wrong time is sufficient to desynchronize peripheral clocks and induce obesity with hyperphagia, physical inactivity and metabolic disorders in mice. *Metabolism* **2016**, *65*, 714–727. [CrossRef]
30. Taheri, S.; Lin, L.; Austin, D.; Young, T.; Mignot, E. Short sleep duration is associated with reduced leptin, elevated ghrelin, and increased body mass index. *PLoS Med.* **2004**, *1*, e62. [CrossRef]
31. Lee, K.W.; Song, W.O.; Cho, M.S. Dietary quality differs by consumption of meals prepared at home vs. outside in Korean adults. *Nutr. Res. Pract.* **2016**, *10*, 294–304. [CrossRef]

32. Research Group on Health and Nutrition Information. The National Health and Nutrition Survey in Japan. 2014. Available online: https://www.mhlw.go.jp/file/04-Houdouhappyou-10904750-Kenkoukyoku-Gantaisakukenkouzoushinka/0000117311.pdf (accessed on 3 September 2020). (In Japanese)
33. Sasaki, S.; Katagiri, A.; Tsuji, T.; Shimoda, T.; Amano, K. Self-reported rate of eating correlates with body mass index in 18-y-old Japanese women. *Int. J. Obes. Relat. Metab. Disord.* **2003**, *27*, 1405–1410. [CrossRef]

Publisher's Note: MDPI stays neutral with regard to jurisdictional claims in published maps and institutional affiliations.

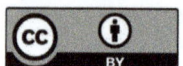

© 2020 by the authors. Licensee MDPI, Basel, Switzerland. This article is an open access article distributed under the terms and conditions of the Creative Commons Attribution (CC BY) license (http://creativecommons.org/licenses/by/4.0/).

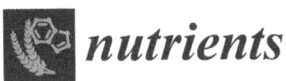

Article

Adherence to a Plant-Based Diet and Consumption of Specific Plant Foods—Associations with 3-Year Weight-Loss Maintenance and Cardiometabolic Risk Factors: A Secondary Analysis of the PREVIEW Intervention Study

Ruixin Zhu [1], Mikael Fogelholm [2], Sally D. Poppitt [3], Marta P. Silvestre [3,4], Grith Møller [1], Maija Huttunen-Lenz [5], Gareth Stratton [6], Jouko Sundvall [7], Laura Råman [7], Elli Jalo [2], Moira A. Taylor [8], Ian A. Macdonald [9], Svetoslav Handjiev [10], Teodora Handjieva-Darlenska [10], J. Alfredo Martinez [11,12,13,14], Roslyn Muirhead [15], Jennie Brand-Miller [15] and Anne Raben [1,16,*]

Citation: Zhu, R.; Fogelholm, M.; Poppitt, S.D.; Silvestre, M.P.; Møller, G.; Huttunen-Lenz, M.; Stratton, G.; Sundvall, J.; Råman, L.; Jalo, E.; et al. Adherence to a Plant-Based Diet and Consumption of Specific Plant Foods—Associations with 3-Year Weight-Loss Maintenance and Cardiometabolic Risk Factors: A Secondary Analysis of the PREVIEW Intervention Study. Nutrients 2021, 13, 3916. https://doi.org/10.3390/nu13113916

Academic Editor: Yoshihiro Fukumoto

Received: 27 September 2021
Accepted: 31 October 2021
Published: 1 November 2021

Publisher's Note: MDPI stays neutral with regard to jurisdictional claims in published maps and institutional affiliations.

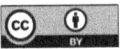

Copyright: © 2021 by the authors. Licensee MDPI, Basel, Switzerland. This article is an open access article distributed under the terms and conditions of the Creative Commons Attribution (CC BY) license (https://creativecommons.org/licenses/by/4.0/).

1. Department of Nutrition, Exercise and Sports, Faculty of Science, University of Copenhagen, Rolighedsvej 30, Frederiksberg C, 1958 Copenhagen, Denmark; ruixinzhu@nexs.ku.dk (R.Z.); gmp@nexs.ku.dk (G.M.)
2. Department of Food and Nutrition, University of Helsinki, P.O. Box 66, 00014 Helsinki, Finland; mikael.fogelholm@helsinki.fi (M.F.); elli.jalo@helsinki.fi (E.J.)
3. Human Nutrition Unit, Department of Medicine, School of Biological Sciences, University of Auckland, Auckland 1042, New Zealand; s.poppitt@auckland.ac.nz (S.D.P.); m.silvestre@auckland.ac.nz (M.P.S.)
4. CINTESIS, NOVA Medical School, NMS, Universidade Nova de Lisboa, 1169-056 Lisboa, Portugal
5. Institute for Nursing Science, University of Education Schwäbisch Gmünd, Oberbettringerstrasse 200, 73525 Schwäbisch Gmünd, Germany; maija.huttunen-lenz@ph-gmuend.de
6. Applied Sports, Technology, Exercise and Medicine (A-STEM) Research Centre, Swansea University, Swansea SA1 8EN, UK; g.stratton@swansea.ac.uk
7. Finnish Institute for Health and Welfare, P.O. Box 30, 00271 Helsinki, Finland; jouko.sundvall@outlook.com (J.S.); laura.raman@thl.fi (L.R.)
8. Division of Physiology, Pharmacology and Neuroscience, School of Life Sciences, Queen's Medical Centre, Nottingham NG7 2UH, UK; moira.taylor@nottingham.ac.uk
9. Division of Physiology, Pharmacology and Neuroscience, School of Life Sciences, Queen's Medical Centre, MRC/ARUK Centre for Musculoskeletal Ageing Research, ARUK Centre for Sport, Exercise and Osteoarthritis, National Institute for Health Research (NIHR) Nottingham Biomedical Research Centre, Nottingham NG7 2RD, UK; ian.macdonald1@nottingham.ac.uk
10. Department of Pharmacology and Toxicology, Medical University of Sofia, 1000 Sofia, Bulgaria; svhandjiev@gmail.com (S.H.); teodorah@abv.bg (T.H.-D.)
11. Department of Nutrition and Physiology, University of Navarra, 31008 Pamplona, Spain; jalfmtz@unav.es
12. Precision Nutrition and Cardiometabolic Health Program, IMDEA-Food Institute (Madrid Institute for Advanced Studies), CEI UAM + CSIC, 28049 Madrid, Spain
13. Centro de Investigacion Biomedica en Red Area de Fisiologia de la Obesidad y la Nutricion (CIBEROBN), 28029 Madrid, Spain
14. IdisNA Instituto for Health Research, 31008 Pamplona, Spain
15. Charles Perkins Centre, School of Life and Environmental Sciences, University of Sydney, Camperdown, Sydney 2006, Australia; roslyn.muirhead@sydney.edu.au (R.M.); jennie.brandmiller@sydney.edu.au (J.B.-M.)
16. Steno Diabetes Center Copenhagen, 2820 Gentofte, Denmark
* Correspondence: ara@nexs.ku.dk; Tel.: +45-21-30-69-12

Abstract: Plant-based diets are recommended by dietary guidelines. This secondary analysis aimed to assess longitudinal associations of an overall plant-based diet and specific plant foods with weight-loss maintenance and cardiometabolic risk factors. Longitudinal data on 710 participants (aged 26–70 years) with overweight or obesity and pre-diabetes from the 3-year weight-loss maintenance phase of the PREVIEW intervention were analyzed. Adherence to an overall plant-based diet was evaluated using a novel plant-based diet index, where all plant-based foods received positive scores and all animal-based foods received negative scores. After adjustment for potential confounders, linear mixed models with repeated measures showed that the plant-based diet index was inversely associated with weight regain, but not with cardiometabolic risk factors. Nut intake was inversely associated with regain of weight and fat mass and increments in total cholesterol and LDL cholesterol. Fruit intake was inversely associated with increments in diastolic blood pressure, total cholesterol, and LDL cholesterol. Vegetable intake was inversely associated with an increment in diastolic blood pressure and triglycerides and was positively associated with an increase in HDL cholesterol. All reported associations with cardiometabolic risk factors were independent of weight change. Long-term consumption of nuts, fruits, and vegetables may be beneficial for weight management and cardiometabolic health, whereas an overall plant-based diet may improve weight management only.

Keywords: plant-based dietary patterns; grains; legumes; nuts; fruits; vegetables; obesity; cardiovascular disease

1. Introduction

Cardiovascular diseases (CVDs) have placed a substantial healthcare and economic burden on governments and individuals [1]. Obesity is a major risk factor for CVDs [1]. Plant-based diets (PBDs) recommended by European food-based dietary guidelines [2] and the EAT-Lancet Commission [3] may be beneficial in terms of environmental sustainability, particularly if plant-based proteins replace animal-based foods such as red meat [2]. PBDs may also assist in weight management and prevention of CVDs [4–9] and improve multiple cardiometabolic risk factors [5].

Many previous randomized controlled trials (RCTs) and observational studies have explored the association of a vegetarian or a PBD with weight loss (WL) [8] or weight gain [6] or BMI [5]. Some prospective cohort studies have explored the association of PBDs with risk of CVDs [10], whereas previous evidence on PBDs and cardiometabolic risk factors was mainly based on cross-sectional studies and small-scale, short- or medium-term RCTs [11–17]. Long-term data on adherence to a PBD and weight regain and cardiometabolic risk factors during weight-loss maintenance (WLM), particularly after diet-induced rapid WL, are largely lacking.

Specific components of a PBD may also have an important role to play in weight management and cardiometabolic health. Certain plant foods such as whole grains, vegetables, fruits, legumes, and nuts are rich in vitamins, minerals, antioxidants, unsaturated fatty acids, and dietary fiber [7]. These plant foods are considered healthy, with improved health outcomes [7]. Other plant foods such as sugar-sweetened beverages, cakes, and cookies have lower nutrient density and higher energy density [7]. These plant foods are regarded as unhealthy and may have negative effects on health [7]. To our knowledge, few long-term studies have to date explored consumption of plant foods and weight regain and cardiometabolic risk factors during WLM.

Therefore, the objective of the current study was to assess the longitudinal associations of adherence to an overall PBD and specific plant foods with WLM and cardiometabolic risk factors in adults with high risk of type 2 diabetes (T2D). Data from the PREVIEW study, a 3-year randomized trial aimed at examining the effects of diet and physical activity (PA) interventions on T2D prevention, were used. We hypothesized that consumption of an overall PBD and healthy plant foods would be inversely associated with weight regain and cardiometabolic risk factors.

2. Materials and Methods
2.1. Study Design

The PREVIEW study was a 3-year, large-scale, 2 × 2 factorial randomized trial. It was conducted at 8 study centers including Denmark, Finland, The Netherlands, the UK, Spain, Bulgaria, New Zealand, and Australia. The detailed information has been described elsewhere [18], and the main results have been published [19,20]. Briefly, the PREVIEW study was designed to examine the effect of a high protein-low glycemic index (GI) diet vs a moderate protein–moderate GI diet (25 E% protein and GI < 50 vs. 15 E% protein and GI > 56) combined with 2 PA programs (high intensity or moderate intensity) on T2D incidence in adults with overweight or obesity and pre-diabetes. The primary endpoint was T2D incidence. The participants underwent an 8-week weight loss (WL) period, and during this period, they were instructed to consume a low energy total meal replacement diet containing 3.4 MJ·day^{-1}. After this period, participants started a 148-week WLM period and received 1 of the 4 diet–PA interventions. The intervention diets were consumed ad libitum during WLM, and the participants were given examples of eating plans, cooking books, and food-exchange lists. Both diet interventions included the recommendation of whole grain cereals. A behavioral modification program (PREMIT) and 17 group visits were conducted throughout the intervention to improve dietary and PA compliance [21]. Dietary compliance was evaluated using 4-day food records. In addition, urinary nitrogen or urea analyses were done on 24 h urine samples to assess compliance to the diets, i.e., protein intake. PA compliance was evaluated using 7-day accelerometry.

The PREVIEW study was designed and conducted in line with the Declaration of Helsinki and its latest amendments. The protocol of the PREVIEW study was reviewed and approved by the following Human Ethics Committees at each intervention center. Denmark: The Research Ethics Committees of the Capital Region, ethical approval code: H-1-2013-052; Finland: Coordinating Ethical Committee of HUS (Helsinki and Uusimaa Hospital District), ethical approval code: HUS/1733/2017; the UK: UK National Research Ethics Service (NRES) and East Midlands (Leicester) Ethics Committee, ethical approval code: 13/EM/0259; the Netherlands: Medical Ethics Committee of the Maastricht University Medical Centre, ethical approval code: NL43054.068.13/METC 13-3-008; Spain: Research Ethics Committee of the University of Navarra, ethical approval code: 71/2013; Bulgaria: Commission on Ethics in Scientific Research with the Medical University-Sofia (KENIMUS), ethical approval code: 4303/13.06.2014; Australia: The University of Sydney, Human Research Ethics Committee (HREC), ethical approval code: 2013/535; and New Zealand: Health and Disability Ethics Committees (HDEC), ethical approval code: X14-0408.

The current analysis was an exploratory analysis based on the secondary outcomes of the PREVIEW study. Given that only 5 study centers (Finland, the UK, Bulgaria, New Zealand, and Australia) provided food intake data in g·day^{-1} or serving size·day^{-1} and full plant food categories, only data from the WLM phase (8–156 weeks) from participants at these 5 study centers were included.

2.2. Study Population

Participants aged 25–70 years with overweight (BMI 25–29.9 kg·m^{-2}) or obesity (BMI $\geq$ 30 kg·m^{-2}) and pre-diabetes were recruited between June 2013 and April 2015. Pre-diabetes was defined as impaired FPG (FPG of 5.6–6.9 mmol·L^{-1}) or impaired glucose tolerance (2-h plasma glucose of 7.8–11.0 mmol·L^{-1} and FPG < 7.0 mmol·L^{-1}) after an oral glucose tolerance test (oral ingestion of 75 g of glucose) [22]. Participants who were diagnosed with diabetes (T2D or type 1 diabetes) prior to the study or who were non-compliant with the intervention were excluded. Eligible participants were enrolled, underwent randomization by gender and age, and started WL. Participants who lost $\geq$8% of initial BW after the WL phase were eligible to continue, entering the 148-week WLM period. In the current analysis, we included those with available plant food data (and full plant food categories) at 26 weeks and plausible energy intake (2520–14700 kJ·day^{-1} for women and 3360–17640 kJ·day^{-1} for men) [23]. All participants provided written informed consent.

2.3. Assessment of Dietary Intake and Adherence to an Overall Plant-Based Diet

Dietary intake was estimated using self-administered 4-day food records on 4 consecutive days, including 3 weekdays and 1 weekend day. The 4-day food records were collected at 26, 52, 104, and 156 weeks. Participants were encouraged to record their diet by weighing foods and drinks using a weigh scale or household measures in the absence of a scale. Standard household measures such as cup, spoon, glass, and portions were explained. Additionally, participants were asked to describe the food in detail (e.g., type of foods, cooking methods, and ingredients). Food records were entered into the national nutrient analysis software, i.e., AivoDiet (Finland), Nutritics (the UK), Nutrition Calculation (Bulgaria), and Foodworks (Australia and New Zealand). Food intake at each time point was calculated as the average of 4 days and expressed in $g \cdot day^{-1}$ or $serving \cdot day^{-1}$. Serving sizes were converted to grams of food [23].

We created 11 food groups according to nutrients and culinary similarities within the larger categories of plant foods and animal-based foods (Table 1). Plant food groups included total grains and potatoes, legumes, nuts, vegetables, and fruits. Animal-based food groups included dairy products, eggs, red meat, processed meat, poultry and fish/seafood. Adherence to an overall PBD was evaluated using a plant-based diet index (PDI), modified from Satija et al. [24]. As conversion from $serving \cdot day^{-1}$ to $g \cdot day^{-1}$ of high-sugar products may introduce bias, they were not included in the PDI. In addition, in our dietary data, there was not a specific potato group. Potatoes and potato products were considered as 1 group. For the PDI calculation, food groups were divided into quintiles of consumption ($g \cdot day^{-1}$) and given positive (between 1 and 5) or negative (between –5 and –1) scores. For positive scores, participants in the highest quintile were assigned a score of 5 and those in the lowest quintile were assigned a score of 1. All plant food groups were given positive scores and all animal food groups were given negative scores. Scores based on the 11 food groups were summed to obtain the index. Higher PDI reflected lower consumption of animal-based foods.

Table 1. Examples of food items in the 11 food groups.

Food Groups	Foods	Plant-Based Diet Index
Plant		
Grains	Bread rolls/baps/bagels, breads, cereal bars, cereal products, cereals, crackers/crispbreads, flours, grains, pastas, pastries/buns, rice, potatoes, potato products, pastry, plain cake, biscuits, and starch-based carbohydrate-rich snacks	Positive scores
Legumes	Pulses, beans, peas, lentils, and soy foods	Positive scores
Nuts	Nuts and seeds	Positive scores
Vegetables	leafy vegetables, dried vegetables, mushrooms, pickles/chutney, roots/tubers/bulbs, sea vegetables/algae, vegetable dishes, and avocado	Positive scores
Fruits	Fruits, canned fruit, and dried fruit	Positive scores
Animal		
Dairy	Milk products, cow's milk, cream, creams, drinking yogurts, milkshakes/smoothies, processed milk/powders, yogurts, chilled desserts, and cheeses	Negative scores
Eggs	Eggs, egg products, and egg dishes	Negative scores
Red meat	Beef, pork, lamb, organ meats, meat dishes, and meat products	Negative scores
Processed meat	Frankfurters, bacon, corned beef, sausage, cured ham, and luncheon meat made from beef, pork, and poultry	Negative scores
Poultry	Poultry and poultry products, chicken, turkey	Negative scores
Fish/seafood	Fatty fish, fish products, low-fat fish, canned fatty fish, canned low-fat fish, seafoods, and crustaceans, including lobster and shrimps	Negative scores

2.4. Assessment of Outcomes

Outcomes including body weight (BW), fat mass (FM), waist circumference (WC), fasting plasma glucose (FPG), fasting insulin, glycosylated hemoglobin A_{1c} (HbA_{1c}), homeostatic model assessment of insulin resistance (HOMA-IR), fasting triglycerides, total cholesterol, high-density lipoprotein cholesterol (HDL cholesterol), low-density lipoprotein cholesterol (LDL cholesterol), systolic blood pressure (SBP), and diastolic blood pressure (DBP) were measured at 8, 26, 52, 104, and 156 weeks. BW was measured in the fasting state (>10 h), with participants wearing light clothing or underwear. FM was determined by dual energy X-ray absorptiometry in the UK, Australia, and New Zealand and by bioelectrical impedance in Finland and Bulgaria. Blood samples were drawn from fasting participants' antecubital veins. FPG, HbA_{1c}, fasting insulin, fasting triglycerides, total cholesterol, HDL cholesterol, and LDL cholesterol were determined at the central laboratory of the Finnish Institute for Health and Welfare, Helsinki, Finland. HOMA-IR was calculated with the formula: fasting insulin $(mU \cdot L^{-1}) \times FPG (mmol \cdot L^{-1})/22.5$ [25]. SBP and DBP were determined using a validated automatic device on participants' right arm after 5–10 min in a resting position.

2.5. Assessment of Covariates

Self-reported questionnaires were used to collect sociodemographic information including age, sex, ethnicity, and smoking status at baseline (0 weeks). PA was determined using 7-day accelerometry (ActiSleep+, ActiGraph LLC, Pensacola, FL, USA) and was expressed as counts·min^{-1}, i.e., mean activity counts during valid wear time.

2.6. Statistical Analysis

For descriptive statistics, the normality of continuous variables was assessed by p–p plots and histograms. Approximately normally distributed variables are presented as means ± standard deviation (SD) and non-normal variables as medians (25th, 75th percentiles). Categorical variables are presented as absolute values and frequencies.

We conducted an available-case analysis and merged all participants into 1 group to assess longitudinal associations of adherence to an overall PBD (evaluated by PDI) and plant food intake with yearly changes in outcomes including BW and cardiometabolic risk factors, using adjusted linear mixed models with repeated measures. Model 1 was adjusted for fixed factors including age (continuous), sex (categorical; women and men), ethnicity (categorical; Caucasian, Asian, Black, Arabic, or other), intervention group (categorical), BMI at 8 weeks, weight or cardiometabolic risk factors at 8 weeks (continuous), and time (categorical) and random factors including study center (categorical) and participant-ID. For adherence to a PBD, model 2 was adjusted for covariates in model 1 plus fixed factors including time-varying PA (continuous), energy intake (kJ·day^{-1}; continuous), and alcohol intake (g·day^{-1}; continuous). For specific plant food intake, model 2 was additionally adjusted for consumption of animal-based foods (g·day^{-1}; continuous) and other plant foods (g·day^{-1}; continuous) as fixed factors. As dietary sodium intake may be associated with blood pressure [26], model 2 was additionally adjusted for sodium intake (g·day^{-1}; continuous) when DBP or SBP was added as a dependent variable. Model 3 was adjusted for covariates in model 2 plus time-varying yearly weight change (continuous) as a fixed factor. Yearly changes were obtained by dividing changes in outcomes from 8 to 26, 52, 104, and 156 weeks by changes in years. To best represent the long-term dietary and PA patterns of participants during WLM, a cumulative average method [24,27] based on all available measurements of self-reported diet and device-measured PA was used. In this calculation, the 26-week diet was related to yearly changes in weight and cardiometabolic risk factors from 8 to 26 weeks; the average of the 26- and 52-week diets was related to yearly changes in weight and cardiometabolic risk factors from 8 to 52 weeks; the average of the 26-, 52-, and 104-week diets was related to yearly changes in weight and cardiometabolic risk factors from 8 to 104 weeks; the average of the 26-, 52-,104-, and 156-week diets was related to yearly changes in weight and cardiometabolic risk factors from 8 to 156 weeks. Cumulative average PA was calculated using the same method. Detailed information is included in Supplementary Materials Table S1. A sensitivity analysis was conducted by adding smoking status (categorical; daily, less than weekly, or no smoking) at 0 weeks in the abovementioned models. As the results were similar, they are not shown.

The associations of adherence to PBD with outcomes of interest are expressed as changes in outcomes per year induced by each 1 SD increment in PDI. To clarify the associations of PDI with BW, we also divided the participants into 2 groups, i.e., higher (n = 344 at 8 weeks) or lower (n = 344 at 8 weeks) adherence to PBD, at each time point separately according to PDI. We examined the difference in change in BW between the 2 groups using linear mixed models adjusted for the covariates in model 2. As the 2 groups were defined afresh at each time point, we compared the 2 groups at each time point regardless of the significance of time and group interaction. The associations of plant foods with outcomes of interest are expressed as changes in outcomes per year associated with each 1-serving size increment in plant food intake. The serving sizes were defined as follows: 75 g·day^{-1} for total grains and potatoes, 10 g·day^{-1} for legumes, 5 g·day^{-1} for nuts, 100 g·day^{-1} for vegetables, 50 g·day^{-1} for fruits, and 150 g·day^{-1} for combined consumption of vegetables and fruit—all based on medians and 25th and 75th percentiles of plant food intakes from dietary records over 3 years.

Missing data were not handled with multiple imputation because this method did not increase precision [28,29]. Data were analyzed using IBM SPSS v26.0 (Chicago, IL, USA). All P values were based on 2-sided tests and $P < 0.05$ was considered significant.

3. Results

In the present available-case analysis, we included 710 participants and 2144–2336 observations of outcomes from available plant food data and full plant food categories at 26 weeks and plausible energy intakes (Figure 1). Of these, 493 participants completed the study. Participants who withdrew during WLM did so for personal reasons, including time constraints, moving away, and illness. The median age of participants (69% women) at the beginning of WLM was 57 years (range: 26–70 years) (Table 2). As there were no poultry and processed meat data from participants in Bulgaria, PDI analysis was based on 688 participants with both complete plant food and animal food data.

Adherence to an overall PBD was inversely associated with weight regain and increment in LDL cholesterol in model 2, whereas after adjustment for weight change, the association of PBD with LDL cholesterol was lost (Figure 2). No associations were observed between PBD and other cardiometabolic risk factors in models 2 and 3 (Table S2). In all participants (n = 688), compared with those with lower adherence to PBD, participants with higher adherence to PBD had less weight regain at 52 and 104 weeks (Figure S1A). In completers (n = 493), compared with those with lower adherence to PBD, participants with higher adherence to PBD had less weight regain at 26, 52, and 104 weeks (Figure S1B).

Total grains and potatoes were not associated with any health outcomes in models 2 and 3 (Table S3). Legumes were positively associated with an increase in HDL cholesterol, whereas after adjustment for weight change, the association was lost (Figure 3). No associations were observed between legumes and weight regain or other cardiometabolic risk factors in models 2 and 3 (Table S4). Nuts were inversely associated with increments in BW, FM, HbA$_{1c}$, total cholesterol, and LDL cholesterol in model 2. After adjustment for weight change, the association of nuts with HbA$_{1c}$ was lost (Figure 3). No associations were observed between nuts and other cardiometabolic risk factors in models 2 and 3 (Table S5).

In the available analysis, fruits were inversely associated with increments in DBP, total cholesterol, and LDL cholesterol after adjustment for weight change in model 3 (Figure 4). No associations were observed between fruits and weight regain or other cardiometabolic risk factors in models 2 and 3 (Table S6). Vegetables were inversely associated with DBP and triglycerides and were positively associated with HDL cholesterol, independent of weight change in model 3 (Figure 4). No associations were observed between vegetables and weight regain or other cardiometabolic risk factors in models 2 and 3 (Table S7). Combined vegetable and fruit intake was inversely associated with an increment in SBP, and DBP and was positively associated with an increase in HDL cholesterol in model 2, whereas after adjustment for weight change, only the associations of DBP and HDL cholesterol with combined vegetable and fruit intake remained significant in model 3 (Figure 4 and Table S8).

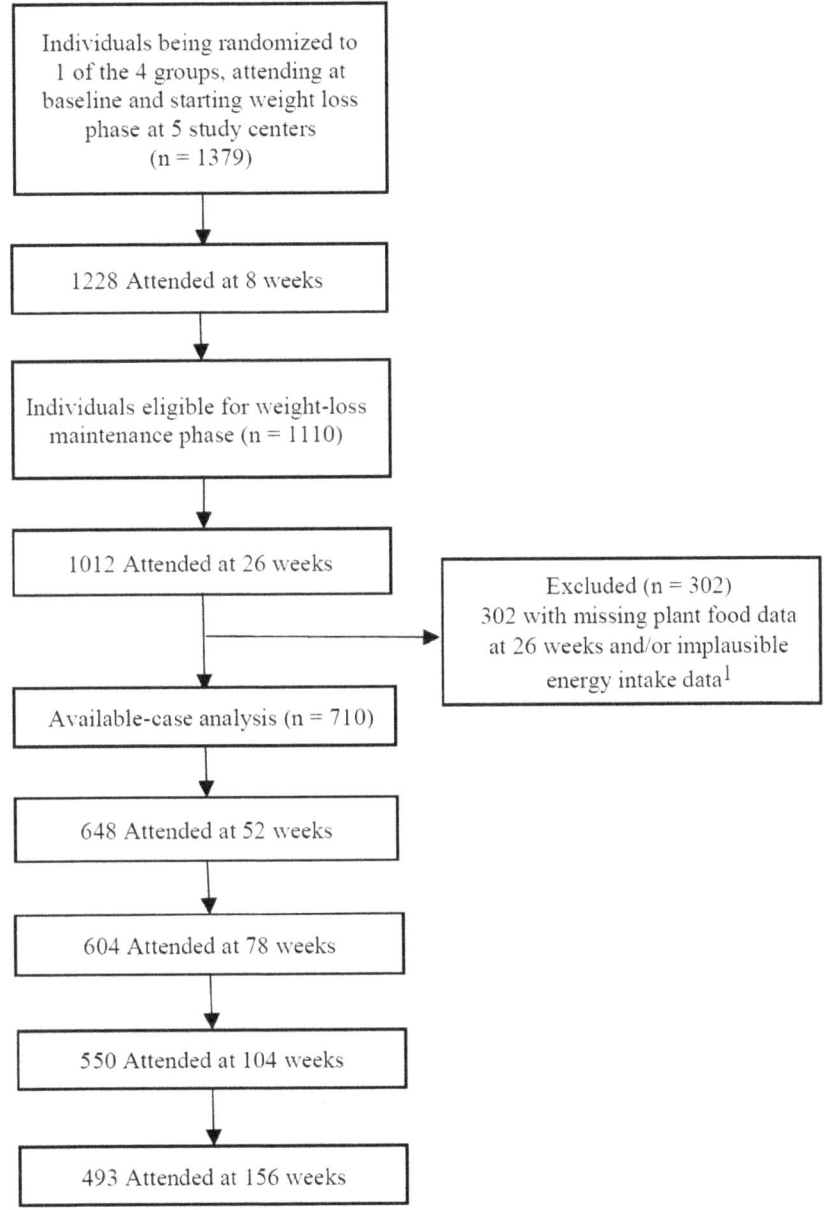

Figure 1. Participant flow diagram. [1] Individuals with missing plant food data at 26 weeks and/or implausible energy intake data (<2520 or >14,700 kJ·day^{-1} for women and <3360 or >17,640 kJ·day^{-1} for men) were excluded.

Table 2. Characteristics of participants at baseline (0 weeks), the start of weight-loss maintenance (8 weeks), or 26 weeks.

Characteristics	
n	710
Socio-demographics [1]	
Female, n (%)	491 (69.2)
Age (years)	57 (46, 63)
Height (m)	1.66 (1.61, 1.73)
Ethnicity, n (%)	
Caucasian	617 (86.9)
Asian	24 (3.4)
Black	19 (2.7)
Arabic	4 (0.6)
Other	46 (6.5)
Smoking, n (%)	
No	659 (92.8)
Yes, but less than weekly	17 (2.4)
Yes, at least daily	30 (4.2)
Missing	4 (0.6)
Anthropometric outcomes and body composition [2]	
Body weight (kg)	86.1 ± 16.6
BMI (kg·m^{-2})	29.5 (26.7, 33.5)
Fat mass (kg)	33.5 ± 12.3
Waist circumference (cm)	100.2 ± 12.6
Cardiometabolic risk factors [2]	
Fasting plasma glucose (mmol·L^{-1})	5.7 ± 0.6
HbA$_{1c}$ (mmol·mol^{-1})	35.0 ± 3.1
HbA$_{1c}$ (%)	5.4 ± 0.3
Fasting insulin (mU·L^{-1})	7.3 (5.3, 9.9)
HOMA-IR	1.8 (1.3, 2.5)
Systolic blood pressure (mmHg)	121.6 ± 15.8
Diastolic blood pressure (mmHg)	72.1 ± 9.5
Triglycerides (mmol·L^{-1})	1.0 (0.8, 1.2)
Total cholesterol (mmol·L^{-1})	4.1 ± 0.9
HDL cholesterol (mmol·L^{-1})	1.1 ± 0.2
LDL cholesterol (mmol·L^{-1})	2.4 (1.9, 3.0)
Energy and food intake [3]	
Energy (kJ·day^{-1})	29,491 ± 7731
Grains (g·day^{-1})	206.1 (144.7, 276.6)
Legumes (g·day^{-1})	0.2 (0, 27.5)
Nuts (g·day^{-1})	3.2 (0, 10.8)
Fruits (g·day^{-1})	169.5 (83.8, 260.5)
Vegetables (g·day^{-1})	185.9 (97.1, 310.7)
Dairy (g·day^{-1})	361.0 (226.4, 501.0)
Eggs (g·day^{-1})	20.8 (5.1, 41.3)
Red meat (g·day^{-1})	35.9 (0, 71.9)
Processed meat (g·day^{-1})	12.0 (0, 29.7)
Poultry (g·day^{-1})	37.2 (9.6, 70.4)
Fish/seafood (g·day^{-1})	30.0 (3.6, 62.7)

Values represent mean ± standard deviation, median (25th, 75th percentiles), and the number of participants (%) [1] Data were collected at 0 weeks. [2] Data were collected at 8 weeks. [3] Data were collected at 26 weeks. BMI, body mass index; HbA$_{1c}$, glycosylated hemoglobin A$_{1c}$; HDL cholesterol, high-density lipoprotein cholesterol; HOMA-IR, homeostatic model assessment of insulin resistance; LDL cholesterol, low-density lipoprotein cholesterol.

Outcomes	Yearly mean change (95%CI)	P-value
ΔBody weight (kg·year^{-1})		
Model 1	−0.15 (−0.33, 0.03)	0.097
Model 2	−0.24 (−0.48, −0.002)	0.048
ΔLDL-cholesterol (mmol·L^{-1}·year^{-1})		
Model 1	−0.02 (−0.04, 0.005)	0.119
Model 2	−0.03 (−0.07, −0.001)	0.044
Model 3	−0.03 (−0.07, 0.001)	0.057

Inverse association   Positive association

Figure 2. Longitudinal associations of adherence to a plant-based diet with yearly weight regain and changes in cardiometabolic risk factors during weight-loss maintenance. Yearly mean change and 95% CI of main effects indicating changes in body weight or cardiometabolic risk factors per year associated with a 1 standard deviation increment in plant-based diet index. Analyses were conducted using a linear mixed model with repeated measures. Model 1 was adjusted for fixed factors including age, sex, ethnicity, BMI at 8 weeks, body weight, or cardiometabolic risk factors at 8 weeks, and time and random factors including study center and participant ID. Model 2 was adjusted for covariates in model 1 plus fixed factors including time-varying physical activity, energy intake (kJ·day^{-1}), alcohol intake (g·day^{-1}). Model 3 was adjusted for covariates in model 2 plus time-varying yearly changes in body weight as a fixed factor. LDL cholesterol, low-density lipoprotein cholesterol.

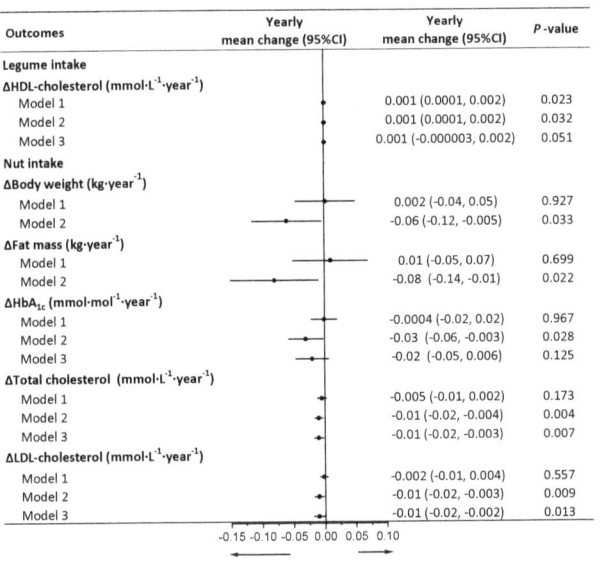

Figure 3. Longitudinal associations of legume (10 g·day^{-1}) or nut (5 g·day^{-1}) intake with yearly weight regain and changes in cardiometabolic risk factors during weight-loss maintenance. Yearly mean change and 95% CI of main effects indicating changes in body weight or cardiometabolic risk factors per year associated with 10 g increment in legume intake or 5 g increment in vegetable intake. Analyses were conducted using a linear mixed model with repeated measures. Model 1 was adjusted for fixed factors including age, sex, ethnicity, BMI at 8 weeks, body weight, or cardiometabolic risk factors at 8 weeks and time and random factors including study center and participant ID. Model 2 was adjusted for covariates in model 1 plus fixed factors including time-varying physical activity, energy intake (kJ·day^{-1}), alcohol intake (g·day^{-1}), animal-based food intake (g·day^{-1}), and other plant food intake (g·day^{-1}). Model 3 was adjusted for covariates in model 2 plus time-varying yearly changes in body weight as a fixed factor. HbA$_{1c}$, glycosylated hemoglobin A$_{1c}$; HDL cholesterol, high-density lipoprotein cholesterol; LDL cholesterol, low-density lipoprotein cholesterol.

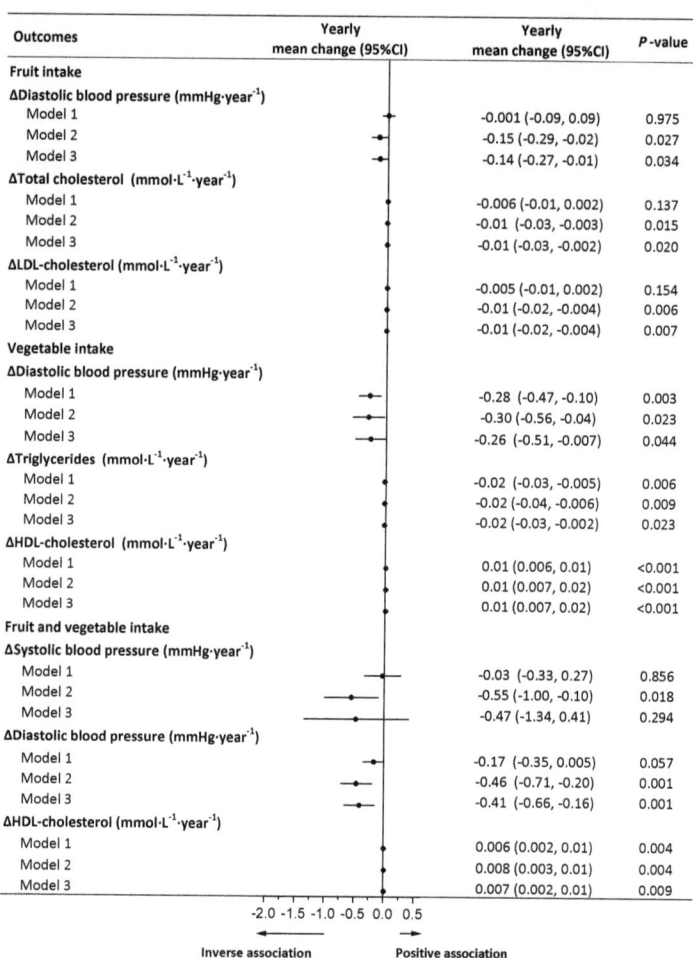

Figure 4. Longitudinal associations of fruit (50 g·day^{-1}) or vegetable (100 g·day^{-1}) or fruit and vegetable intake (150 g·day^{-1}) with yearly changes in cardiometabolic risk factors during weight-loss maintenance. Yearly mean change and 95% CI of main effects indicating changes in cardiometabolic risk factors per year associated with 50 g increment in fruit intake or 100 g increment in vegetable intake or 150 g increment in fruit and vegetable intake. Analyses were conducted using a linear mixed model with repeated measures. Model 1 was adjusted for fixed factors including age, sex, ethnicity, BMI at 8 weeks, cardiometabolic risk factors at 8 weeks, and time and random factors including study center and participant ID. Model 2 was adjusted for covariates in model 1 plus fixed factors including time-varying physical activity, energy intake (kJ·day^{-1}), alcohol intake (g·day^{-1}), animal-based food intake (g·day^{-1}), and other plant food intake (g·day^{-1}); for systolic blood pressure and diastolic blood pressure, model 2 was additionally adjusted for dietary sodium intake (g·day^{-1}). Model 3 was adjusted for covariates in model 2 plus time-varying yearly changes in body weight as a fixed factor. HDL cholesterol, high-density lipoprotein cholesterol; LDL cholesterol, low-density lipoprotein cholesterol.

4. Discussion

In this 3-year, multi-center study, we examined the longitudinal associations of an overall PBD and specific plant foods with WLM and cardiometabolic risk factors in individuals with a high risk of developing T2D. We found that adherence to an overall PBD diet improved weight management. Consumption of nuts, fruits, and vegetables and fruits and vegetables was inversely associated with weight regain or cardiometabolic risk factors. Importantly, the reported associations with cardiometabolic risk factors were independent of weight change.

In the present analysis, we found that an overall PBD was inversely associated with weight regain, which is in agreement with findings from meta-analyses of RCTs [5,8,30] and prospective studies. Satija et al. [31] and Choi et al. [6] found inverse associations between adherence to a PBD and long-term weight gain. We did not find any associations between an overall PBD and cardiometabolic risk factors including glycemic markers, lipids, and blood pressure, after adjustment for weight change. On the contrary, Satija et al. [24,27,31] and Chen et al. [32] showed that an overall PDI was associated with smaller weight change or lower risk of T2D and coronary heart disease in three US prospective cohort studies. In addition, Glenn et al. [33] found that a plant-based Portfolio Diet was associated with a reduced CVD risk in the Women's Health Initiative Prospective Cohort.

The mixed findings may be partly explained by differences in assessment of adherence to a PBD. In observational studies, compliance to a PBD was commonly assessed by dietary indices such as PDI (including 18 food groups) [24,27] and A Priori Diet Quality Score (including 46 food groups) [6]. Specifically, the PDI created by Satija et al. [27] included vegetable oils, tea, and coffee (as healthy plant foods) and sugar-sweetened beverages and sweets and desserts (as unhealthy plant foods). However, in our PDI version, we did not include these food groups. In addition, some prospective studies showed that compared with overall PDI, healthy PDI emphasizing whole grains, fruits, vegetables, nuts, legumes, and vegetable oils showed stronger associations with smaller weight change and lower risk of T2D and coronary heart disease [24,27,31]. Furthermore, we did not calculate healthy PDI by giving positive scores to whole grains, vegetable oils, and tea and coffee and giving negative scores to refined grains, sugar sweetened beverages, and sweets and desserts. Compared with healthy PBDs or vegetarian diets in the abovementioned studies, our PDI captured a "less healthy" diet. PBDs rich in healthy components have higher dietary fiber and micronutrients as well as lower energy, GI, and glycemic load [27]. In a previous secondary analysis of the PREVIEW study, we found positive associations between GI, glycemic load, and weight regain during WLM [34].

In terms of specific components of PBDs, we found that nuts were linked with improved weight management and cardiometabolic risk factors during WLM. Similar to our findings, meta-analyses of prospective studies and RCTs also showed that nuts improved weight management [35–37] and cardiometabolic risk factors including HOMA-IR and fasting insulin [38]. In a study based on a cross-sectional nutrition survey, compared with non-nut consumers, nut consumers had lower BW, BMI, and WC, whereas there were no differences in cardiometabolic risk factors including blood pressure, total cholesterol, HDL cholesterol, and HbA_{1c} [13]. The results, however, were limited by cross-sectional design, and causal inferences could not be drawn. Our study stands out because it used long-term, repeatedly measured, and updated dietary records and health outcomes, which not only provided a large number of observations, but also deeper insights into the causally relevant associations compared with cross-sectional studies and prospective studies with diet measured at baseline only.

We also observed that fruits, vegetables, and combined consumption of vegetables and fruits were associated with improved cardiometabolic risk factors. Similarly, in a population-based cross-sectional study, Mirmiran et al. [39] showed that consumption of fruits and vegetables was associated with lower concentrations of total cholesterol and LDL cholesterol. However, in a 12-week RCT, McEvoy et al. [40] did not find dose–response effects of fruit and vegetable intake on cardiometabolic risk factors including ambulatory blood pressure and plasma lipids. For grains, several RCTs and observational studies suggested that whole grains showed inverse effects on cardiometabolic risk factors [41–43], whereas refined grains showed positive effects [44,45]. However, there are conflicting reports of the associations of whole grains with obesity measures [46,47]. In the current study, total grains were not associated with any favorable change in health outcome. This may be because the grain group in the PREVIEW dietary dataset was not strictly based on whole grains, although whole grains were recommended to participants in each intervention arms during WLM.

The strengths of the current study are that this is the first multi-center, international study to explore associations of consumption of a PBD and specific plant foods with weight gain and cardiometabolic risk factors during 3-year WLM after diet-induced WL. Additionally, our study included individuals who met the pre-diabetes criteria (not just overweight/obesity) at the start. Furthermore, long-term, repeated dietary records were collected, which provided a large number of observations and a sufficient statistical power to adjust for important and multiple confounding factors including animal-based food intake and PA measured by accelerometry.

The current study also has some limitations. First, the attrition rate, especially at the end of the study, was higher than expected, which may affect the generalization of our findings. Second, the dietary data were obtained via 4-day food records, and misreporting, overreporting, or underreporting were inevitable [48]. Third, specific food groups such as refined grains, whole grains, and sugar sweetened beverages were not included in PDI calculation, which made this index less accurate when describing adherence to an overall PBD. It was not possible for us to investigate unhealthy PDI or specific unhealthy plant foods because these foods were specifically excluded in the dietary instructions. Furthermore, in order to make the results easy to understand, we divided the participants into higher or lower plant-based diet adherence groups according to PDI at each time point. Unlike RCTs, however, in the present analysis the participants were not randomly allocated to one of the two groups, which means that their baseline characteristics may be unbalanced. The statistical phenomenon "regression toward the mean" may have affected the two groups differently, making the natural variation in BW appear as true change [49]. Finally, residual and unmeasured confounders are possible in any observational analysis, which may create bias. Hyperuricemia, an independent risk factor for major CVD [50] and an important confounding factor, was not included in the current analysis. As we collected smoking status at baseline only (not at each time point), it was not possible to adjust for smoking status as a time-varying variable in the models. Adjustment for baseline values only may introduce bias because smokers may quit smoking during a long-term healthy lifestyle intervention.

5. Conclusions

This secondary analysis showed that long-term consumption of specific healthy plant foods including nuts, fruits, and vegetables improved weight management and cardiometabolic health, whereas adherence to an overall PBD benefited weight management only. Our findings support the hypothesis that specific components in a PBD are important as well. Although healthy and high-quality plant foods are currently recommended to individuals for reducing weight regain and the risk of developing CVDs, the observational nature of our analysis cannot establish a cause-and-effect relationship. The findings should be treated with caution because misreporting of food intake and unmeasured confounders are common.

Supplementary Materials: The following are available online at https://www.mdpi.com/article/10.3390/nu13113916/s1, Table S1: Calculations for cumulative average dietary intake, physical activity, and yearly changes in body weight and cardiometabolic risk factors, Table S2. Longitudinal associations of adherence to healthy plant-based diet with yearly changes in weight outcomes and cardiometabolic risk factors during weight-loss maintenance (n = 688), Table S3. Longitudinal associations of total grain and potato intake with yearly weight regain and changes in cardiometabolic risk factors during weight-loss maintenance (n = 710), Table S4. Longitudinal associations of legume intake with yearly weight regain and changes in cardiometabolic risk factors during weight-loss maintenance (n = 710), Table S5. Longitudinal associations of nut intake with yearly changes in waist circumference and cardiometabolic risk factors during weight-loss maintenance (n = 710), Table S6.

Longitudinal associations of fruit intake with yearly weight regain and changes in cardiometabolic risk factors during weight-loss maintenance (n = 710), Table S7. Longitudinal associations of vegetable intake with yearly weight regain and changes in cardiometabolic risk factors during weight-loss maintenance (n = 710), Table S8. Longitudinal associations of vegetable and fruit intake with yearly weight regain and changes in cardiometabolic risk factors during weight-loss maintenance (n = 710), Figure S1. Changes in body weight during weight-loss maintenance in all participants (n = 688) (A) or completers (n = 493) (B) with lower or higher adherence to the plant-based diet.

Author Contributions: Conceptualization for the secondary analysis, R.Z. and A.R.; methodology, A.R., J.B.-M., M.F., S.D.P., I.A.M., J.A.M., G.S. and S.H.; sample analysis, J.S. and L.R.; writing—original draft preparation, R.Z.; writing—review and editing, R.Z., A.R., J.B.-M., M.F., S.D.P., J.A.M., G.M., M.H.-L., E.J., R.M., M.A.T., M.P.S., T.H.-D., I.A.M., G.S., S.H., J.S. and L.R. A.R. attests that all listed authors meet authorship criteria and that no others meeting the criteria have been omitted. The funders had no role in the design of the study; in the collection, analyses, or interpretation of data; in the writing of the manuscript; or in the decision to publish the results. All authors have read and agreed to the published version of the manuscript.

Funding: EU framework programme 7 (FP7/2007-2013) grant agreement # 312057. National Health and Medical Research Council—EU Collaborative Grant, AUS 8, ID 1067711). The Glycemic Index Foundation Australia through royalties to the University of Sydney. The New Zealand Health Research Council (grant #14/191) and University of Auckland Faculty Research Development Fund. The Cambridge Weight Plan© donated all products for the 8-week LED period. The Danish Agriculture & Food Council. The Danish Meat and Research Institute. National Institute for Health Research Biomedical Research Centre (NIHR BRC) (UK). Engineering and Physical Sciences Research Council (EPSRC) (UK). Nutritics (Dublin) donated all dietary analyses software used by UNOTT. Juho Vainio Foundation (FIN), Academy of Finland (grant numbers: 272376, 314383, 266286, 314135), Finnish Medical Foundation, Gyllenberg Foundation, Novo Nordisk Foundation, Finnish Diabetes Research Foundation, University of Helsinki, Government Research Funds for Helsinki University Hospital (FIN), Jenny and Antti Wihuri Foundation (FIN), Emil Aaltonen Foundation (FIN). China Scholarship Council.

Institutional Review Board Statement: The PREVIEW study was conducted according to the guidelines of the Declaration of Helsinki, and the study was approved by the Human Ethics Committees at each intervention center (Denmark: The Research Ethics Committees of the Capital Region, ethical approval code: H-1-2013-052; Finland: Coordinating Ethical Committee of HUS (Helsinki and Uusimaa Hospital District), ethical approval code: HUS/1733/2017; the UK: UK National Research Ethics Service (NRES) and East Midlands (Leicester) Ethics Committee, ethical approval code: 13/EM/0259; the Netherlands: Medical Ethics Committee of the Maastricht University Medical Centre, ethical approval code: NL43054.068.13/METC 13–3-008; Spain: Research Ethics Committee of the University of Navarra, ethical approval code: 71/2013; Bulgaria: Commission on Ethics in Scientific Research with the Medical University-Sofia (KENIMUS), ethical approval code: 4303/13.06.2014; Australia: The University of Sydney, Human Research Ethics Committee (HREC), ethical approval code: 2013/535; and New Zealand: Health and Disability Ethics Committees (HDEC), ethical approval code: X14-0408).

Informed Consent Statement: Written informed consent was obtained from all participants.

Data Availability Statement: The dataset for this study is available from the corresponding author on reasonable request.

Acknowledgments: The PREVIEW consortium would like to thank all study participants at every intervention center for their time and commitment and all scientists, advisors, and students for their dedication and contributions to the study. Specially, we would like to thank Thomas Meinert Larsen (University of Copenhagen), Margriet Westerterp-Plantenga (Maastricht University), Edith Feskens (Wageningen University), and Wolfgang Schlicht (University of Stuttgart).

Conflicts of Interest: A.R. has received honorariums from Unilever and the International Sweeteners Association. J.B.-M. is President and Director of the Glycemic Index Foundation, oversees a glycemic index testing service at the University of Sydney, and is a co-author of books about diet and diabetes. She is a member of the Scientific Advisory Board of the Novo Foundation and of ZOE Global. I.A.M. was a member of the UK Government Scientific Advisory Committee on Nutrition, Treasurer of the Federation of European Nutrition Societies, Treasurer of the World Obesity Federation, member of the Mars Scientific Advisory Council, member of the Mars Europe Nutrition Advisory Board, and Scientific Adviser to the Waltham Centre for Pet Nutrition. He was also a member of the Nestle Research Scientific Advisory Board and of the Novozymes Scientific Advisory Board. He withdrew from all of these roles in 2020 and on 1 August 2020 became Professor Emeritus at the University of Nottingham and took up the post of Scientific Director of the Nestle Institute of Health Sciences in Lausanne, Switzerland. S.D.P. was the Fonterra Chair in Human Nutrition during the PREVIEW intervention.

References

1. Timmis, A.; Townsend, N.; Gale, C.P.; Torbica, A.; Lettino, M.; Petersen, S.E.; Mossialos, E.A.; Maggioni, A.P.; Kazakiewicz, D.; May, H.T.; et al. European Society of Cardiology: Cardiovascular Disease Statistics 2019. *Eur. Heart J.* **2020**, *41*, 12–85. [CrossRef] [PubMed]
2. Bechthold, A.; Boeing, H.; Tetens, I.; Schwingshackl, L.; Nothlings, U. Perspective: Food-Based Dietary Guidelines in Europe-Scientific Concepts, Current Status, and Perspectives. *Adv. Nutr.* **2018**, *9*, 544–560. [CrossRef]
3. Willett, W.; Rockstrom, J.; Loken, B.; Springmann, M.; Lang, T.; Vermeulen, S.; Garnett, T.; Tilman, D.; DeClerck, F.; Wood, A.; et al. Food in the Anthropocene: The EAT-Lancet Commission on healthy diets from sustainable food systems. *Lancet* **2019**, *393*, 447–492. [CrossRef]
4. Aune, D. Plant Foods, Antioxidant Biomarkers, and the Risk of Cardiovascular Disease, Cancer, and Mortality: A Review of the Evidence. *Adv. Nutr.* **2019**, *10*, S404–S421. [CrossRef]
5. Dinu, M.; Abbate, R.; Gensini, G.F.; Casini, A.; Sofi, F. Vegetarian, vegan diets and multiple health outcomes: A systematic review with meta-analysis of observational studies. *Crit. Rev. Food Sci. Nutr.* **2017**, *57*, 3640–3649. [CrossRef]
6. Choi, Y.; Larson, N.; Gallaher, D.D.; Odegaard, A.O.; Rana, J.S.; Shikany, J.M.; Steffen, L.M.; Jacobs, D.R., Jr. A Shift toward a Plant-Centered Diet from Young to Middle Adulthood and Subsequent Risk of Type 2 Diabetes and Weight Gain: The Coronary Artery Risk Development in Young Adults (CARDIA) Study. *Diabetes Care* **2020**, *43*, 2796–2803. [CrossRef] [PubMed]
7. Hemler, E.C.; Hu, F.B. Plant-Based Diets for Personal, Population, and Planetary Health. *Adv. Nutr.* **2019**, *10*, S275–S283. [CrossRef] [PubMed]
8. Huang, R.Y.; Huang, C.C.; Hu, F.B.; Chavarro, J.E. Vegetarian Diets and Weight Reduction: A Meta-Analysis of Randomized Controlled Trials. *J. Gen. Intern. Med.* **2016**, *31*, 109–116. [CrossRef] [PubMed]
9. Kim, H.; Caulfield, L.E.; Garcia-Larsen, V.; Steffen, L.M.; Coresh, J.; Rebholz, C.M. Plant-Based Diets Are Associated With a Lower Risk of Incident Cardiovascular Disease, Cardiovascular Disease Mortality, and All-Cause Mortality in a General Population of Middle-Aged Adults. *J. Am. Heart Assoc.* **2019**, *8*, e012865. [CrossRef] [PubMed]
10. Satija, A.; Hu, F.B. Plant-based diets and cardiovascular health. *Trends Cardiovasc. Med.* **2018**, *28*, 437–441. [CrossRef]
11. Bielefeld, D.; Grafenauer, S.; Rangan, A. The Effects of Legume Consumption on Markers of Glycaemic Control in Individuals with and without Diabetes Mellitus: A Systematic Literature Review of Randomised Controlled Trials. *Nutrients* **2020**, *12*, 2123. [CrossRef]
12. Abbaspour, N.; Roberts, T.; Hooshmand, S.; Kern, M.; Hong, M.Y. Mixed nut consumption may improve cardiovascular disease risk factors in overweight and obese adults. *Nutrients* **2019**, *11*, 1488. [CrossRef]
13. Brown, R.C.; Tey, S.L.; Gray, A.R.; Chisholm, A.; Smith, C.; Fleming, E.; Parnell, W. Association of Nut Consumption with Cardiometabolic Risk Factors in the 2008/2009 New Zealand Adult Nutrition Survey. *Nutrients* **2015**, *7*, 7523–7542. [CrossRef]
14. Carter, P.; Gray, L.J.; Talbot, D.; Morris, D.H.; Khunti, K.; Davies, M.J. Fruit and vegetable intake and the association with glucose parameters: A cross-sectional analysis of the Let's Prevent Diabetes Study. *Eur. J. Clin. Nutr.* **2013**, *67*, 12–17. [CrossRef] [PubMed]
15. Fisk, P.S., II; Middaugh, A.L.; Rhee, Y.S.; Brunt, A.R. Few favorable associations between fruit and vegetable intake and biomarkers for chronic disease risk in American adults. *Nutr. Res.* **2011**, *31*, 616–624. [CrossRef] [PubMed]
16. Toumpanakis, A.; Turnbull, T.; Alba-Barba, I. Effectiveness of plant-based diets in promoting well-being in the management of type 2 diabetes: A systematic review. *BMJ Open Diabetes Res. Care* **2018**, *6*, e000534. [CrossRef] [PubMed]
17. Yokoyama, Y.; Barnard, N.D.; Levin, S.M.; Watanabe, M. Vegetarian diets and glycemic control in diabetes: A systematic review and meta-analysis. *Cardiovasc. Diagn. Ther.* **2014**, *4*, 373–382. [CrossRef]
18. Fogelholm, M.; Larsen, T.M.; Westerterp-Plantenga, M.; Macdonald, I.; Martinez, J.A.; Boyadjieva, N.; Poppitt, S.; Schlicht, W.; Stratton, G.; Sundvall, J.; et al. PREVIEW: Prevention of diabetes through lifestyle intervention and population studies in Europe and around the world. design, methods, and baseline participant description of an adult cohort enrolled into a three-year randomised clinical trial. *Nutrients* **2017**, *9*, 632. [CrossRef]
19. Christensen, P.; Meinert Larsen, T.; Westerterp-Plantenga, M.; Macdonald, I.; Martinez, J.A.; Handjiev, S.; Poppitt, S.; Hansen, S.; Ritz, C.; Astrup, A.; et al. Men and women respond differently to rapid weight loss: Metabolic outcomes of a multi-centre intervention study after a low-energy diet in 2500 overweight, individuals with pre-diabetes (PREVIEW). *Diabetes Obes. Metab.* **2018**, *20*, 2840–2851. [CrossRef]
20. Raben, A.; Vestentoft, P.S.; Brand-Miller, J.; Jalo, E.; Drummen, M.; Simpson, L.; Martinez, J.; Handjieva-Darlenska, T.; Stratton, G.; Huttunen-Lenz, M.; et al. PREVIEW-Results from a 3-year randomised 2 x 2 factorial multinational trial investigating the role of protein, glycemic index and physical activity for prevention of type-2 diabetes. *Diabetes Obes. Metab.* **2020**, *23*, 324–337. [CrossRef]

21. Kahlert, D.; Unyi-Reicherz, A.; Stratton, G.; Meinert Larsen, T.; Fogelholm, M.; Raben, A.; Schlicht, W. PREVIEW behavior modification intervention toolbox (PREMIT): A study protocol for a psychological element of a multicenter project. *Front. Psychol.* **2016**, *7*, 1136. [CrossRef]
22. American Diabetes Association. 2. Classification and Diagnosis of Diabetes. *Diabetes Care* **2017**, *40*, S11–S24. [CrossRef] [PubMed]
23. National Health and Medical Research Council. *Australian Dietary Guidelines*; National Health and Medical Research Council: Canberra, Australia, 2013.
24. Satija, A.; Bhupathiraju, S.N.; Rimm, E.B.; Spiegelman, D.; Chiuve, S.E.; Borgi, L.; Willett, W.C.; Manson, J.E.; Sun, Q.; Hu, F.B. Plant-Based Dietary Patterns and Incidence of Type 2 Diabetes in US Men and Women: Results from Three Prospective Cohort Studies. *PLoS Med.* **2016**, *13*, e1002039. [CrossRef] [PubMed]
25. Wallace, T.M.; Levy, J.C.; Matthews, D.R. Use and abuse of HOMA modeling. *Diabetes Care* **2004**, *27*, 1487–1495. [CrossRef] [PubMed]
26. He, F.J.; Tan, M.; Ma, Y.; MacGregor, G.A. Salt Reduction to Prevent Hypertension and Cardiovascular Disease: JACC State-of-the-Art Review. *J. Am. Coll. Cardiol.* **2020**, *75*, 632–647. [CrossRef]
27. Satija, A.; Bhupathiraju, S.N.; Spiegelman, D.; Chiuve, S.E.; Manson, J.E.; Willett, W.; Rexrode, K.M.; Rimm, E.B.; Hu, F.B. Healthful and Unhealthful Plant-Based Diets and the Risk of Coronary Heart Disease in U.S. Adults. *J. Am. Coll. Cardiol.* **2017**, *70*, 411–422. [CrossRef]
28. Peters, S.A.; Bots, M.L.; den Ruijter, H.M.; Palmer, M.K.; Grobbee, D.E.; Crouse III, J.R.; O'Leary, D.H.; Evans, G.W.; Raichlen, J.S.; Moons, K.G. Multiple imputation of missing repeated outcome measurements did not add to linear mixed-effects models. *J. Clin. Epidemiol.* **2012**, *65*, 686–695. [CrossRef]
29. Twisk, J.; de Boer, M.; de Vente, W.; Heymans, M. Multiple imputation of missing values was not necessary before performing a longitudinal mixed-model analysis. *J. Clin. Epidemiol.* **2013**, *66*, 1022–1028. [CrossRef]
30. Wang, F.; Zheng, J.; Yang, B.; Jiang, J.; Fu, Y.; Li, D. Effects of Vegetarian Diets on Blood Lipids: A Systematic Review and Meta-Analysis of Randomized Controlled Trials. *J. Am. Heart Assoc.* **2015**, *4*, e002408. [CrossRef]
31. Satija, A.; Malik, V.; Rimm, E.B.; Sacks, F.; Willett, W.; Hu, F.B. Changes in intake of plant-based diets and weight change: Results from 3 prospective cohort studies. *Am. J. Clin. Nutr.* **2019**, *110*, 574–582. [CrossRef]
32. Chen, Z.; Drouin-Chartier, J.P.; Li, Y.; Baden, M.Y.; Manson, J.E.; Willett, W.C.; Voortman, T.; Hu, F.B.; Bhupathiraju, S.N. Changes in Plant-Based Diet Indices and Subsequent Risk of Type 2 Diabetes in Women and Men: Three U.S. Prospective Cohorts. *Diabetes Care* **2021**, *44*, 663–671. [CrossRef]
33. Glenn, A.J.; Lo, K.; Jenkins, D.J.A.; Boucher, B.A.; Hanley, A.J.; Kendall, C.W.C.; Manson, J.E.; Vitolins, M.Z.; Snetselaar, L.G.; Liu, S.; et al. Relationship Between a Plant-Based Dietary Portfolio and Risk of Cardiovascular Disease: Findings From the Women's Health Initiative Prospective Cohort Study. *J. Am. Heart Assoc.* **2021**, *10*, e021515. [CrossRef]
34. Zhu, R.; Larsen, T.M.; Fogelholm, M.; Poppitt, S.; Vestentoft, P.S.; Silvestre, M.P.; Jalo, E. Dose-dependent associations of dietary glycemic index, glycemic load and fiber with 3-year weight-loss maintenance and glycemic status in a high-risk population: A secondary analysis of the PREVIEW diabetes prevention study. *Diabetes Care* **2021**, *44*, 1672–1681. [CrossRef]
35. Schlesinger, S.; Neuenschwander, M.; Schwedhelm, C.; Hoffmann, G.; Bechthold, A.; Boeing, H.; Schwingshackl, L. Food Groups and Risk of Overweight, Obesity, and Weight Gain: A Systematic Review and Dose-Response Meta-Analysis of Prospective Studies. *Adv. Nutr.* **2019**, *10*, 205–218. [CrossRef]
36. Li, H.; Li, X.; Yuan, S.; Jin, Y.; Lu, J. Nut consumption and risk of metabolic syndrome and overweight/obesity: A meta-analysis of prospective cohort studies and randomized trials. *Nutr. Metab.* **2018**, *15*, 46. [CrossRef]
37. Eslami, O.; Shidfar, F.; Dehnad, A. Inverse association of long-term nut consumption with weight gain and risk of overweight/obesity: A systematic review. *Nutr. Res.* **2019**, *68*, 1–8. [CrossRef]
38. Tindall, A.M.; Johnston, E.A.; Kris-Etherton, P.M.; Petersen, K.S. The effect of nuts on markers of glycemic control: A systematic review and meta-analysis of randomized controlled trials. *Am. J. Clin. Nutr.* **2019**, *109*, 297–314. [CrossRef]
39. Ibarrola-Jurado, N.; Bulló, M.; Guasch-Ferré, M.; Ros, E.; Martínez-González, M.A.; Corella, D.; Fiol, M.; Wärnberg, J.; Estruch, R.; Román, P. Cross-sectional assessment of nut consumption and obesity, metabolic syndrome and other cardiometabolic risk factors: The PREDIMED study. *PLoS ONE* **2013**, *8*, e57367. [CrossRef] [PubMed]
40. McEvoy, C.T.; Wallace, I.R.; Hamill, L.L.; Hunter, S.J.; Neville, C.E.; Patterson, C.C.; Woodside, J.V.; Young, I.S.; McKinley, M.C. Increasing fruit and vegetable intake has no dose-response effect on conventional cardiovascular risk factors in overweight adults at high risk of developing cardiovascular disease. *J. Nutr.* **2015**, *145*, 1464–1471. [CrossRef] [PubMed]
41. Marshall, S.; Petocz, P.; Duve, E.; Abbott, K.; Cassettari, T.; Blumfield, M.; Fayet-Moore, F. The Effect of Replacing Refined Grains with Whole Grains on Cardiovascular Risk Factors: A Systematic Review and Meta-Analysis of Randomized Controlled Trials with GRADE Clinical Recommendation. *J. Acad. Nutr. Diet.* **2020**, *120*, 1859–1883.E31. [CrossRef] [PubMed]
42. Tieri, M.; Ghelfi, F.; Vitale, M.; Vetrani, C.; Marventano, S.; Lafranconi, A.; Godos, J.; Titta, L.; Gambera, A.; Alonzo, E.; et al. Whole grain consumption and human health: An umbArella review of observational studies. *Int. J. Food Sci. Nutr.* **2020**, *71*, 668–677. [CrossRef]
43. Reynolds, A.; Mann, J.; Cummings, J.; Winter, N.; Mete, E.; Te Morenga, L. Carbohydrate quality and human health: A series of systematic reviews and meta-analyses. *Lancet* **2019**, *393*, 434–445. [CrossRef]

44. Musa-Veloso, K.; Poon, T.; Harkness, L.S.; O'Shea, M.; Chu, Y. The effects of whole-grain compared with refined wheat, rice, and rye on the postprandial blood glucose response: A systematic review and meta-analysis of randomized controlled trials. *Am. J. Clin. Nutr.* **2018**, *108*, 759–774. [CrossRef]
45. Schwingshackl, L.; Hoffmann, G.; Lampousi, A.M.; Knuppel, S.; Iqbal, K.; Schwedhelm, C.; Bechthold, A.; Schlesinger, S.; Boeing, H. Food groups and risk of type 2 diabetes mellitus: A systematic review and meta-analysis of prospective studies. *Eur. J. Epidemiol.* **2017**, *32*, 363–375. [CrossRef] [PubMed]
46. Sadeghi, O.; Sadeghian, M.; Rahmani, S.; Maleki, V.; Larijani, B.; Esmaillzadeh, A. Whole-grain consumption does not affect obesity measures: An updated systematic review and meta-analysis of randomized clinical trials. *Adv. Nutr.* **2020**, *11*, 280–292. [CrossRef] [PubMed]
47. Ye, E.Q.; Chacko, S.A.; Chou, E.L.; Kugizaki, M.; Liu, S. Greater whole-grain intake is associated with lower risk of type 2 diabetes, cardiovascular disease, and weight gain. *J. Nutr.* **2012**, *142*, 1304–1313. [CrossRef]
48. Park, Y.; Dodd, K.W.; Kipnis, V.; Thompson, F.E.; Potischman, N.; Schoeller, D.A.; Baer, D.J.; Midthune, D.; Troiano, R.P.; Bowles, H.; et al. Comparison of self-reported dietary intakes from the Automated Self-Administered 24-h recall, 4-d food records, and food-frequency questionnaires against recovery biomarkers. *Am. J. Clin. Nutr.* **2018**, *107*, 80–93. [CrossRef]
49. Barnett, A.G.; Van Der Pols, J.C.; Dobson, A.J. Regression to the mean: What it is and how to deal with it. *Int. J. Epidemiol.* **2005**, *34*, 215–220. [CrossRef]
50. Capuano, V.; Marchese, F.; Capuano, R.; Torre, S.; Iannone, A.G.; Capuano, E.; Lamaida, N.; Sonderegger, M.; Capuano, E. Hyperuricemia as an independent risk factor for major cardiovascular events: A 10-year cohort study from Southern Italy. *J. Cardiovasc. Med.* **2017**, *18*, 159–164. [CrossRef]

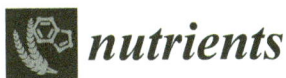

Article

Milk Intake and Stroke Mortality in the Japan Collaborative Cohort Study—A Bayesian Survival Analysis

Chaochen Wang [1,*], Hiroshi Yatsuya [2], Yingsong Lin [1], Tae Sasakabe [1], Sayo Kawai [1], Shogo Kikuchi [1], Hiroyasu Iso [3] and Akiko Tamakoshi [4]

1. Department of Public Health, Aichi Medical University School of Medicine, 480-1195 Aichi, Japan; linys@aichi-med-u.ac.jp (Y.L.); tsasa@aichi-med-u.ac.jp (T.S.); ksayo@aichi-med-u.ac.jp (S.K.); kikuchis@aichi-med-u.ac.jp (S.K.)
2. Department of Public Health, Fujita Health University School of Medicine, Toyoake 470-1192, Japan; yatsuya@fujita-hu.ac.jp
3. Public Health, Department of Social Medicine, Osaka University Graduate School of Medicine, Osaka 565-0871, Japan; iso@pbhel.med.osaka-u.ac.jp
4. Department of Public Health, Hokkaido University, Faculty of Medicine, Sapporo 002-8501, Japan; tamaa@med.hokudai.ac.jp
* Correspondence: chaochen@wangcc.me; Tel.: +81-561-62-3311

Received: 1 August 2020; Accepted: 3 September 2020; Published: 9 September 2020

Abstract: The aim of this study was to further examine the relationship between milk intake and stroke mortality among the Japanese population. We used data from the Japan Collaborative Cohort (JACC) Study (total number of participants = 110,585, age range: 40–79) to estimate the posterior acceleration factors (AF) as well as the hazard ratios (HR) comparing individuals with different milk intake frequencies against those who never consumed milk at the study baseline. These estimations were computed through a series of Bayesian survival models that employed a Markov Chain Monte Carlo simulation process. In total, 100,000 posterior samples were generated separately through four independent chains after model convergency was confirmed. Posterior probabilites that daily milk consumers had lower hazard or delayed mortality from strokes compared to non-consumers was 99.0% and 78.0% for men and women, respectively. Accordingly, the estimated posterior means of AF and HR for daily milk consumers were 0.88 (95% Credible Interval, CrI: 0.81, 0.96) and 0.80 (95% CrI: 0.69, 0.93) for men and 0.97 (95% CrI: 0.88, 1.10) and 0.95 (95% CrI: 0.80, 1.17) for women. In conclusion, data from the JACC study provided strong evidence that daily milk intake among Japanese men was associated with delayed and lower risk of mortality from stroke especially cerebral infarction.

Keywords: milk intake; mortality; stroke; Bayesian survival anlysis; time-to-event data; JACC study

1. Introduction

Eastern Asian populations were reported to have a higher burden from both mortality and morbidity from stroke than populations in European or American regions [1]. Dairy foods, especially milk, have been suggested to relate with decreased stroke risk by nearly 7% for each 200 g increment of daily consumption [2]. Although two daily servings of milk or dairy products is recommended in Japan [3], the actual per capita intake (≈63 g/day) of these food groups is much lower and less frequent than that in Western countries [4]. Given that previous reports have also indicated no significant [5–7] or even positive associations [8], it would be of interest to provide information on the association within a context where most individuals have much lower range of milk intake compared to most of the previous studies. Whether people with such a low level intake of milk can still benefit against stroke would requires elucidation.

Moreover, a more intuitive or straightforward interpretation would be available if we were able to show the probabilities and the certainty that the existing data can provide evidence about whether drinking milk can delay or lower the hazard of dying from stroke. This would require the transformation of the research question into "Do individuals with milk intake habit have lower hazard of dying from a stroke event?" Another way of asking the same research question would be "Can an event of dying from stroke be postponed by forming a milk intake habit?" The later question directly compares the length of times before events or the speed from the same departure point (entry of the study) to a fatal stroke event. Accelerated failure time (AFT) models under the Bayesian framework are convenient tools that would help to avoid worrying about the assumptions of repeatability of a large scale prospective study, and can calculate the exact proportion of posterior estimates (hazard ratios, HR) that are lower than 1. AFT model is helpful in estimating acceleration factors (AF) which can be interpreted as the velocity for developing an event of interest. This velocity parameter shows how faster/slower individuals in one exposure group might have an event compared to others in different exposure groups [9,10].

Our aim was to provide a more straightforward answer to the primary research question that, whether someone answering that he/she drank milk at the baseline of study, had lower hazard of dying from stroke compared with his/her counterparts who said they never consumed milk. If the answer to the primary objective was yes, then the probabilities that individuals with different frequencies of milk intake may have lower risk compared with those who never drank milk were calculated through a Markov Chain Monte Carlo (MCMC) simulation process. A Bayesian survival analysis method was applied on an existing database and through which we provided estimates about whether drinking milk could delay a stroke mortality event from happening after controlling for the other potential confounders.

2. Materials and Methods

2.1. The Database

We used data from the Japan Collaborative Cohort (JACC) study, which was sponsored by the Ministry of Education, Sports, Science, and Technology of Japan. Sampling methods and details about the JACC study have been described extensively in the literature [11–13]. Participants in the JACC study completed self-administered questionnaires about their lifestyles, food intake (food frequency questionnaire, FFQ), and medical histories of cardiovascular disease or cancer. In the final follow-up of the JACC study, data from a total of 110,585 individuals (46,395 men and 64,190 women) who, aged between 40–79 at the baseline, were successfully retained for the current analysis. We further excluded samples if they met one of the following criteria: (1) with any disease history of stroke, cancer, myocardial infarction, ischemic heart disease, or other types heart disease (n = 6655, 2931 men and 3724 women); (2) did not answer the question regarding their milk consumption in the baseline FFQ survey (n = 9545, 3593 men and 5952 women). Finally, 94,385 (39,386 men and 54,999 women) were left in the database. The study design and informed consent procedure were approved by the Ethics Review Committee of Hokkaido University School of Medicine.

2.2. Exposure and the Outcome of Interest

Frequency of milk intake during the preceding year of the baseline was assessed by FFQ as "never", "1–2 times/month", "1–2 times/week", "3–4 times/week", and "Almost daily". The exact amount of milk consumption was difficult to assess here. However, good reproducibility and validity were confirmed previously (Spearman rank correlation coefficient between milk intake frequency and weighed dietary record for 12 days was 0.65) [14]. From the same validation study [14] on the FFQ, daily consumers of milk were found to have a median intake of 146 g. At the baseline of the JACC study (between 1988 and 1990), most "milk and dairy product" consumption (92.1%) was in the form of whole milk [15].

In the study area, investigators conducted a systematic review of death certificates till the end of 2009. Date and cause of death were confirmed with the permission of the Director-General of the Prime Minister's Office. The follow-up period was defined as from the time the baseline survey was completed, which was between 1988–1990, until the end of 2009 (administrative censor), the date when they moved out of the study area, or the date of death from stroke was recorded—whichever occurred first. Other causes of death were treated as censored and assumed not informative. The causes of death were coded by the 10th Revision of the International Statistical Classification of Diseases and Related Health Problems (ICD-10); therefore, stroke was defined as I60–I69. We further classified these deaths into hemorrhagic stroke (I60, I61 and I62) or cerebral infarction (I63) when subtypes of stroke in their death certificates were available.

2.3. Statistical Approach

Analyses were stratified by sex as difference in milk consumption levels and mortality rate were suggested previously [16,17]. We calculated sex-specific means (standard deviation, SD) and proportion of selected baseline characteristics according to the frequency of milk intake. Age-adjusted stroke mortality rate were expressed as per 1000 person-year, predicted through poisson regression models.

Full parametric proportional hazard models under Bayesian framework with Weibull distribution were fitted using Just Another Gibbs Sampler (JAGS) program [18], version 4.3.0 in R, version 4.0.1 [19]. JAGS program is similar to the OpenBUGS [20] project that uses a Gibbs sampling engine for MCMC simulation. In the current analysis, we specified non-informative prior distributions for each of the parameters in our models ($\beta_n \sim N(0, 1000)$, and $\kappa_{shape} \sim \Gamma(0.001, 0.001)$). The Brooks–Gelman–Rubin diagnostic [21] was used to refine the approximate point of convergence, the point when the ratio of the chains is stable around 1 and the within and between chain variability start to reach stability, was visually checked. The auto-correlation tool further identified if convergence has been achieved or if a high degree of auto-correlation exists in the sample. Then, the number of iterations discarded as "burn-in" was chosen. All models had a posterior sample size of 100,000 from four separated chains with a "burn-in" of 2500 iterations. Posterior means (SD) and 95% Credible Intervals (CrI) of the estimated hazard ratios (HRs), as well as acceleration factors (AFs), were presented for each category of milk intake frequency taking the "never" category as the reference. Posterior probabilities that the estimated hazard of dying from stroke for the milk intake for frequency that higher or equal to "1–2 times/month" were smaller compared with those who chose "never" for their milk intake frequency, and were calculated as $Pr(HR < 1)$.

The parametric forms of the models fitted in the Bayesian survival analyses included three models: (1) the crude model, (2) the age-centered adjusted model, (3) and a model further adjusted for potential confounders which includes: age (centered, continuous), smoking habit (never, current, former), alcohol intake (never or past, <4 times/week, Daily), body mass index (<18.5, ≥18.5 and <25, ≥25 and <30, ≥30 kg/m^2), history of hypertension, diabetes, kidney/liver diseases (yes/no), exercise (more than 1 h/week, yes/no), sleep duration (<7, ≥7 and <8, ≥8 and <9, ≥9, hours), quartiles of total energy intake, coffee intake (never, <3–4 times/week, almost daily), and education level (attended school till age 18, yes/no).

3. Results

The total follow-up was 1,555,073 person-year (median = 19.3 years), during which 2675 deaths from stroke were confirmed (1352 men and 1323 women). Among these stroke mortalities, 952 were hemorrhagic stroke (432 men and 520 women), and 957 were cerebral infarction (520 men and 437 women). The number of deaths from causes other than stroke was 18,868 (10,731 men and 8137 women); 5493 (2022 men and 3471 women) dropped out from the follow-up (5.8%); 67,349 (25,281 men and 42,068 women) were censored at the end of follow-up (71.4%). The medians (interquartile range, IQR) of follow-up years for hemorrhagic stroke mortality were 9.9 (5.4, 12.3) in men and 10.9 (5.9, 15.1) in women; the medians (IQR) of follow-up years for cerebral infarction mortality were 11.2 (7.1, 15.3) and 11.8 (7.9, 16.4) in men and women, respectively. Age-adjusted stroke mortality rates for each category of milk intake frequency was estimated to be 1.8, 2.0, 1.7, 1.6, an 1.5 per 1000 person-year for men and 1.3, 1.4, 1.2, 1.1, and 1.2 per 1000 person-year for women.

As listed in Table 1, compared with those who chose "never" as their milk intake frequency at baseline, milk drinkers were less likely to be a current smoker or a daily alcohol consumer in both men and women. Furthermore, people who consumed milk more than 1–2 times/month were more likely to be a daily consumers of vegetables and fruit, as well as coffee, and were more likely to perform exercise more than 1 h/week among both sexes.

Table 1. Sex-specific baseline characteristics according to the frequency of milk intake (JACC study, 1988–2009).

			Milk Drinkers			
	Never	Drinkers	1–2 Times/ Month	1–2 Times/ Week	3–4 Times/ Week	Almost Daily
Men (n = 39,386)						
Number of subjects	8508	30,878	3522	5928	5563	15,865
Age, year (mean (SD))	56.8 (9.9)	56.8 (10.2)	55.2 (10.1)	55.4 (10.1)	55.4 (9.9)	58.1 (10.1)
Current smoker, %	58.7	49.8	57.4	55.9	51.1	45.4
Daily alcohol drinker, %	51.9	47.8	50.9	48.4	48.6	46.5
BMI, kg/m^2 (mean (SD))	22.6 (3.4)	22.7 (3.4)	22.8 (2.8)	22.8 (2.8)	22.9 (5.4)	22.6 (2.8)
Exercise (>1 h/week), %	19.0	27.6	26.5	25.0	25.5	29.5
Sleep duration, 8–9 h, %	35.6	35.9	34.6	36.2	35.1	36.3
Energy intake, kcal/day (mean (SD))	1611 (505)	1764 (504)	1606 (496)	1679 (495)	1772 (509)	1830 (495)
Vegetable intake, daily, %	21.3	25.4	20.1	20.4	20.8	30.1
Fruit intake, daily, %	14.8	22.4	15.4	16.3	17.3	28.1
Green tea intake, daily, %	76.5	79.2	79.9	78.3	77.9	79.8
Coffee intake, daily, %	43.8	50.7	50.5	48.0	47.5	52.9
Educated over 18 years old, %	9.9	14.1	12.4	12.8	11.1	15.9
History of diabetes, %	5.0	6.3	4.5	4.2	5.5	7.7
History of hypertension, %	18.4	17.9	17.5	17.1	16.8	18.7
History of kidney diseases, %	3.0	3.4	3.8	3.0	3.0	3.5
History of liver diseases, %	5.8	6.5	6.3	6.0	5.4	7.2
Women (n = 54,999)						
number of subjects	10,407	44,592	3640	7590	8108	25,254
Age, year (mean (SD))	58.0 (10.2)	56.9 (9.9)	56.5 (10.2)	55.6 (10.1)	55.6 (9.9)	57.9 (9.9)
Current smoker, %	6.9	4.2	6.1	5.5	4.3	3.5
Daily alcohol drinker, %	4.3	4.5	5.5	4.3	4.2	4.6
BMI, kg/m^2 (mean (SD))	23.0 (3.4)	22.9 (3.7)	23.0 (3.8)	23.1 (4.4)	23.1 (3.1)	22.8 (3.6)
Exercise (>1 h/week), %	13.6	20.8	17.1	18.5	18.8	22.6
Sleep duration, 8–9 h, %	27.7	25.6	25.1	25.9	25.4	25.7
Energy intake, kcal/day (mean (SD))	1519 (451)	1690 (449)	1522 (447)	1596 (443)	1661 (432)	1752 (443)
Vegetable intake, daily, %	24.7	30.4	25.0	24.6	24.2	34.8
Fruit intake, daily, %	25.0	35.7	26.6	29.2	29.2	41.1
Green tea intake, daily, %	73.8	76.8	77.0	76.4	75.8	77.3
Coffee intake, daily, %	39.6	48.2	46.2	46.4	44.4	50.2
Educated over 18 years old, %	4.8	8.3	6.7	7.2	6.5	9.4
History of diabetes, %	2.6	3.7	3.2	2.7	2.7	4.4
History of hypertension, %	21.5	19.7	20.5	19.1	18.9	20.0
History of kidney diseases, %	3.6	4.1	3.9	3.7	3.7	4.4
History of liver diseases, %	3.5	4.6	4.9	3.9	3.9	5.0

Note: Abbreviations: JACC: Japan Collaborative Cohort; SD: standard deviation; BMI: body mass index.

Detailed results from the Bayesian survival models (crude, age-adjusted and multivariable-adjusted) according to the frequency of milk intake separated by sex are listed in Table 2 (men) and Table 3 (women). Compared to those who never had milk, both men and women had slower speed and lower hazard of dying from total stroke in crude models. Velocities that milk consumers dying from stroke were slowed down by a crude acceleration factor (AF) between 0.79 (SD = 0.05; 95% CrI: 0.74, 0.90) and 0.93 (SD = 0.04; 95% CrI: 0.85, 1.02) compared with non-consumers. Chances that the posterior crude HRs were estimated to be lower than 1 for those who had at least 1–2 times/month was higher than 86.5% in men and greater than 94.6% in women. However, lower hazard and delayed time-to-event was observed to remain after age or multivariable adjustment only among daily male milk consumers. Specifically, the means (SD; 95% CrI) of posterior multivariable-adjusted AF and HR for daily male consumers of milk were 0.88 (SD = 0.05; 95% CrI: 0.81, 0.96) and 0.80 (SD = 0.07; 95% CrI: 0.69, 0.93) with a probability of 99.0% to be smaller than the null value (=1). Daily female milk consumers had posterior AFs and HRs that were distributed with means of 0.97 (SD = 0.09; 95% CrI: 0.88, 1.10) and 0.95 (SD = 0.12; 95% CrI: 0.80, 1.17) which had about a 78.0% chance that their HRs could be smaller than 1.

Table 2. Summary of posterior Acceleration Factors (AF) and Hazard Ratios (HR) of mortality from total stroke, stroke types according to the frequency of milk intake in men (JACC study, 1988–2009).

	Never	1–2 Times/Month	1–2 Times/Week	3–4 Times/Week	Almost Daily
Person-year	135,704	56,551	97,098	92,153	252,364
N	8508	3522	5928	5563	15,865
Total Stroke	326	122	181	177	546
Model 0					
Mean AF (SD)	1	0.93 (0.07)	0.83 (0.05)	0.85 (0.05)	0.93 (0.04)
95% CrI	-	(0.81, 1.06)	(0.73, 0.94)	(0.74, 0.96)	(0.85, 1.02)
Mean HR (SD)	1	0.89 (0.09)	0.77 (0.07)	0.79 (0.07)	0.90 (0.06)
95% CrI	-	(0.73, 1.08)	(0.63, 0.91)	(0.66, 0.94)	(0.79, 1.03)
Pr(HR < 1)	-	86.5%	99.9%	99.7%	93.5%
Model 1					
Mean AF (SD)	1	0.99 (0.06)	0.90 (0.05)	0.91 (0.05)	0.85 (0.04)
95% CrI	-	(0.87, 1.11)	(0.81, 1.00)	(0.82, 1.01)	(0.78, 0.92)
Mean HR (SD)	1	0.98 (0.11)	0.84 (0.08)	0.86 (0.08)	0.76 (0.05)
95% CrI	-	(0.79, 1.19)	(0.70, 1.00)	(0.71, 1.02)	(0.66, 0.87)
Pr(HR < 1)	-	58.7%	97.3%	96.1%	100.0%
Model 2					
Mean AF (SD)	1	1.00 (0.07)	0.92 (0.06)	0.94 (0.06)	0.88 (0.05)
95% CrI	-	(0.88, 1.14)	(0.82, 1.03)	(0.84, 1.05)	(0.81, 0.96)
Mean HR (SD)	1	1.01 (0.12)	0.87 (0.09)	0.90 (0.09)	0.80 (0.07)
95% CrI	-	(0.81, 1.24)	(0.72, 1.05)	(0.74, 1.08)	(0.69, 0.93)
Pr(HR < 1)	-	50.6%	93.7%	89.6%	99.0%
Hemorrhagic stroke	100	42	58	56	176
Model 0					
Mean AF (SD)	1	1.03 (0.17)	0.85 (0.12)	0.87 (0.13)	0.98 (0.11)
95% CrI	-	(0.74, 1.38)	(0.63, 1.12)	(0.65, 1.14)	(0.78, 1.22)
Mean HR (SD)	1	1.03 (0.19)	0.82 (0.14)	0.84 (0.15)	0.97 (0.13)
95% CrI	-	(0.70, 1.46)	(0.56, 1.14)	(0.60, 1.17)	(0.75, 1.26)
Pr(HR < 1)	-	47.2%	88.4%	86.3%	63.1%
Model 1					
Mean AF (SD)	1	1.08 (0.17)	0.91 (0.13)	0.92 (0.13)	0.90 (0.10)
95% CrI	-	(0.80, 1.45)	(0.70, 1.20)	(0.71, 1.19)	(0.74, 1.11)
Mean HR (SD)	1	1.11 (0.21)	0.88 (0.16)	0.90 (0.16)	0.88 (0.12)
95% CrI	-	(0.75, 1.58)	(0.63, 1.25)	(0.63, 1.24)	(0.67, 1.14)
Pr(HR < 1)	-	31.6%	79.7%	76.6%	87.6%
Model 2					
Mean AF (SD)	1	1.11 (0.18)	0.93 (0.15)	0.96 (0.16)	0.96 (0.13)
95% CrI	-	(0.79, 1.58)	(0.70, 1.25)	(0.71, 1.34)	(0.76, 1.25)
Mean HR (SD)	1	1.14 (0.22)	0.92 (0.17)	0.95 (0.18)	0.95 (0.14)
95% CrI	-	(0.75, 1.61)	(0.63, 1.29)	(0.65, 1.37)	(0.71, 1.27)
Pr(HR < 1)	-	28.8%	72.4%	64.4%	69.3%
Cerebral infarction	151	41	64	66	198
Model 0					
Mean AF (SD)	1	0.76 (0.09)	0.71 (0.07)	0.74 (0.08)	0.79 (0.06)
95% CrI	-	(0.59, 0.94)	(0.58, 0.86)	(0.61, 0.89)	(0.68, 0.93)
Mean HR (SD)	1	0.65 (0.12)	0.59 (0.09)	0.64 (0.09)	0.71 (0.09)
95% CrI	-	(0.46, 0.92)	(0.43, 0.79)	(0.47, 0.85)	(0.56, 0.89)
Pr(HR < 1)	-	99.1%	99.9%	99.7%	99.5%

Table 2. Cont.

	Never	1–2 Times/Month	1–2 Times/Week	3–4 Times/Week	Almost Daily
Model 1					
Mean AF (SD)	1	0.83 (0.08)	0.79 (0.07)	0.82 (0.07)	0.74 (0.05)
95% CrI	-	(0.68, 1.01)	(0.67, 0.93)	(0.69, 0.96)	(0.66, 0.84)
Mean HR (SD)	1	0.73 (0.13)	0.65 (0.10)	0.70 (0.11)	0.58 (0.07)
95% CrI	-	(0.49, 1.02)	(0.48, 0.88)	(0.51, 0.94)	(0.46, 0.72)
Pr(HR < 1)	-	96.9%	99.8%	98.9%	100.0%
Model 2					
Mean AF (SD)	1	0.84 (0.09)	0.80 (0.08)	0.83 (0.08)	0.75 (0.06)
95% CrI	-	(0.67, 1.02)	(0.67, 0.95)	(0.69, 0.99)	(0.66, 0.85)
Mean HR (SD)	1	0.73 (0.14)	0.67 (0.11)	0.72 (0.12)	0.61 (0.08)
95% CrI	-	(0.50, 1.04)	(0.48, 0.91)	(0.52, 0.99)	(0.48, 0.79)
Pr(HR < 1)	-	96.1%	99.1%	97.5%	99.8%

Note: Abbreviations: N, number of subjects,; SD, standard deviation; CrI, credible interval. Pr(HR < 1) indicates the probability for posterior HR to be smaller than 1. Model 0 = Crude model; Model 1 = age-adjusted model; Model 2 = multivariable adjusted model. Covariates included in Model 2: age, smoking habit, alcohol intake, body mass index, history of hypertension, diabetes, kidney/liver diseases, exercise, sleep duration, quartiles of total energy intake, coffee intake, and education level.

Table 3. Summary of posterior Acceleration Factors (AF) and Hazard Ratios (HR) of mortality from total stroke and stroke types according to the frequency of milk intake in women (JACC study, 1988–2009).

	Never	1–2 Times/Month	1–2 Times/Week	3–4 Times/Week	Almost Daily
Person-year	173,222	59,904	129,233	139,919	418,925
N	10,407	3640	7590	8108	25,254
Total Stroke	300	84	182	172	585
Model 0					
Mean AF (SD)	1	0.88 (0.07)	0.87 (0.05)	0.79 (0.05)	0.88 (0.04)
95% CrI	-	(0.75, 1.03)	(0.78, 0.98)	(0.71, 0.90)	(0.80, 0.96)
Mean HR (SD)	1	0.83 (0.10)	0.81 (0.08)	0.70 (0.07)	0.81 (0.07)
95% CrI	-	(0.64, 1.05)	(0.68, 0.97)	(0.58, 0.85)	(0.71, 0.93)
Pr(HR < 1)	-	94.6%	98.7%	99.9%	99.6%
Model 1					
Mean AF (SD)	1	0.99 (0.09)	1.11 (0.08)	1.02 (0.08)	0.95 (0.06)
95% CrI	-	(0.85, 1.17)	(0.97, 1.26)	(0.89, 1.16)	(0.86, 1.06)
Mean HR (SD)	1	1.00 (0.14)	1.18 (0.14)	1.03 (0.12)	0.92 (0.09)
95% CrI	-	(0.76, 1.31)	(0.95, 1.47)	(0.82, 1.28)	(0.78, 1.09)
Pr(HR < 1)	-	52.3%	6.3%	42.0%	86.8%
Model 2					
Mean AF (SD)	1	1.01 (0.12)	1.11 (0.14)	1.02 (0.12)	0.97 (0.09)
95% CrI	-	(0.85, 1.20)	(0.97, 1.30)	(0.89, 1.19)	(0.88, 1.10)
Mean HR (SD)	1	1.01 (0.17)	1.19 (0.15)	1.03 (0.15)	0.95 (0.12)
95% CrI	-	(0.75, 1.36)	(0.96, 1.52)	(0.81, 1.31)	(0.80, 1.17)
Pr(HR < 1)	-	52.8%	6.4%	44.4%	78.0%
Hemorrhagic stroke	108	27	78	76	231
Model 0					
Mean AF (SD)	1	0.78 (0.13)	0.98 (0.12)	0.90 (0.11)	0.92 (0.09)
95% CrI	-	(0.55, 1.06)	(0.76, 1.25)	(0.70, 1.13)	(0.76, 1.12)
Mean HR (SD)	1	0.73 (0.16)	0.98 (0.15)	0.87 (0.14)	0.89 (0.11)
95% CrI	-	(0.47, 1.08)	(0.71, 1.31)	(0.64, 1.16)	(0.71, 1.15)
Pr(HR < 1)	-	94.7%	58.1%	83.1%	83.0%
Model 1					
Mean AF (SD)	1	0.88 (0.13)	1.12 (0.13)	1.04 (0.13)	0.95 (0.09)
95% CrI	-	(0.63, 1.17)	(0.90, 1.41)	(0.82, 1.32)	(0.80, 1.14)
Mean HR (SD)	1	0.84 (0.18)	1.17 (0.18)	1.06 (0.17)	0.93 (0.12)
95% CrI	-	(0.54, 1.24)	(0.86, 1.58)	(0.76, 1.45)	(0.73, 1.19)
Pr(HR < 1)	-	81.6%	16.9%	38.9%	74.6%

Table 3. *Cont.*

	Never	1–2 Times/Month	1–2 Times/Week	3–4 Times/Week	Almost Daily
Model 2					
Mean AF (SD)	1	0.93 (0.24)	1.23 (0.38)	1.14 (0.33)	1.04 (0.25)
95% CrI	-	(0.64, 1.33)	(0.93, 1.98)	(0.87, 1.83)	(0.83, 1.55)
Mean HR (SD)	1	0.89 (0.22)	1.26 (0.26)	1.15 (0.23)	1.02 (0.19)
95% CrI	-	(0.55, 1.39)	(0.90, 1.90)	(0.83, 1.74)	(0.78, 1.51)
Pr(HR < 1)	-	73.2%	9.5%	24.8%	53.3%
Cerebral infarction	102	35	63	50	187
Model 0					
Mean AF (SD)	1	1.01 (0.13)	0.90 (0.09)	0.75 (0.08)	0.86 (0.06)
95% CrI	-	(0.79, 1.27)	(0.75, 1.10)	(0.60, 0.91)	(0.75, 0.99)
Mean HR (SD)	1	1.03 (0.20)	0.85 (0.14)	0.61 (0.11)	0.78 (0.10)
95% CrI	-	(0.69, 1.48)	(0.60, 1.13)	(0.43, 0.84)	(0.59, 0.99)
Pr(HR < 1)	-	51.9%	75.6%	97.6%	96.1%
Model 1					
Mean AF (SD)	1	1.21 (0.32)	1.16 (0.30)	0.98 (0.19)	0.97 (0.14)
95% CrI	-	(0.95, 2.08)	(0.93, 1.95)	(0.79, 1.48)	(0.84, 1.43)
Mean HR (SD)	1	1.37 (0.33)	1.25 (0.28)	0.94 (0.22)	0.92 (0.17)
95% CrI	-	(0.89, 2.18)	(0.87, 1.95)	(0.63, 1.52)	(0.69, 1.40)
Pr(HR < 1)	-	8.5%	14.2%	70.1%	79.4%
Model 2					
Mean AF (SD)	1	1.19 (0.19)	1.12 (0.15)	0.96 (0.12)	0.97 (0.09)
95% CrI	-	(0.94, 1.62)	(0.92, 1.49)	(0.78, 1.21)	(0.83, 1.18)
Mean HR (SD)	1	1.38 (0.29)	1.21 (0.22)	0.91 (0.18)	0.94 (0.14)
95% CrI	-	(0.89, 2.02)	(0.85, 1.70)	(0.62, 1.34)	(0.69, 1.25)
Pr(HR < 1)	-	7.3%	15.6%	72.8%	70.0%

Note: Abbreviations: N, number of subjects; SD, standard deviation; CrI, credible interval. Pr(HR < 1) indicates the probability for posterior HR to be smaller than 1. Model 0 = Crude model; Model 1 = age-adjusted model; Model 2 = multivariable adjusted model. Covariates included in Model 2: age, smoking habit, alcohol intake, body mass index, history of hypertension, diabetes, kidney/liver diseases, exercise, sleep duration, quartiles of total energy intake, coffee intake, and education level.

Posterior distributions of AFs and HRs for mortality from hemorrhagic stroke were found to contain the null value for either men or women among all fitted models. In contrast, men who a had milk intake frequency higher than 1–2 times/week were found to be associated with an average of 17–20% slower velocity or 28–39% lower risk of dying from cerebral infarction compared to men who never drank milk (Model 2 in Table 2). Probability that the posterior HRs distributed below the null value was greater or equal to 97.5%. No evidence was found about the associations between milk intake and risk of cerebral infarction mortality among women.

4. Discussion

In the JACC study cohort, our analyses showed that men in Japan who consumed milk almost daily had lower hazard of dying from stroke especially from cerebral infarction. Our evidence also suggested that stroke mortality events were delayed among Japanese male daily milk consumers compared with non-consumers.

These findings showed similar negative effect estimates that were reported previously [16] using data from the same cohort, in which the outcomes of interest were focused on cardiovascular diseases and all-cause mortality. Moreover, we have further updated the results with more comprehensive and straightforward evidence about whether and how certain the data shown about the daily consumption of milk were contributing to a postponed stroke (mostly cerebral infarction) mortality event among Japanese men. A recent dose-response meta-analysis of 18 prospective cohort studies showed a similar negative association [2] between milk consumption and risk of stroke. The same meta-analysis also reported a greater reduction in risk of stroke (18%) for East Asian populations in contrast with the 7% less risk in the pooled overall finding for all populations combined. Benefits of increased milk intake might be particularly noticeable in East Asian countries where strokes are relatively more common, and milk consumption is much lower than those studies conducted among European or American populations [22]. However, the Life Span Study [6], which was conducted about 10 years earlier than the JACC Study, reported a null association between milk intake and fatal stroke among men and women combined who survived the Hiroshima and Nagasaki atomic bomb. The difference could be largely explained by the different targeting populations between the two studies. Kondo et al. [23] also reported a null association in both men or women from the NIPPON DATA80 study. In fact, the exact number of stroke mortality events was about 85% less and the number of participants in the NIPPON DATA80 study was about 90% less than those in the JACC study database—their null association might likely due to its limited statistical power. Umesawa et al. [24] reported that dairy calcium intake was inversely associated with ischemic stroke mortality risk, which could be considered as one of the potential pieces of evidence that supported our findings. Furthermore, a stronger inverse association between milk consumption and stroke mortality in men rather than in women was found in the Singapore Chinese Health Study [17] as well. The reasons for this gender difference is currently unknown. This might be due to generally better/healthier lifestyles (such as much less smokers and alcohol drinkers) in women regardless of milk intake frequency, or maybe due to other factors that were not available in/considered by our models, such as intake of calcium or other supplements. The probably existing beneficial effect of milk intake might be less evident in women than in men. Further investigation is needed.

Possible reasons for a protective effect of milk consumption against stroke could be interpreted, as such an association might be mediated by its content in calcium, magnesium, potassium, and other bioactive compounds, as recommended by Iacoviello et al. [25]. Apart from the inorganic minerals in milk that would be helpful with health effects, recent studies on animal models also indicated key evidence that stroke-associated morbidity was delayed in stroke-prone rats who were fed with milk-protein enriched diets [26,27]. More precisely, Singh et al. [28] found that whey protein and its components—lactalbumin and lactoferrin—improved energy balance and glycemic control against the onset of neurological deficits associated with stroke. Bioactive peptides from milk proteins were also responsible for the limitation of thrombosis [29] through their angiotensin convertase enzyme inhibitory potential, which might partly explain why the effect was found mainly for mortality from cerebral infarction in the current study.

Strength and Limitations

Some limitations are worth mentioning here. First, the milk intake frequency, as well as other lifestyle information, was collected only once at the baseline and was self-reported. Apparently, life habits are possible to alter over time and these would result in misclassification and residual confounding. Second, despite the fact that the reasonable validity of FFQ in the JACC study cohort was assessed and confirmed, measurement errors are inevitable. Therefore, we did not try to compute the amount of consumption by multiplying an average volume per occasion with the frequency of intake, since the random error might be exaggerated and the observed associations may have attenuated. Third, the Bayesian way of conducting the survival analysis using a large sample size is computationally expensive. However, the classic maximum likelihood estimations are based on unrealistic assumptions, such as repeatability of the study, and fixed but unknown values of parameters, which are unfulfilled in a large cohort study in the current setting. The strengths of our analyses included that we transformed the research questions to more transparent ones that are easier for interpretation. Direct probabilities that daily milk intake is associated with lower hazard or delayed stroke mortality event were provided here after thorough computer simulations.

5. Conclusions

In conclusion, the JACC study database provided evidence that Japanese men who consumed milk daily had a lower risk of dying from stroke, particularly cerebral infarction, compared with their counterparts who never consumed milk. The time before an event of stroke mortality occurred was slowed down among men who drank milk regularly.

Author Contributions: Conceived and designed the JACC study (maintaining the database, organization of the cohort project): H.I., A.T. and S.K. (Shogo Kikuchi); conceived and designed the current analysis: C.W. and H.Y.; data analysis: C.W.; manuscript (including tables) preparation: C.W.; revised the manuscript critically: H.Y., Y.L., T.S., S.K. (Sayo Kawai), S.K. (Shogo Kikuchi), H.I., A.T. All authors have read and agreed to the published version of the manuscript.

Funding: The funding sponsors had no role in the design of the study; in the collection, analyses, or interpretation of data; in the writing of the manuscript, or in the decision to publish the results. This study has been supported by Grants-in-Aid for Scientific Research from the Ministry of Education, Culture, Sports, Science and Technology of Japan (MEXT) (MonbuKagaku-sho); Grants-in-Aid for Scientific Research on Priority Areas of Cancer; Grants-in-Aid for Scientific Research on Priority Areas of Cancer Epidemiology from MEXT (nos. 61010076, 62010074, 63010074, 1010068, 2151065, 3151064, 4151063, 5151069, 6279102, 11181101, 17015022, 18014011, 20014026, 20390156, 26293138); and a JSPS KAKENHI (16H06277). This research was also supported by Grants-in-Aid from the Ministry of Health, Labour and Welfare, Health and Labor sciences research grants, Japan (Comprehensive Research on Cardiovas- cular Disease and Life-Style Related Diseases: H20– Junkankitou [Seishuu]–Ippan–013; H23–Junkankitou [Seishuu]–Ippan–005); an Intramural Research Fund (22-4-5) for Cardiovascular Diseases of the National Cerebral and Cardiovascular Center; Comprehensive Research on Cardiovascular Diseases and Life-Style- Related Diseases (H26-Junkankitou [Seisaku]-Ippan-001) and H29–Junkankitou [Seishuu]–Ippan–003).

Acknowledgments: The authors would like to express their sincere appreciation to Kunio Aoki and Yoshiyuki Ohno, Professors Emeritus at Nagoya University School of Medicine and former chairpersons of the JACC Study. All members of JACC Study Group can be found at https://publichealth.med.hokudai.ac.jp/jacc/index.html.

Conflicts of Interest: The authors declare no conflict of interest.

Abbreviations

The following abbreviations are used in this manuscript:

JACC	Japan Collaborative Cohort
FFQ	Food Frequency Questionnaire
MCMC	Markov Chain Monte Carlo
JAGS	Just Another Gibbs Samplers
AFT	accelerated failure time
HR	hazard ratio
AF	acceleration factor
SD	standard deviation
CrI	credible interval

References

1. Kim, J.S. Stroke in Asia: A global disaster. *Int. J. Stroke* **2014**, *9*, 856–857. [CrossRef]
2. De Goede, J.; Soedamah-Muthu, S.S.; Pan, A.; Gijsbers, L.; Geleijnse, J.M. Dairy consumption and risk of stroke: A systematic review and updated dose–response meta-analysis of prospective cohort studies. *J. Am. Heart Assoc.* **2016**, *5*, e002787. [CrossRef] [PubMed]
3. Yoshiike, N.; Hayashi, F.; Takemi, Y.; Mizoguchi, K.; Seino, F. A new food guide in Japan: The Japanese food guide Spinning Top. *Nutr. Rev.* **2007**, *65*, 149–154. [CrossRef] [PubMed]
4. Saito, A.; Okada, E.; Tarui, I.; Matsumoto, M.; Takimoto, H. The Association between Milk and Dairy Products Consumption and Nutrient Intake Adequacy among Japanese Adults: Analysis of the 2016 National Health and Nutrition Survey. *Nutrients* **2019**, *11*, 2361. [CrossRef]
5. Iso, H.; Stampfer, M.J.; Manson, J.E.; Rexrode, K.; Hennekens, C.H.; Colditz, G.A.; Speizer, F.E.; Willett, W.C. Prospective study of calcium, potassium, and magnesium intake and risk of stroke in women. *Stroke* **1999**, *30*, 1772–1779. [CrossRef] [PubMed]

6. Sauvaget, C.; Nagano, J.; Allen, N.; Grant, E.J.; Beral, V. Intake of animal products and stroke mortality in the Hiroshima/Nagasaki Life Span Study. *Int. J. Epidemiol.* **2003**, *32*, 536–543. [CrossRef] [PubMed]
7. Elwood, P.C.; Pickering, J.E.; Fehily, A.; Hughes, J.; Ness, A. Milk drinking, ischaemic heart disease and ischaemic stroke I. Evidence from the Caerphilly cohort. *Eur. J. Clin. Nutr.* **2004**, *58*, 711–717. [CrossRef] [PubMed]
8. Larsson, S.C.; Männistö, S.; Virtanen, M.J.; Kontto, J.; Albanes, D.; Virtamo, J. Dairy foods and risk of stroke. *Epidemiology* **2009**, *20*, 355. [CrossRef]
9. Wei, L.J. The accelerated failure time model: A useful alternative to the Cox regression model in survival analysis. *Stat. Med.* **1992**, *11*, 1871–1879. [CrossRef]
10. Ibrahim, J.G.; Chen, M.H.; Sinha, D. Bayesian Survival Analysis. In *Wiley StatsRef: Statistics Reference Online*; John Wiley & Sons: Hoboken, NJ, USA, 2014.
11. Ohno, Y.; Tamakoshi, A.; JACC Study Group. Japan collaborative cohort study for evaluation of cancer risk sponsored by monbusho (JACC study). *J. Epidemiol.* **2001**, *11*, 144–150. [CrossRef]
12. Tamakoshi, A.; Yoshimura, T.; Inaba, Y.; Ito, Y.; Watanabe, Y.; Fukuda, K.; Iso, H. Profile of the JACC study. *J. Epidemiol.* **2005**, *15*, S4–S8. [CrossRef] [PubMed]
13. Tamakoshi, A.; Ozasa, K.; Fujino, Y.; Suzuki, K.; Sakata, K.; Mori, M.; Kikuchi, S.; Iso, H. Cohort profile of the Japan Collaborative Cohort Study at final follow-up. *J. Epidemiol.* **2013**. [CrossRef] [PubMed]
14. Date, C.; Fukui, M.; Yamamoto, A.; Wakai, K.; Ozeki, A.; Motohashi, Y.; Adachi, C.; Okamoto, N.; Kurosawa, M.; Tokudome, Y.; et al. Reproducibility and validity of a self-administered food frequency questionnaire used in the JACC study. *J. Epidemiol.* **2005**, *15*, S9–S23. [CrossRef] [PubMed]
15. Ministry of Health and Welfare. *Kokumin Eiyo No Genjyo (The National Nutrition Survey in Japan, 1990)*; Daiichi Shuppan: Tokyo, Japan, 1992.
16. Wang, C.; Yatsuya, H.; Tamakoshi, K.; Iso, H.; Tamakoshi, A. Milk drinking and mortality: Findings from the Japan collaborative cohort study. *J. Epidemiol.* **2015**, *25*, 66–73. [CrossRef]
17. Talaei, M.; Koh, W.P.; Yuan, J.M.; Pan, A. The association between dairy product intake and cardiovascular disease mortality in Chinese adults. *Eur. J. Nutr.* **2016**, *56*, 2343–2352. [CrossRef]
18. Plummer, M. JAGS: A program for analysis of Bayesian graphical models using Gibbs sampling. In Proceedings of the 3rd international workshop on distributed statistical computing, Vienna, Austria, 20–22 March 2003.
19. R Core Team. *R: A Language and Environment for Statistical Computing*; R Foundation for Statistical Computing: Vienna, Austria, 2020.
20. Lunn, D.; Spiegelhalter, D.; Thomas, A.; Best, N. The BUGS project: Evolution, critique and future directions. *Stat. Med.* **2009**, *28*, 3049–3067. [CrossRef]
21. Brooks, S.P.; Gelman, A. General methods for monitoring convergence of iterative simulations. *J. Comput. Graph. Stat.* **1998**, *7*, 434–455.
22. Dehghan, M.; Mente, A.; Rangarajan, S.; Sheridan, P.; Mohan, V.; Iqbal, R.; Gupta, R.; Lear, S.; Wentzel-Viljoen, E.; Avezum, A.; et al. Association of dairy intake with cardiovascular disease and mortality in 21 countries from five continents (PURE): A prospective cohort study. *Lancet* **2018**, *392*, 2288–2297. [CrossRef]
23. Kondo, I.; Ojima, T.; Nakamura, M.; Hayasaka, S.; Hozawa, A.; Saitoh, S.; Ohnishi, H.; Akasaka, H.; Hayakawa, T.; Murakami, Y.; et al. Consumption of dairy products and death from cardiovascular disease in the Japanese general population: The NIPPON DATA80. *J. Epidemiol.* **2013**, *23*, 47–54. [CrossRef]
24. Umesawa, M.; Iso, H.; Ishihara, J.; Saito, I.; Kokubo, Y.; Inoue, M.; Tsugane, S. Dietary calcium intake and risks of stroke, its subtypes, and coronary heart disease in Japanese: The JPHC Study Cohort I. *Stroke* **2008**, *39*, 2449–2456. [CrossRef]
25. Iacoviello, L.; Bonaccio, M.; Cairella, G.; Catani, M.V.; Costanzo, S.; D'Elia, L.; Giacco, R.; Rendina, D.; Sabino, P.; Savini, I.; et al. Diet and primary prevention of stroke: Systematic review and dietary recommendations by the ad hoc Working Group of the Italian Society of Human Nutrition. *Nutr. Metab. Cardiovasc. Dis.* **2018**, *28*, 309–334. [CrossRef] [PubMed]
26. Chiba, T.; Itoh, T.; Tabuchi, M.; Ooshima, K.; Satou, T.; Ezaki, O. Delay of stroke onset by milk proteins in stroke-prone spontaneously hypertensive rats. *Stroke* **2012**, *43*, 470–477. [CrossRef] [PubMed]

27. Singh, A.; Pezeshki, A.; Zapata, R.C.; Yee, N.J.; Knight, C.G.; Tuor, U.I.; Chelikani, P.K. Diets enriched in whey or casein improve energy balance and prevent morbidity and renal damage in salt-loaded and high-fat-fed spontaneously hypertensive stroke-prone rats. *J. Nutr. Biochem.* **2016**, *37*, 47–59. [CrossRef] [PubMed]
28. Singh, A.; Zapata, R.C.; Pezeshki, A.; Knight, C.G.; Tuor, U.I.; Chelikani, P.K. Whey Protein and Its Components Lactalbumin and Lactoferrin Affect Energy Balance and Protect against Stroke Onset and Renal Damage in Salt-Loaded, High-Fat Fed Male Spontaneously Hypertensive Stroke-Prone Rats. *J. Nutr.* **2020**, *150*, 763–774. [CrossRef] [PubMed]
29. Tokajuk, A.; Zakrzeska, A.; Chabielska, E.; Car, H. Whey protein concentrate limits venous thrombosis in rats. *Appl. Physiol. Nutr. Metab.* **2019**, *44*, 907–910. [CrossRef]

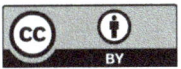

© 2020 by the authors. Licensee MDPI, Basel, Switzerland. This article is an open access article distributed under the terms and conditions of the Creative Commons Attribution (CC BY) license (http://creativecommons.org/licenses/by/4.0/).

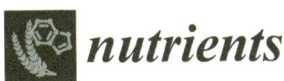

Article

Dietary Supplementation with Selenium and Coenzyme Q_{10} Prevents Increase in Plasma D-Dimer While Lowering Cardiovascular Mortality in an Elderly Swedish Population

Urban Alehagen [1,*], Jan Aaseth [2], Tomas L. Lindahl [3], Anders Larsson [4] and Jan Alexander [5]

1. Division of Cardiovascular Medicine, Department of Health, Medicine and Caring Sciences, Linköping University, SE-581 85 Linköping, Sweden
2. Research Department, Innlandet Hospital Trust, N-2381 Brumunddal, Norway; jaol-aas@online.no
3. Division of Clinical Chemistry and Pharmacology, Department of Biomedical and Clinical Sciences, Linköping University, SE-581 85 Linköping, Sweden; tomas.lindahl@liu.se
4. Department of Medical Sciences, Uppsala University, SE-751 85 Uppsala, Sweden; anders.larsson@medsci.uu.se
5. Norwegian Institute of Public Health, N-0403 Oslo, Norway; Jan.Alexander@fhi.no
* Correspondence: Urban.Alehagen@liu.se; Tel.: +46-10-103-0000

Abstract: A low intake of selenium is associated with increased cardiovascular mortality. This could be reduced by supplementation with selenium and coenzyme Q_{10}. D-dimer, a fragment of fibrin mirroring fibrinolysis, is a biomarker of thromboembolism, increased inflammation, endothelial dysfunction and is associated with cardiovascular mortality in ischemic heart disease. The objective was to examine the impact of selenium and coenzyme Q_{10} on the level of D-dimer, and its relationship to cardiovascular mortality. D-dimer was measured in 213 individuals at the start and after 48 months of a randomised double-blind placebo-controlled trial with selenium yeast (200 µg/day) and coenzyme Q_{10} (200 mg/day) (n = 106) or placebo (n = 107). The follow-up time was 4.9 years. All included individuals were low in selenium (mean 67 µg/L, SD 16.8). The differences in D-dimer concentration were evaluated by the use of T-tests, repeated measures of variance and ANCOVA analyses. At the end, a significantly lower D-dimer concentration was observed in the active treatment group in comparison with those on placebo ($p = 0.006$). Although D-dimer values at baseline were weakly associated with high-sensitive CRP, while being more strongly associated with soluble tumour necrosis factor receptor 1 and sP-selectin, controlling for these in the analysis there was an independent effect on D-dimer. In participants with a D-dimer level above median at baseline, the supplementation resulted in significantly lower cardiovascular mortality compared to those on placebo ($p = 0.014$). All results were validated with a persisting significant difference between the two groups. Therefore, supplementation with selenium and coenzyme Q_{10} in a group of elderly low in selenium and coenzyme Q_{10} prevented an increase in D-dimer and reduced the risk of cardiovascular mortality in comparison with the placebo group. The obtained results also illustrate important associations between inflammation, endothelial function and cardiovascular risk.

Keywords: D-dimer; intervention; elderly; cardiovascular mortality; selenium; coenzyme Q_{10}

1. Introduction

D-dimer is a fragment of degraded fibrin and reflects the activation of fibrinolysis and thrombosis, but also the activity of peripheral artery disease [1]. It is thus an indicator of the fibrin turnover [2]. The most common indications for use of D-dimer are in the diagnosis of venous thromboembolism [3–7], for the exclusion of pulmonary embolism [8] and in the evaluation of recanalisation of pulmonary emboli after anticoagulation [9]. D-dimer is one of the most commonly used biomarkers in clinical medicine [10]. The assay is mainly based on antibodies against D-dimer [11], and as different antibodies are used in commercial kits, there is some variability in the obtained measurements [12].

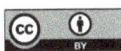

After successful electro-conversion, the level of D-dimer is reduced in patients with atrial fibrillation; hence, it is believed that the velocity and turbulence of the blood flow is important for the level of D-dimer as well [13–15]. However, the occurrence of emboli in atrial fibrillation as a reason for the increased level of D-dimer cannot be ignored. An increased level of D-dimer has also been associated with increased mortality in patients with heart failure [16] and ischaemic heart disease [17,18]. In patients with myocardial infarction, an association between an increased level of D-dimer and increased risk of mortality after a percutaneous coronary intervention has been reported [19,20]. This relation between D-dimer and mortality risk could be explained by the thrombus area in patients with concomitant pulmonary emboli, but there is also a reported association between the myocardial infarct area and level of D-dimer and mortality risk [21]. Hence, D-dimer also could contribute to prognostic cardiovascular risk information, as has also been reported by Bai et al. [22].

Clinical interpretation of D-dimer-values is complicated by the fact that D-dimer increases with age for patients over 50 years [23]. Furthermore, elevated levels of D-dimer could also be the result of inflammatory activity in the absence of thromboembolism [24]. It has been reported that D-dimer and C-reactive protein (CRP) both provide prognostic information in patients with acute coronary syndromes [25], probably based on the close relation between inflammation and ischaemic heart disease. Recently, a matter of discussion has been the intimate relation between D-dimer and endothelial function, where a dysfunction is an important step in the development of inflammation and structural damage [26]. Therefore, it is of interest to more broadly investigate the inflammatory response by examining the D-dimer response following supplementation with selenium and coenzyme Q_{10}. In this context, it is interesting to note that several reports have demonstrated the prognostic properties of D-dimer in patients with COVID-19 disease [22–24] emphasising the important association between D-dimer and inflammation and disease prognosis [27–29].

Our group has previously reported that in an elderly population with symptoms that could be interpreted as heart failure, D-dimer had prognostic information regarding risk of cardiovascular mortality during a follow-up time of more than five years [30]. Even if exclusion of those with atrial fibrillation or dilated atria as seen on echocardiography, or development of malignant disease during the follow-up time [31,32], the prognostic information remained. Therefore, we assume that an association between D-dimer concentration and cardiovascular disease exists, due for example to increases in atherosclerosis again resulting in a hypercoagulable state [33,34].

Selenium is an essential trace element needed for any human cell in order to fulfil normal cellular functions [35,36]. However, because of soil low in selenium, the dietary intake of selenium is low in European regions, with an estimated intake in European countries of <50 µg/day [37]. In order to obtain an optimal cellular function, the required intake of selenium is at least 75 µg/day of selenium for adult Caucasians [38]. However, to obtain an optimal expression of one of the important selenoproteins; for selenoprotein P, which distributes selenium from the liver to peripheral tissues, a daily intake of 100–150 µg/day of selenium is required [39]. Moreover, in conditions with increased oxidative stress and during inflammation, the need for selenium is increased [40]. These requirements can be met for persons living in regions with an adequate selenium content of the soil, as in the USA. However, in healthy, elderly community-living persons in Sweden, our group has previously reported increased cardiovascular mortality associated with a low intake of selenium [41].

Coenzyme Q_{10} is present in all human cells, where it is active in the mitochondrial respiratory chain, but it is also an important lipid soluble antioxidant. The endogenous production of coenzyme Q_{10} declines with age, and at the age of 80, the endogenous myocardial production of coenzyme Q_{10} is about half that at 20 years of age [42,43].

Cytosolic selenoenzyme thioreductase1 plays a major role in reducing ubiquinone (the oxidised form of coenzyme Q_{10}) to ubiquinol, the active, reduced form of coenzyme Q_{10}.

For an optimal functioning, the cell is both dependent on an adequate supply of coenzyme Q_{10} and synthesis of selenoproteins. An insufficiency in selenium and reduced thioredoxin reductase activity could therefore result in decreased concentrations of active coenzyme Q_{10} (ubiquinol) in the cell. This important relationship between selenium and coenzyme Q_{10} has been known about for a long time [44,45].

Our group has previously observed effects by combined intervention with selenium and coenzyme Q_{10} on several biomarkers for inflammation in a randomised clinical trial on an elderly Swedish population. Thus, the levels of sP-selectin, CRP, osteopontin, osteoprotegerin, soluble tumour necrosis factor receptor 1 (TNFr1) and soluble tumour necrosis factor receptor 2 (TNFr2) were significantly lowered in those receiving active treatment, as compared with those in the placebo group [46,47]. We also observed effects on the biomarker levels of the von Willebrand factor and plasminogen activator inhibitor-1 indicating improved endothelial function in the verum group [48]. With this in mind, we wanted to evaluate if an association between D-dimer levels and supplementation of selenium and coenzyme Q_{10} exists, as D-dimer has also been reported to be associated with endothelial function [26].

Apart from a small study from the former Eastern Germany on 61 patients with myocardial infarction [49], we did not find any other report in the literature using the combined supplementation with selenium and coenzyme Q_{10}, which is why the presented results are novel and interesting.

The aim of the present sub-study was to investigate a possible influence of supplementation for four years with selenium and coenzyme Q_{10} on the level of D-dimer, with emphasis on its role in cardiovascular mortality during 4.9 years of follow-up, in an elderly Swedish population.

2. Methods

2.1. Subjects

From a rural municipality, all individuals living in the age between 69 and 88 years were invited to participate in a study on epidemiology in 1998 ($n = 1320$). Out of those 876 decided to participate in the main project. In 2003, those still alive ($n = 675$) were invited to participate in an intervention project with selenium and coenzyme Q_{10} as a dietary supplement. Due to the fact that some individuals regarded the transportation distance to the Health Center for inclusion as being too long, the number who agreed to participate were 589 individuals. Out of those, 443 individuals in the age 70–88 years agreed to participate in the intervention project. The supplementation consisted of selenium and coenzyme Q_{10}, or placebo given over four years, and where blood samples were drawn every 6 months [50]. All participants in the intervention study had a suboptimal pre-intervention serum selenium level, mean 67 µg/L (SD 16.8) (equivalent to an estimated daily intake of 35 µg/day), and this is below what is regarded as an adequate selenium concentration of ≥ 100 µg/L [51].

In the present sub-analysis on impact on D-dimer, from the group of 443 participants in the intervention, we excluded individuals with conditions known to influence the concentration of D-dimer: atrial fibrillation and/or on treatment with anticoagulants ($n = 50$), participants with malignancies ($n = 17$) or the dimension of the left atrium > 40 mm ($n = 163$). The final population consisted of 213 individuals. Of those, 106 individuals were on active treatment, and 107 individuals were on placebos.

In the main project, the participants received supplementation of 200 mg/day of coenzyme Q_{10} capsules (Bio-Quinon 100 mg B.I.D, Pharma Nord, Vejle, Denmark) and 200 µg/day of organic selenium yeast tablets (SelenoPrecise 100 µg B.I.D, Pharma Nord, Vejle, Denmark) ($n = 221$), or a similar placebo ($n = 222$) over 48 months. After this time, the intervention was finished. The study tablets were taken in addition to any regular medication. All study medications (active drug and placebo) not consumed were returned and counted. One of three experienced cardiologists examined all study participants at the inclusion. Besides a new clinical history, a clinical examination was performed at inclusion and after the study period, including blood pressure, there was an assessment using the New York Heart Association functional class (NYHA class) as well as an electrocardiogram (ECG) and Doppler-echocardiography. Echocardiographic examinations were performed with the participant in the left lateral position. The ejection fraction (EF) readings were categorised into four classes: 30%, 40% and 50% [52,53]. Normal systolic function was defined as EF ≥ 50%, while severely impaired systolic function was defined as EF < 30%. Only the systolic function was evaluated. The inclusion started in January 2003 and finished in February 2010.

The exclusion criteria for the main project were: recent myocardial infarction (within four weeks); planned cardiovascular operative procedure within four weeks; hesitation concerning whether the candidate could decide for him/herself to participate in the study or not, or doubt about whether he/she understood the consequences of participation; serious disease that substantially reduced survival or when it was not expected that the participant could cooperate for the full four-year period; other factors making participation unreasonable, or drug/alcohol abuse [50]. Cardiovascular mortality (CV mortality) was registered for all study participants for a follow-up period of 4.9 years. Information regarding mortality was obtained from the National Board of Health and Welfare in Sweden. It registers all deaths of Swedish citizens based on death certificates or autopsy reports. All patients obtained written informed consent.

Cardiovascular mortality was defined as mortality due to myocardial infarctions, cerebrovascular lesions, fatal cardiac arrythmias, heart failure and aortic aneurysms.

The result of the main study was that the actively treated group showed a significantly increased cardiac systolic function, a reduced concentration of the cardiac peptide N-terminal fragment of B-type natriuretic peptide (NT-proBNP), and significantly reduced cardiovascular mortality [50]. As the result of the main study was surprising, several sub studies were performed. This sub study is one of the different steps in order to obtain better understanding of the mechanisms between supplementation as clinical results.

2.2. Biochemical Analyses

All blood samples were collected at start of the study, and after 48 months, and were drawn with the participants resting and in a supine position. Pre-chilled, EDTA vials for plasma were used. The vials were centrifuged at $3000 \times g$, +4 °C, and were then frozen at −70 °C. No sample was thawed more than once.

2.3. Determination of D-Dimer

Blood was collected in Vacutainer tubes containing 1/10 volume sodium citrate 0.11 mol/L and stored at −70 °C until analysis. The samples were analysed utilising an automated micro-latex D-dimer reagent, MRX-143, from Medirox (Nyköping, Sweden) using ACL Top analyser (Instrumentation Laboratories, Milan, Italy). The precision was good; for a low control at mean concentrations of 0.39 mg/L (n = 917) and a high control at 0.96 mg/L (n = 526), the total imprecision was 7.3% and 2.9%, respectively.

2.4. Statistical Methods

Descriptive data are presented as percentages or mean ± standard deviation (SD). A Student's unpaired two-sided T-test was used for continuous variables and the chi-square test was used for analysis of one discrete variable. Kaplan–Meier evaluations of all-cause and cardiovascular mortality were made for both the active treatment and placebo groups. The term 'censored participants' refers to those still living at the end of the study, or who had died for reasons other than cardiovascular disease. 'Completed participants' refers to those who had died due to cardiovascular disease. Repeated measures of variance were used in order to obtain better information on the individual changes in the concentration of the biomarker analysed, compared to group mean values.

In the analysis of covariance (ANCOVA) evaluation, both transformed and non-transformed data were applied, with no significant difference in the results.

In the ANCOVA evaluation, the D-dimer concentration after 48 months was used as an independent variable. In the model, adjustments were made for smoking, hypertension, diabetes, ischaemic heart disease (IHD), NYHA class III, Hb < 120 g/L, statin treatment, P-selectin at inclusion, endostatin at inclusion, soluble tumor necrosis factor receptor 1 (sTNF-r1) at inclusion, sTNF-r2 at inclusion, Growth differentiation factor 15 (GDF-15) at inclusion, D-dimer at inclusion and supplementation with selenium and coenzyme Q_{10}.

p-values < 0.05 were considered significant, based on a two-sided evaluation. All data were analysed using standard software (Statistica v. 13.2, Dell Inc., Tulsa, OK, USA).

3. Results

In Table 1 the baseline characteristics for the active treatment and the placebo groups are presented. It is seen that the two groups are reasonably well balanced with regard to the co-variates analysed.

Table 1. Baseline characteristics of the study population receiving dietary supplementation of selenium and coenzyme Q_{10} combined or placebo during four years.

	Active Treatment Group $n = 106$	Placebo Group $n = 107$	p-Value
Age years, mean (SD)	77.0 (3.7)	77.0 (3.3)	0.36
Gender, Males/Females	43/64	46/61	
History			
Diabetes, n (%)	25 (23.6)	21 (19.6)	0.51
Smoking, n (%)	9 (8.5)	12 (11.2)	0.50
Hypertension, n (%)	75 (70.8)	75 (70.1)	0.92
IHD, n (%)	18 (17.0)	22 (20.6)	0.50
NYHA class I, n (%)	54 (50.9)	57 (53.3)	0.73
NYHA class II, n (%)	33 (31.1)	26 (24.3)	0.27
NYHA class III, n (%)	19 (17.9)	23 (21.5)	0.51
NYHA class IV, n (%)	0	0	
Medications			
ACEI/ARB, n (%)	18 (17.0)	20 (18.7)	0.74
Beta blockers, n (%)	32 (30.2)	24 (22.4)	0.20
Diuretics, n (%)	29 (27.4)	32 (29.9)	0.68
Statins, n (%)	20 (18.9)	20 (18.7)	0.97
Examinations			
EF < 40%, n (%)	2 (1.9)	7 (6.5)	0.20
s-selenium pre-intervention µg/L, mean (SD)	67.6 (14.8)	66.3 (15.8)	0.98

Note: ACEI: ACE- inhibitors; ARB: Angiotension receptor blockers; EF: Ejection fraction; IHD: Ischemic heart disease; NYHA: New York Heart Association functional class; SD: Standard Deviation. Note: Values are means ± SDs or frequency (percent). Note: Student's unpaired two-sided t-test was used for continuous variables and the chi-square test was used for analysis of one discrete variable.

From the evaluations, 46 out of 213 (22%) had diabetes, 150 out of 213 (70%) had hypertension, 40 out of 213 (19%) had ischaemic heart disease and nine out of 213 (4%) had impaired systolic cardiac function defined as an EF of less than 40%. The population evaluated could be considered as representative for an elderly Swedish population. Upon analysing the association between D-dimer and age at the study start, a significant association was noted (r = 0.20; p = 0.003). The mean concentration of D-dimer did not differ between males and females (females: 0.32 mg/L (SD 0.31) vs. males: 0.32 mg/L (SD 0.58); p = 0.98). The sub-population studied was followed for 4.9 years from 2003 regarding mortality.

3.1. Relation between D-Dimer and Biomarkers for Inflammation at Study Start

As D-dimer has been reported to be associated with biomarkers of inflammation, we examined whether D-dimer was associated with hs-CRP (high sensitive CRP). A weak non-significant association was seen (r = 0.10; p = 0.17). However, the size of the association found is as reported by Folsom et al. (r = 0.13) [18]. Stronger associations were seen between D-dimer and soluble tumour necrosis factor (TNF) receptor 1, (r = 0.35; p > 0.0001), and soluble TNF receptor 2 (r = 0.24; p = 0.01). We also found a significant association with sP-selectin (r = 0.17; p = 0.01), another biomarker for inflammation, which is also a marker for platelet activation.

3.2. Effect of Supplementation on the Concentration of D-Dimer

At inclusion, there was no significant difference in the mean concentration of D-dimer between the two groups (active: 0.29 mg/L vs. placebo: 0.36 mg/L; p = 0.27). However, after 48 months, a significant difference in the concentration of D-dimer between the two groups could be seen (active: 0.22 mg/L vs. 0.34 mg/L; T-value: 2.80; p = 0.006).

As a validation of the results obtained, we performed a repeated measures of variance analysis (Figure 1). From this evaluation, the difference between the two groups, active vs. placebo, was still significant (F (1, 111) = 5.11; p = 0.026).

As a second step in the validation of the obtained results, an ANCOVA analysis was performed (Table 2).

Table 2. Analysis of covariance using D-dimer after 48 months as dependent variable.

Effects	Mean Squares	Degrees of Freedom	F	p
Intercept	0.24	1	6.35	0.01
Smoker	0.01	1	0.39	0.53
Hypertension	0.11	1	2.92	0.09
Diabetes	0.02	1	0.66	0.42
IHD	0.001	1	0.03	0.86
NYHA III	0.005	1	0.13	0.72
Hb < 120g/L	0.02	1	0.47	0.49
Statin treatment	0.08	1	2.16	0.15
p-selectin incl	0.002	1	0.04	0.84
hsCRP incl	0.0002	1	0.004	0.95
Endostatin incl	0.30	1	8.08	0.006
sTNF-r1 incl	0.009	1	0.23	0.63
sTNF-r2 incl	0.25	1	6.73	0.01
GDF-15 incl	0.12	1	3.14	0.08
D-dimer incl	0.95	1	25.6	0.000002
Active treatment	0.37	1	9.89	0.002
Error	0.04	1		

Note: GDF-15: Growth/differentiation factor 15; HsCRP: High sensitivity assay of CRP; IHD: Ischemic heart disease; NYHA: New York Heart Association functional class III; sTNF-r1: Tumor necrosis factor receptor 1; sTNF-r2: Tumor necrosis factor receptor 2.

We found a significantly lower concentration of D-dimer (p = 0.002) in those supplemented with selenium and coenzyme Q_{10}, also after adjusting for co-variates that might influence the concentration of D-dimer, like the CRP, sP-selectin, TNF-r1, TNf-r2, endostatin and GDF-15, all of which being biomarkers of inflammation.

3.3. Effect of Supplementation with Selenium and Coenzyme Q_{10} on Mortality

This sub-study population was followed during a median follow-up period of 4.9 years from 2003. As the study population was relatively small, we chose to evaluate the groups where the risk of mortality was highest. As it has been shown that an increased level of

D-dimer increases this risk, we chose to include those with a concentration of D-dimer above the median (0.21 mg/L) at baseline for an evaluation of CV mortality. A significantly lower fraction suffering from CV mortality was seen in those on active treatment, compared with those on placebo (active treatment: one out of 53 vs. placebo: eight out of 52; χ^2: 6.10; $p = 0.014$). When comparing all-cause mortality in the two groups, the mortality in the placebo group was twice that in the active treatment group, but this difference did not reach statistical significance (active treatment: five out of 53 vs. placebo: 10 out of 52; χ^2: 2.06; $p = 0.15$). Of note, the groups were small, which probably contributed to the non-significance of the latter difference.

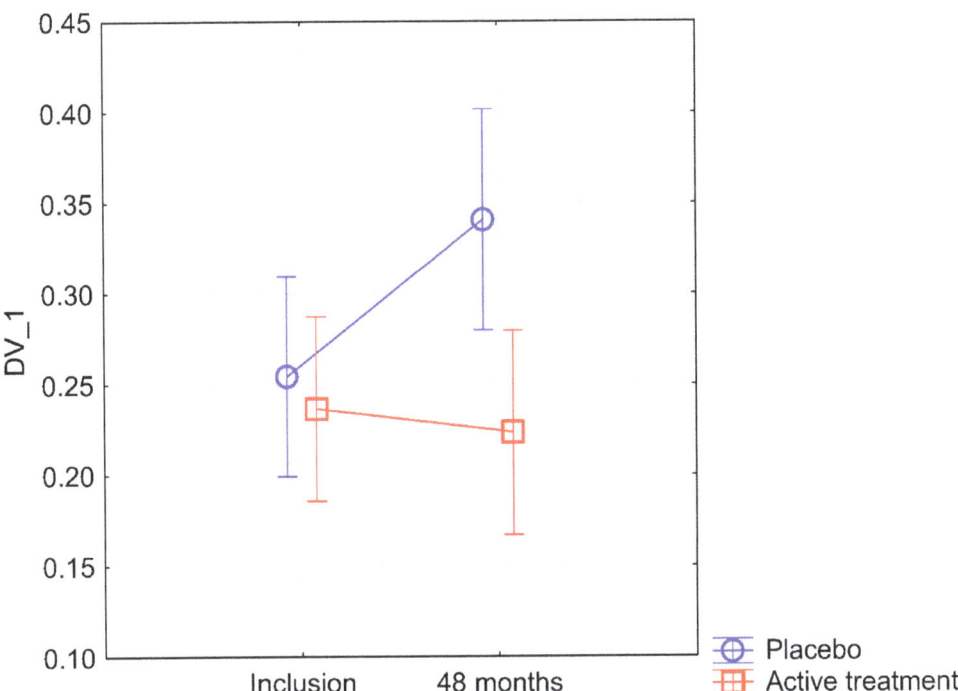

Figure 1. Concentration of D-dimer at the start of the project and after 48 months in the selenium and coenzyme Q_{10} treatment group compared to the placebo group in the study population. Evaluation performed by use of repeated measures of variance methodology. Current effect: ($F (1, 111) = 5.11; p = 0.026$). Vertical bars denote 0.95 confidence intervals. Blue curve: Placebo; Red curve: Active treatment group. Bars indicate ±95% CI.

In order to validate the obtained differences in CV mortality between those on active treatment versus those on placebo, a Kaplan–Meier analysis was performed (Figure 2). From that, it could be seen that significantly fewer participants suffered from CV mortality among those who were given active treatment, as compared to those on placebo ($z = 2.39$; $p = 0.017$).

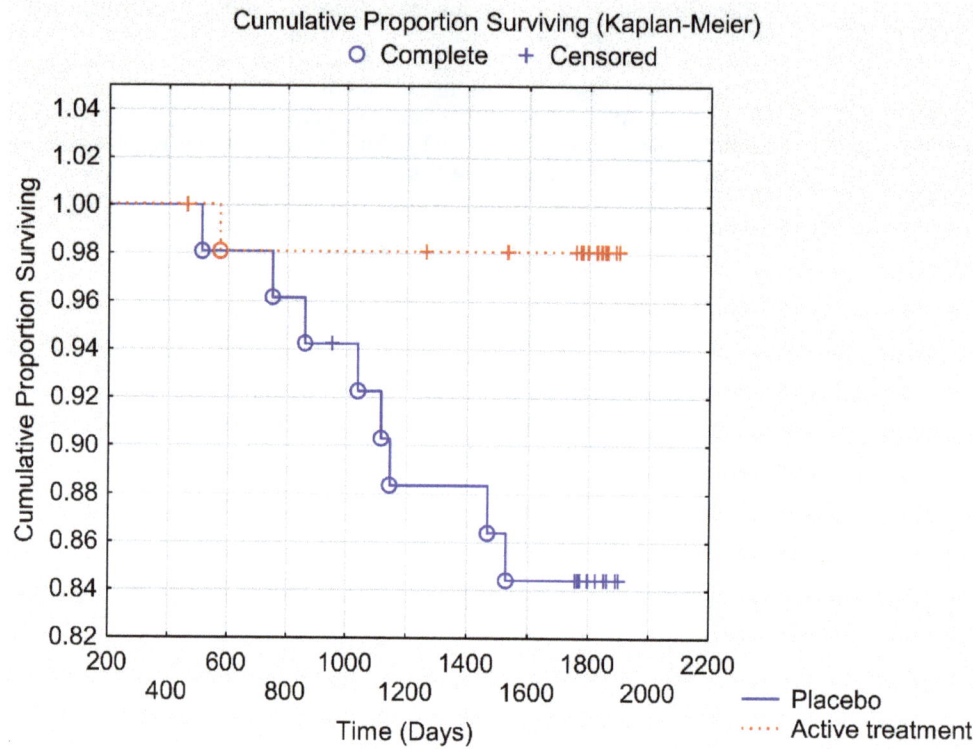

Figure 2. Kaplan–Meier graph illustrating cardiovascular mortality in participants with a D-dimer level above median (0.21 mg/L) and given selenium and coenzyme Q_{10} treatment versus those on placebo during a follow-up period of 4.9 years. Note: Censored participants were those still living at the end of the study period, or who had died for reasons other than cardiovascular disease. Completed participants were those who had died due to cardiovascular disease.

3.4. Impact of Supplementation on D-Dimer Levels in Participants with Hypertension or Ischaemic Heart Disease

We conducted a sub-group analysis on participants with hypertension, and/or with ischaemic heart disease, diseases where inflammation is an inseparable part of the picture. In this sub-population, we evaluated the group with a D-dimer concentration above the median (>0.21 mg/L) at baseline. Also in this group, we found a significant difference in impact of the treatment on D-dimer concentration between those on active treatment and those on placebo, when applying the repeated measures of variance methodology ($F_{(1, 75)} = 6.23$; $p = 0.015$) (Figure 3).

Upon analysing mortality, we found that those on active treatment had a significantly lower CV mortality, compared with those on placebo (active: one out of 46 vs. placebo: six out of 41; χ^2: 4.55; $p = 0.033$). There was no significant difference in all-cause mortality (active: four out of 46 vs. placebo: eight out of 41: χ^2: 2.13; $p = 0.14$). However, these groups were small, and consequently the results should be interpreted with caution.

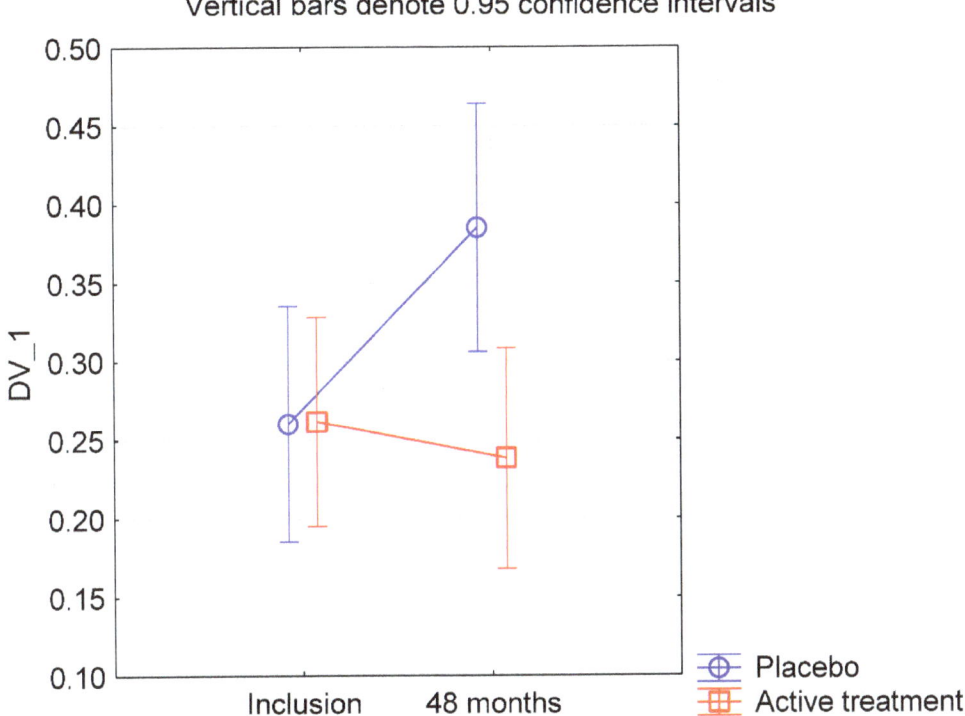

Figure 3. Concentration of D-dimer at the start of the project and after 48 months in the selenium and coenzyme Q_{10} treatment group compared to the placebo group in a sub-group of the study population consisting of participants with hypertension or ischaemic heart disease. Evaluation performed by use of repeated measures of variance methodology. Current effect: (F (1, 75) = 6.23; p = 0.015). Vertical bars denote 0.95 confidence intervals. Blue curve: Placebo; Red curve: Active treatment group. Bars indicate ±95% CI.

4. Discussion

The present evaluations of the effect of supplementation with selenium and coenzyme Q_{10} on the level of D-dimer in an elderly community-living population in Sweden has shown that this treatment prevented an increase in D-dimer levels, as compared with the placebo group in which the levels appeared to increase. Also, in a sub-group analysis of patients with hypertension or ischemic heart disease, a significantly lower concentration of D-dimer as a result of the supplementation was observed. In those with a D-dimer level above the median at baseline, the supplementation resulted in significantly lower cardiovascular mortality compared with those on placebo. Although the studied subjects had a low serum selenium at inclusion (mean 67 µg/L, SD 16.8), which is lower than recommended [51], we consider the studied group to be representative for an elderly Swedish population.

From the main study (referred to as the KiSel-10 project), we have previously disclosed that intervention with selenium and coenzyme Q_{10} caused reduced levels of biomarkers of inflammation [34,35]. As regards this elderly population with a suboptimal selenium status, our group has also observed a significant reducing effect on von Willebrand factor, and plasminogen activator inhibitor-1, by the supplementation with selenium and coenzyme Q_{10} [48]. These latter biomarkers, which are indicators of endothelial function, suggest development of dysfunction in non-supplemented elderly controls. In the present study, we aimed at focusing on D-dimer as an additional biomarker for endothelial dysfunction.

The sub-population included here was selected with the aim of eliminating clinical conditions (atrial fibrillation, increased left atrium size, treatment with anticoagulants and malignancies) known to increase the level of D-dimer. As a result, the sample size was reduced by about 50%. To compensate for the increased uncertainty of the results based on the small study samples, we performed a two-step validation process; first through repeated measures of variance, and then through ANCOVA evaluation, and for mortality through Kaplan–Meier survival analyses. From these analyses, it remained clear that in the elderly Swedish population under investigation with supplementation of selenium and coenzyme Q_{10} had a significantly lower D-dimer concentration than those on placebo by preventing the increase in D-dimer concentration that seemed to take place among those on placebo.

An important issue is whether the elevated level of D-dimer in the studied cohort is a result of thromboembolism—which secondarily results in an increased level of inflammation, or whether inflammation per se resulted in an increased level of D-dimer in the absence of thrombus formation. Previous studies have indicated that an increased level of D-dimer could result from an increased non-specific inflammation without any on-going thromboembolism [54,55]. Our present results could thus be explained by the previously reported increase in inflammatory activity in elderly populations [34,35]. However, it is to be noted that even if adjusted for biomarkers of inflammation as co-variates, an independent reduction in the level of D-dimer persisted as a result of the supplementation with selenium and coenzyme Q_{10}. This indicates an association between D-dimer and the supplementation beyond the role of D-dimer as a biomarker solely of inflammation.

In accordance with previous observations [56,57], we found a significant positive association between age and D-dimer in our population. Thus, the participants on placebo showed a substantial increase in the D-dimer level. This association could be a result of an increased level of inflammation as part of the normal ageing process in "healthy" subjects or could be an indicator on pathological inflammatory activity in the apparently selenium-deficient population evaluated [35]. It appears that an increase in D-dimer besides a reported positive association with inflammation, also is positively associated with endothelial dysfunction. Therefore, in those with a low baseline selenium concentration supplementation with selenium and coenzyme Q_{10} could prevent the increase in D-dimer observed in the placebo group and thereby inflammation and endothelial dysfunction, and also decrease the cardiovascular risk.

5. Limitations

The population analysed in this study was of a relatively small size. This increases therefore the uncertainty of the obtained results. However, as we used a two-step validation process, we argue that the results are likely to be correct. Even if the size of the study population is small, we regard the results as being interesting from a scientific point of view, and for hypothesis-generating.

The included participants represented a relatively narrow age stratum, so it is not possible to extrapolate the results to other age groups without uncertainty.

Finally, as the evaluated population consisted of Caucasians who were low in selenium and coenzyme Q_{10}, it is not necessarily true that the obtained results could be extrapolated to another population.

6. Conclusions

D-dimer, a fragment of cleaved fibrin, reflects the fibrinolytic process, which is why it is used in clinical routines to rule out a possible thromboembolic process. However, D-dimer is also intimately related to inflammatory activity and also to endothelial dysfunction. In this report, an elderly community-living population with a relative selenium deficiency was given a dietary supplement consisting of selenium and coenzyme Q_{10}. While the level of D-dimer in the placebo group increased during the intervention period, it remained unchanged or was slightly reduced in those on active treatment. After 48 months, D-dimer was significantly lower in the active treatment group in comparison with those on placebo. The results were validated through repeated measures of variance methodology and ANCOVA analyses.

We observed a significantly reduced CV mortality among those with a high D-dimer level when given selenium and coenzyme Q_{10}, as compared to those on placebo. In a subgroup analysis of patients with hypertension or ischemic heart disease, the significantly lower concentration of D-dimer as a result of the supplementation could be demonstrated. High D-dimer levels in the present elderly population may reflect age-related inflammatory activity, although D-dimer may impact cardiovascular pathology beyond its role as a biomarker of inflammation.

The demonstrated results might be of interest for follow-up studies, although the present sample size was small. The results should be regarded as hypothesis-generating and it is hoped they will stimulate more research within the same area.

Author Contributions: Conceived and designed the research project, U.A. and A.L.; conducted the research, U.A. and A.L.; provided the essential reagents, T.L.L. and the analyses were performed in his lab; analysed data and performed the statistical analyses, U.A. and A.L.; wrote the paper, U.A., J.A. (Jan Aaseth), J.A. (Jan Alexander), T.L.L. and A.L.; had the final responsibility for the final content, U.A. All authors have read and approved the final manuscript.

Funding: Part of the analysis cost was supported by grants from Pharma Nord Aps, Denmark, the County Council of Östergötland, Linköping University. The funding organisations had no role in the design, management, analysis or interpretation of the data, nor in the preparation, review or approval of the manuscript. No economic compensation was distributed.

Institutional Review Board Statement: Not applicable.

Ethical Approval: The study was approved by the Regional Ethical Committee (Forskningsetikkommitten, Hälsouniversitetet, SE-581 85 Linköping, Sweden; No. D03-176), and conforms to the ethical guidelines of the 1975 Declaration of Helsinki. (As the Medical Product Agency considered the trial as a trial of one food supplement and not a medication, it declined to review the study protocol). This study has been registered retrospectively at Clinicaltrials.gov, and has the identifier NCT01443780, as it was not mandatory to register at the time the study began.

Informed Consent Statement: Informed consent was obtained from each patient.

Data Availability Statement: Under Swedish Law, the authors cannot share the data used in this study and cannot conduct any further research other than what is specified in the ethical permissions application. For inquiries about the data, researchers should first contact the owner of the database, the University of Linköping. Please contact the corresponding author with requests for and assistance with data. If the university approves the request, researchers can submit an application to the Regional Ethical Review Board for the specific research question that the researcher wants to examine.

Conflicts of Interest: The authors declare no conflict of interest.

Abbreviations

ACEI: ACE inhibitors; ANCOVA: Analysis of covariance, ARB; Angiotension receptor blockers, CRP: C-reactive protein; CV: Cardiovascular; EF: Ejection fraction, ECG: Electrocardiogram, Hs-CRP: High sensitivity analysis of C-reactive protein, IHD: Ischaemic heart disease, NT-proBNP: N-terminal fragment of B-type natriuretic peptide; NYHA class: New York Heart Association functional class, SD: Standard deviation.

References

1. Adam, S.S.; Key, N.S.; Greenberg, C.S. D-dimer antigen: Current concepts and future prospects. *Blood* **2009**, *113*, 2878–2887. [CrossRef]
2. Marder, V.J. Identification and purification of fibrinogen degradation products produced by plasmin: Considerations on the structure of fibrinogen. *Scand. J. Haematol.* **2009**, *8*, 21–36. [CrossRef] [PubMed]
3. Rosendaal, F. Venous thrombosis: A multicausal disease. *Lancet* **1999**, *353*, 1167–1173. [CrossRef]

4. Van der Graaf, F.; van den Borne, H.; van der Kolk, M.; de Wild, P.J.; Janssen, G.W.; van Uum, S.H. Exclusion of deep venous thrombosis with D-dimer testing—Comparison of 13 D-dimer methods in 99 outpatients suspected of deep venous thrombosis using venography as reference standard. *Thromb. Haemost.* **2000**, *83*, 191–198.
5. Wells, P.S.; Brill-Edwards, P.; Stevens, P.; Panju, A.; Patel, A.; Douketis, J.; Massicotte, M.P.; Hirsh, J.; Weitz, J.I.; Kearon, C.; et al. A Novel and Rapid Whole-Blood Assay for D-Dimer in Patients with Clinically Suspected Deep Vein Thrombosis. *Circulation* **1995**, *91*, 2184–2187. [CrossRef]
6. Kearon, C.; Ginsberg, J.S.; Douketis, J.; Crowther, M.; Brill-Edwards, P.; Weitz, J.I.; Hirsh, J. Management of suspected deep venous thrombosis in outpatients by using clinical assessment and D-dimer testing. *Ann. Intern. Med.* **2001**, *135*, 108–111. [CrossRef]
7. Wells, P.S. Integrated strategies for the diagnosis of venous thromboembolism. *J. Thromb. Haemost.* **2007**, *5*, 41–50. [CrossRef]
8. Kearon, C.; De Wit, K.; Parpia, S.; Schulman, S.; Afilalo, M.; Hirsch, A.; Spencer, F.A.; Sharma, S.; D'Aragon, F.; Deshaies, J.-F.; et al. Diagnosis of Pulmonary Embolism with d-Dimer Adjusted to Clinical Probability. *N. Engl. J. Med.* **2019**, *381*, 2125–2134. [CrossRef]
9. Kaczyńska, A.; Kostrubiec, M.; Pacho, R.; Kunikowska, J.; Pruszczyk, P. Elevated D-dimer concentration identifies patients with incomplete recanalization of pulmonary artery thromboemboli despite 6 months anticoagulation after the first episode of acute pulmonary embolism. *Thromb. Res.* **2008**, *122*, 21–25. [CrossRef]
10. Lowe, G.D.O. Fibrin D-Dimer and Cardiovascular Risk. *Semin. Vasc. Med.* **2005**, *5*, 387–398. [CrossRef] [PubMed]
11. Dempfle, C.-E. Validation, Calibration, and Specificity of Quantitative D-Dimer Assays. *Semin. Vasc. Med.* **2005**, *5*, 315–320. [CrossRef]
12. Dempfle, C.; Zips, S.; Ergül, H.; Heene, D.L. The Fibrin Assay Comparison Trial (FACT): Evaluation of 23 quantitative D-dimer assays as basis for the development of D-dimer calibrators. FACT study group. *Thromb. Haemost.* **2001**, *85*, 671–678.
13. Lip, G.Y.; Rumley, A.; Dunn, F.G.; Lowe, G.D. Plasma fibrinogen and fibrin D-dimer in patients with atrial fibrillation: Effects of cardioversion to sinus rhythm. *Int. J. Cardiol.* **1995**, *51*, 245–251. [CrossRef]
14. Kamath, S.; Chin, B.S.P.; Blann, A.D.; Lip, G.Y.H. A study of platelet activation in paroxysmal, persistent and permanent atrial fibrillation. *Blood Coagul. Fibrinolysis* **2002**, *13*, 627–636. [CrossRef]
15. Giansante, C.; Fiotti, N.; Miccio, M.; Altamura, N.; Salvi, R.; Guarnieri, G. Coagulation indicators in patients with paroxysmal atrial fibrillation: Effects of electric and pharmacologic cardioversion. *Am. Heart J.* **2000**, *140*, 423–429. [CrossRef] [PubMed]
16. Zorlu, A.; Yilmaz, M.B.; Yücel, H.; Bektasoglu, G.; Ege, M.R.; Tandogan, I.; Tandoğan, I. Increased d-dimer levels predict cardiovascular mortality in patients with systolic heart failure. *J. Thromb. Thrombolysis* **2011**, *33*, 322–328. [CrossRef]
17. Morange, P.E.; Bickel, C.; Nicaud, V.; Schnabel, R.; Rupprecht, H.J.; Peetz, D.; Lackner, K.J.; Cambien, F.; Blankenberg, S.; Tiret, L.; et al. Haemostatic factors and the risk of cardiovascular death in patients with coronary artery disease: The AtheroGene study. *Arterioscler. Thromb. Vasc. Biol.* **2006**, *26*, 2793–2799. [CrossRef]
18. Folsom, A.R.; Delaney, J.A.C.; Lutsey, P.L.; Zakai, N.A.; Jenny, N.S.; Polak, J.F.; Cushman, M. For the Multiethnic Study of Atherosclerosis Investigators Associations of factor VIIIc, D-dimer, and plasmin-antiplasmin with incident cardiovascular disease and all-cause mortality. *Am. J. Hematol.* **2009**, *84*, 349–353. [CrossRef]
19. Tataru, M.-C.; Heinrich, J.; Junker, R.; Schulte, H.; Von Eckardstein, A.; Assmann, G.; Koehler, E. D-dimers in relation to the severity of arteriosclerosis in patients with stable angina pectoris after myocardial infarction. *Eur. Heart J.* **1999**, *20*, 1493–1502. [CrossRef]
20. Huang, D.; Gao, W.; Wu, R.; Zhong, X.; Qian, J.; Ge, J. D-dimer level predicts in-hospital adverse outcomes after primary PCI for ST-segment elevation myocardial infarction. *Int. J. Cardiol.* **2020**, *305*, 1–4. [CrossRef] [PubMed]
21. Choi, S.; Jang, W.J.; Bin Song, Y.; Lima, J.A.C.; Guallar, E.; Choe, Y.H.; Hwang, J.K.; Kim, E.K.; Yang, J.H.; Hahn, J.-Y.; et al. D-Dimer Levels Predict Myocardial Injury in ST-Segment Elevation Myocardial Infarction: A Cardiac Magnetic Resonance Imaging Study. *PLoS ONE* **2016**, *11*, e0160955. [CrossRef] [PubMed]
22. Bai, Y.; Zheng, Y.-Y.; Tang, J.-N.; Yang, X.-M.; Guo, Q.-Q.; Zhang, J.-C.; Cheng, M.-D.; Song, F.-H.; Wang, K.; Zhang, Z.-L.; et al. D-Dimer to Fibrinogen Ratio as a Novel Prognostic Marker in Patients After Undergoing Percutaneous Coronary Intervention: A Retrospective Cohort Study. *Clin. Appl. Thromb.* **2020**, *26*. [CrossRef] [PubMed]
23. Urban, K.; Kirley, K.; Stevermer, J.J. PURLs: It's time to use an age-based approach to D-dimer. *J. Fam. Pract.* **2014**, *63*, 155–158.
24. Bruinstroop, E.; Van De Ree, M.; Huisman, M. The use of D-dimer in specific clinical conditions: A narrative review. *Eur. J. Intern. Med.* **2009**, *20*, 441–446. [CrossRef]
25. Mjelva, Ø.R.; Pönitz, V.; Brügger-Andersen, T.; Grundt, H.; Staines, H.; Nilsen, D.W. Long-term prognostic utility of pentraxin 3 and D-dimer as compared to high-sensitivity C-reactive protein and B-type natriuretic peptide in suspected acute coronary syndrome. *Eur. J. Prev. Cardiol.* **2016**, *23*, 1130–1140. [CrossRef] [PubMed]
26. Zhang, J.; Tecson, K.M.; McCullough, P.A. Endothelial dysfunction contributes to COVID-19-associated vascular inflammation and coagulopathy. *Rev. Cardiovasc. Med.* **2020**, *21*, 315–319. [CrossRef]
27. Long, H.; Nie, L.; Xiang, X.; Li, H.; Zhang, X.; Fu, X.; Ren, H.; Liu, W.; Wang, Q.; Wu, Q. D-Dimer and Prothrombin Time Are the Significant Indicators of Severe COVID-19 and Poor Prognosis. *BioMed Res. Int.* **2020**, *2020*, 6159720. [CrossRef] [PubMed]
28. Hodges, G.; Pallisgaard, J.; Olsen, A.-M.S.; Mcgettigan, P.; Andersen, M.; Krogager, M.; Kragholm, K.; Køber, L.; Gislason, G.H.; Torp-Pedersen, C.; et al. Association between biomarkers and COVID-19 severity and mortality: A nationwide Danish cohort study. *BMJ Open* **2020**, *10*, e041295. [CrossRef]

29. Yang, L.; Jin, J.; Luo, W.; Gan, Y.; Chen, B.; Li, W. Risk factors for predicting mortality of COVID-19 patients: A systematic review and meta-analysis. *PLoS ONE* **2020**, *15*, e0243124. [CrossRef]
30. Dahlström, U.; Lindahl, T.L.; Alehagen, U. Elevated D-dimer level is an independent risk factor for cardiovascular death in out-patients with symptoms compatible with heart failure. *Thromb. Haemost.* **2004**, *92*, 1250–1258. [CrossRef]
31. Buccheri, G.; Torchio, P.; Ferrigno, D. Plasma levels of D-dimer in lung carcinoma: Clinical and prognostic significance. *Cancer* **2003**, *97*, 3044–3052. [CrossRef]
32. Xu, G.; Zhang, Y.-L.; Huang, W. Relationship between plasma D-dimer levels and clinicopathologic parameters in resectable colorectal cancer patients. *World J. Gastroenterol.* **2004**, *10*, 922–923. [CrossRef] [PubMed]
33. Sato, T.; Yoshimura, M.; Sanda, T.; Hyodo, K.; Yamamoto, J.; Ishii, H.; Yamashita, T. Changes in spontaneous thrombolytic activity during progression of atherosclerosis in Apo(-/-) and LDLR(-/-) double knockout mice. *Int. J. Clin. Exp. Pathol.* **2018**, *11*, 4521–4528.
34. Kremers, B.M.M.; Cate, H.T.; Spronk, H.M.H. Pleiotropic effects of the hemostatic system. *J. Thromb. Haemost.* **2018**, *16*, 1464–1473. [CrossRef] [PubMed]
35. Fairweather-Tait, S.J.; Bao, Y.; Broadley, M.R.; Collings, R.; Ford, D.; Hesketh, J.E.; Hurst, R. Selenium in Human Health and Disease. *Antioxid. Redox Signal.* **2011**, *14*, 1337–1383. [CrossRef] [PubMed]
36. Selenius, M.; Rundlöf, A.-K.; Olm, E.; Fernandes, A.P.; Björnstedt, M. Selenium and the Selenoprotein Thioredoxin Reductase in the Prevention, Treatment and Diagnostics of Cancer. *Antioxid. Redox Signal.* **2010**, *12*, 867–880. [CrossRef] [PubMed]
37. Rayman, M.P. Selenium and human health. *Lancet* **2012**, *379*, 1256–1268. [CrossRef]
38. Xia, Y.; Hill, K.; Li, P.; Xu, J.; Zhou, D.; Motley, A.K.; Wang, L.; Byrne, D.W.; Burk, R.F. Optimization of selenoprotein P and other plasma selenium biomarkers for the assessment of the selenium nutritional requirement: A placebo-controlled, double-blind study of selenomethionine supplementation in selenium-deficient Chinese subjects. *Am. J. Clin. Nutr.* **2010**, *92*, 525–531. [CrossRef]
39. Brodin, O.; Hackler, J.; Misra, S.; Wendt, S.; Sun, Q.; Laaf, E.; Stoppe, C.; Björnstedt, M.; Schomburg, L. Selenoprotein P as Biomarker of Selenium Status in Clinical Trials with Therapeutic Dosages of Selenite. *Nutrients* **2020**, *12*, 1067. [CrossRef]
40. Manzanares, W.; Biestro, A.; Galusso, F.; Torre, M.H.; Manay, N.; Pittini, G.; Facchin, G.; Hardy, G. Serum selenium and glutathione peroxidase-3 activity: Biomarkers of systemic inflammation in the critically ill? *Intensive Care Med.* **2009**, *35*, 882–889. [CrossRef]
41. Alehagen, U.; Johansson, P.; Björnstedt, M.; Rosén, A.; Post, C.; Aaseth, J. Relatively high mortality risk in elderly Swedish subjects with low selenium status. *Eur. J. Clin. Nutr.* **2015**, *70*, 91–96. [CrossRef] [PubMed]
42. Kalén, A.; Appelkvist, E.-L.; Dallner, G. Age-related changes in the lipid compositions of rat and human tissues. *Lipids* **1989**, *24*, 579–584. [CrossRef]
43. Gutierrez-Mariscal, F.M.; Yubero-Serrano, E.M.; Villalba, J.M.; Lopez-Miranda, J. Coenzyme Q_{10}: From bench to clinic in aging diseases, a translational review. *Crit. Rev. Food Sci. Nutr.* **2019**, *59*, 2240–2257. [CrossRef] [PubMed]
44. Xia, L.; Nordman, T.; Olsson, J.M.; Damdimopoulos, A.; Björkhem-Bergman, L.; Nalvarte, I.; Eriksson, L.C.; Arnér, E.S.J.; Spyrou, G.; Björnstedt, M. The Mammalian Cytosolic Selenoenzyme Thioredoxin Reductase Reduces Ubiquinone. *J. Biol. Chem.* **2003**, *278*, 2141–2146. [CrossRef] [PubMed]
45. Norman, J.A.; Little, D.; Bolgar, M.; Di Donato, G. Degradation of brain natriuretic peptide by neutral endopeptidase: Species specific sites of proteolysis determined by mass spectrometry. *Biochem. Biophys. Res. Commun.* **1991**, *175*, 22–30. [CrossRef]
46. Alehagen, U.; Alexander, J.; Aaseth, J.; Larsson, A. Decrease in inflammatory biomarker concentration by intervention with selenium and coenzyme Q_{10}: A subanalysis of osteopontin, osteoprotergerin, TNFr1, TNFr2 and TWEAK. *J. Inflamm.* **2019**, *16*, 5. [CrossRef]
47. Alehagen, U.; Lindahl, T.L.; Aaseth, J.; Svensson, E.; Johansson, P. Levels of sP-selectin and hs-CRP Decrease with Dietary Intervention with Selenium and Coenzyme Q_{10} Combined: A Secondary Analysis of a Randomized Clinical Trial. *PLoS ONE* **2015**, *10*, e0137680. [CrossRef] [PubMed]
48. Alehagen, U.; Alexander, J.; Aaseth, J.; Larsson, A.; Lindahl, T.L. Significant decrease of von Willebrand factor and plasminogen activator inhibitor-1 by providing supplementation with selenium and coenzyme Q_{10} to an elderly population with a low selenium status. *Eur. J. Nutr.* **2020**, *59*, 3581–3590. [CrossRef]
49. Kuklinski, B.; Weissenbacher, E.; Fähnrich, A. Coenzyme Q_{10} and antioxidants in acute myocardial infarction. *Mol. Asp. Med.* **1994**, *15*, s143–s147. [CrossRef]
50. Alehagen, U.; Johansson, P.; Bjornstedt, M.; Rosen, A.; Dahlstrom, U. Cardiovascular mortality and N-terminal-proBNP reduced after combined selenium and coenzyme Q_{10} supplementation: A 5-year prospective randomized double-blind placebo-controlled trial among elderly Swedish citizens. *Int. J. Cardiol.* **2013**, *167*, 1860–1866. [CrossRef]
51. Alexander, J.; Alehagen, U.; Larsson, A.; Aaseth, J. Selenium in clinical medicine and medical biochemistry. *Klin. Biokem. I Nord.* **2019**, *31*, 12–19.
52. Jensen-Urstad, K.; Bouvier, F.; Höjer, J.; Ruiz, H.; Hulting, J.; Samad, B.; Thorstrand, C.; Jensen-Urstad, M. Comparison of Different Echocardiographic Methods With Radionuclide Imaging for Measuring Left Ventricular Ejection Fraction During Acute Myocardial Infarction Treated by Thrombolytic Therapy. *Am. J. Cardiol.* **1998**, *81*, 538–544. [CrossRef]
53. Van Royen, N.; Jaffe, C.C.; Krumholz, H.M.; Johnson, K.M.; Lynch, P.J.; Natale, D.; Atkinson, P.; Deman, P.; Wackers, F.J. Comparison and reproducibility of visual echocardiographic and quantitative radionuclide left ventricular ejection fractions. *Am. J. Cardiol.* **1996**, *77*, 843–850. [CrossRef]

54. Zhang, M.; Zhang, J.; Zhang, Q.; Yang, X.; Shan, H.; Ming, Z.; Chen, H.; Liu, Y.; Yin, J.; Li, Y. D-dimer as a potential biomarker for the progression of COPD. *Clin. Chim. Acta* **2016**, *455*, 55–59. [CrossRef] [PubMed]
55. Ge, Y.L.; Liu, C.H.; Wang, N.; Xu, J.; Zhu, X.Y.; Su, C.S.; Li, H.L.; Zhang, H.F.; Li, Z.Z.; Li, H.L.; et al. Elevated Plasma D-Dimer in Adult Community-Acquired Pneumonia Patients is Associated with an Increased Inflammatory Reaction and Lower Survival. *Clin. Lab.* **2019**, *65*. [CrossRef]
56. Franchini, M.; Lippi, G.; Favaloro, E.J. Aging Hemostasis: Changes to Laboratory Markers of Hemostasis As We Age—A Narrative Review. *Semin. Thromb. Hemost.* **2014**, *40*, 621–633. [CrossRef]
57. Haase, C.; Joergensen, M.; Ellervik, C.; Joergensen, M.K.; Bathum, L. Age- and sex-dependent reference intervals for D-dimer: Evidence for a marked increase by age. *Thromb. Res.* **2013**, *132*, 676–680. [CrossRef] [PubMed]

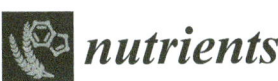

Article

Glucose Fluctuation and Severe Internal Carotid Artery Siphon Stenosis in Type 2 Diabetes Patients

Futoshi Eto [1], Kazuo Washida [1,*], Masaki Matsubara [2], Hisashi Makino [2], Akio Takahashi [1], Kotaro Noda [1], Yorito Hattori [1], Yuriko Nakaoku [3], Kunihiro Nishimura [3], Kiminori Hosoda [2] and Masafumi Ihara [1]

[1] Department of Neurology, National Cerebral and Cardiovascular Center, Suita 564-8565, Japan; eto.futoshi@gmail.com (F.E.); oremonox@gmail.com (A.T.); noda.kotaro@ncvc.go.jp (K.N.); yoh2019@ncvc.go.jp (Y.H.); ihara@ncvc.go.jp (M.I.)

[2] Division of Diabetes and Lipid Metabolism, National Cerebral and Cardiovascular Center, Suita 564-8565, Japan; matsubara.m@ncvc.go.jp (M.M.); makinoh@ncvc.go.jp (H.M.); kiminorihosoda@ncvc.go.jp (K.H.)

[3] Department of Preventive Medicine and Epidemiology, National Cerebral and Cardiovascular Center, Suita 564-8565, Japan; yurikon@ncvc.go.jp (Y.N.); knishimu@ncvc.go.jp (K.N.)

* Correspondence: washida@ncvc.go.jp; Tel.: +81-6-6170-1070

Abstract: The impact of glucose fluctuation on intracranial artery stenosis remains to be elucidated. This study aimed to investigate the association between glucose fluctuation and intracranial artery stenosis. This was a cross-sectional study of type 2 diabetes mellitus (T2DM) patients equipped with the FreeStyle Libre Pro continuous glucose monitoring system (Abbott Laboratories) between February 2019 and June 2020. Glucose fluctuation was evaluated according to the standard deviation (SD) of blood glucose, coefficient of variation (%CV), and mean amplitude of glycemic excursions (MAGE). Magnetic resonance angiography was used to evaluate the degree of intracranial artery stenosis. Of the 103 patients, 8 patients developed severe internal carotid artery (ICA) siphon stenosis ($\geq$70%). SD, %CV, and MAGE were significantly higher in the severe stenosis group than in the non-severe stenosis group (<70%), whereas there was no significant intergroup difference in the mean blood glucose and HbA1c. Multivariable logistic regression analysis adjusted for sex showed that SD, %CV, and MAGE were independent factors associated with severe ICA siphon stenosis. In conclusion, glucose fluctuation is significantly associated with severe ICA siphon stenosis in T2DM patients. Thus, glucose fluctuation can be a target of preventive therapies for intracranial artery stenosis and ischemic stroke.

Keywords: continuous glucose monitoring; glucose fluctuation; intracranial artery stenosis; mean amplitude of glycemic excursions; standard deviation

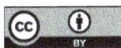

1. Introduction

It was estimated that 451 million individuals globally have diabetes mellitus (DM) in 2017 [1]. DM is a major cause of blindness, kidney failure, heart attacks, stroke, and lower limb amputation. Long-term management of DM can prevent atherosclerotic cardiovascular disease (ASCVD) such as ischemic stroke or acute coronary syndrome. Patients with severe intracranial artery stenosis have the highest rate of recurrent stroke [2,3]. There have been various reports on the relationship between DM and intracranial artery stenosis [4,5], but the findings have been conflicting. Although some studies reported that elevated hemoglobin A1c (HbA1c) and fasting blood glucose levels are associated with intracranial artery stenosis [6], others showed no correlations [7]. Thus, the usefulness of HbA1c and fasting blood glucose levels as predictors of intracranial artery stenosis remains unclear.

There are various indicators for blood glucose control in patients with DM; these include hemoglobin A1c (HbA1c) and glycoalbumin. However, these indicators only reflect the mean blood glucose level for a certain period and cannot reflect glucose fluctuation.

Atherosclerotic stenosis such as intracranial artery stenosis and coronary artery stenosis are major complications of DM. Glucose fluctuation can cause atherosclerosis because it induces chronic inflammation and oxidative stress in the vasculature [8]. Thus, prevention of atherosclerosis in patients with DM requires targeting glucose fluctuation. Continuous glucose monitoring (CGM) systems, such as the FreeStyle Libre Pro, have been recently approved for use in clinical practice. In contrast to self-monitoring of blood glucose (SMBG) where up to 80% of hypoglycemia and hyperglycemia can be missed [9], CGM enables a continuous monitoring of blood glucose levels and fluctuations.

Recent clinical studies have shown that blood glucose fluctuation is related to ASCVD [7,10–12]. Furthermore, glucose fluctuation could predict prognosis after acute coronary syndrome [13]. However, although blood glucose fluctuation is associated with the risk of many cardiovascular diseases, the relationship between blood glucose fluctuation and intracranial artery stenosis remains unclear. Therefore, this study aimed to investigate the relationship between glucose fluctuation and intracranial artery stenosis in type 2 DM (T2DM) patients who are using the FreeStyle Libre Pro continuous glucose monitoring system.

2. Materials and Methods

2.1. Study Design and Patients

This retrospective, observational, cross-sectional study was performed at the National Cerebral and Cardiovascular Center (NCVC), Suita, Osaka, Japan. This study is part of an ongoing prospective longitudinal study on the relationship between glucose fluctuation and cognitive function in T2DM (PROPOSAL Study: Trial Registration, University Hospital Medical Information Network Clinical Trial Registry (UMIN000038546)) [14].

T2DM patients with mild cognitive impairment (MCI) were enrolled in the registry between February 2019 and June 2020. The PROPOSAL Study is aimed at evaluating the relationships between glucose fluctuation indices assessed by CGM and cognitive function among elderly patients with T2DM. Therefore, patients are limited to those aged 65–85 years. T2DM was diagnosed according to the Japan Diabetes Society criteria. MCI was diagnosed based on the clinical course and a score of 17–25 on the Japanese version of Montreal Cognitive Assessment scale [14–16]. Carotid artery stenosis was evaluated according to the North American Symptomatic Carotid Endarterectomy Trial method [17]. Patients with ≥80% carotid artery stenosis [18] or those undergoing renal replacement therapy [19] were excluded because these conditions could affect cognitive function. Additionally, those taking antidementia drugs or having underlying comorbidities affecting cognitive function (depression, thyroid dysfunction, and vitamin B1, vitamin B12, and folate deficiency) were excluded. Sex, age, baseline patient characteristics including current smoking status, medical history such as hypertension or active use of antihypertensive medications, dyslipidemia or active use of lipid-lowering agents, T2DM or antidiabetic treatment, atrial fibrillation or antidiabetic treatment, medical history of percutaneous coronary intervention or coronary artery bypass grafting (PCI/CABG), and former ischemic stroke episode, were collected from the registry.

All subjects gave their informed consent for inclusion before they participated in the study. The study was conducted in accordance with the Declaration of Helsinki, and the protocol was approved by the Ethics Committee of NCVC (Project identification code M30-110-3).

2.2. Imaging Protocol

Magnetic resonance imaging (MRI) was performed with a 3-Tesla system. The vessels constituting the intracranial artery were defined as shown in Figure 1: (i) the A1 or A2 segment of the anterior cerebral arteries (ACA), (ii) the C1 to C5 segment of the intracranial internal carotid arteries (ICA) categorized according to Fischer's classification [20], (iii) the P1 or P2 segment of the posterior cerebral arteries (PCA), and (iv) the M1 or M2 segment of the middle cerebral arteries (MCA).

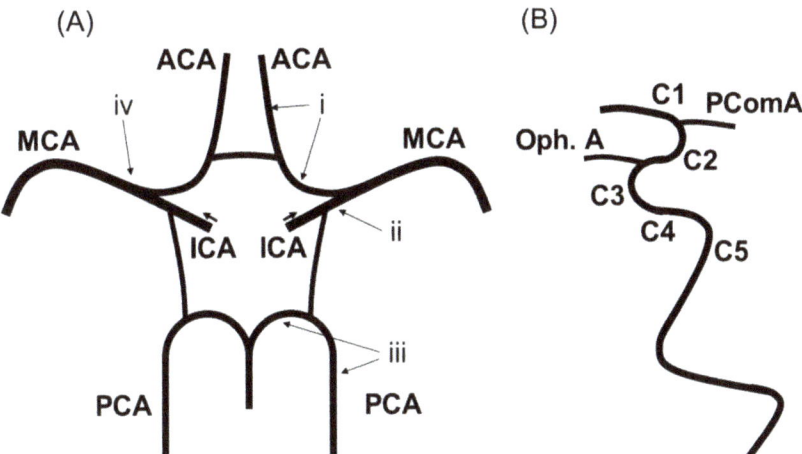

Figure 1. Evaluated vessels comprising the intracranial arteries. Schematic of the intracranial arteries evaluated in this study. (**A**) (i) The A1 or A2 segment of the ACA, (ii) the C1 to C5 segment of intracranial ICA, (iii) the P1 or P2 segment of the PCA, and (iv) the M1 or M2 segment of the MCA. (**B**) Classification of intracranial ICA according to Fischer's classification: C1, from the ACA branch to the PComA branch; C2, from the proximal PComA branch to the ophthalmic artery branch; C3, from the ophthalmic artery branch to the genu of the internal carotid artery; C4, in the cavernous sinus; and C5, from the proximal cavernous sinus to the orifice of the carotid canal. Abbreviations: ACA, anterior cerebral artery; ICA, internal carotid artery; MCA, middle cerebral artery; Oph.A, ophthalmic artery; PCA, posterior cerebral artery; PComA, posterior communicating artery.

Magnetic resonance angiography (MRA) findings of the vessels constituting the intracranial artery were independently read by two stroke neurologists (F.E. and A.T.) blinded to the clinical information, to determine the anatomical variations. Disagreements were resolved through a joint assessment until consensus was reached. The percentage of stenosis for each vessel was listed in 5% increments.

Percent stenosis was measured using the Warfarin-Aspirin Symptomatic Intracranial Disease (WASID) method [21]. The percentage was calculated by MRA using a previous method as follows: (1) the most severe stenosis spot on the maximum-intensity projection or axial source images was measured using the time-of-flight method; then, (2) we measured at the widest, non-tortuous, normal portion of the petrous ICA parallel to the site of stenosis [22]. Intracranial artery stenosis was evaluated on the side with the stronger stenosis. The degree of stenosis was categorized into two categories as severe stenosis (i.e., ≥70% stenosis [3] at specific segments of the intracranial artery: A1 or A2 segment of the ACA, C1-C5 segment of the ICA, P1 or P2 segment of the PCA, and M1 or M2 segment of the MCA) and non-severe stenosis (i.e., <70% stenosis), based on a previous report [23].

2.3. Continuous Glucose Monitoring

The FreeStyle Libre Pro continuous glucose monitoring (FLP-CGM) system (Abbott Laboratories, Chicago, IL, USA) is an interstitial glucose monitoring device with an established accuracy [24]. The FLP sensor is disposable and inserted on the back of an upper extremity for up to 14 days. A unique feature of the sensor is that calibration is not required using SMBG, and after it is removed, data can be downloaded, and glucose profiles evaluated. In this study, the mean glucose, standard deviation (SD), percent coefficient of variation (%CV) [25], and the mean amplitude of glycemic excursions (MAGE) [26] were calculated to evaluate glucose fluctuation. Considering the concerns about the lack of the accuracy of the date at day 1 [24], we used the data from day 2 to the end of recording (maximally, day 14). Additionally, patients in whom blood glucose fluctuations were not measured by CGM within 7 days were excluded according to former protocols [27].

2.4. Statistical Analyses

Continuous variables are shown as the mean ± standard deviation and compared using a *t*-test if data were normally distributed. Meanwhile, categorical variables are shown as frequencies and percentages and compared using Fisher's exact test. Agreement in stenosis assessments between the two physicians was assessed using weighted kappa statistics. These statistics are appropriate when there are more than two ordered categories and adjust for chance agreement and degree of disagreement between raters. Logistic regression models were used to evaluate the associations of each glucose fluctuation factor with severe and non-severe intracranial stenosis. Univariable logistic regression models were used to calculate odds ratios (ORs) and 95% confidence intervals (CIs). Sex, age, current smoking, duration years of T2DM, medical history of hypertension, dyslipidemia, atrial fibrillation, former ischemic stroke episode, and PCI/CABG were entered in the univariable models. Multivariable logistic regression analyses were performed using covariates significantly associated with intracranial stenosis in univariable models.

All statistical analyses were conducted by two physicians (F.E. and Y.N.) using JMP 14.0.0 statistical software (SAS Institute Inc., Cary, NC, USA) and Stata 15.1 software (StataCorp, College Station, TX, USA). A *p* value of <0.05 was considered statistically significant.

3. Results

3.1. Baseline Patient Characteristics

The patient inclusion flow chart is shown in Figure 2. Of the 109 T2DM patients enrolled in the registry, 103 patients with a mean age of 76 ± 5 years (females, 30%) were included in the current analysis. Six patients were excluded due to missing baseline data (*n* = 4), non-availability for MRI (*n* = 1), and evaluation with 1.5 Tesla system for MRI (*n* = 1). CGM data of all 103 patients were obtained.

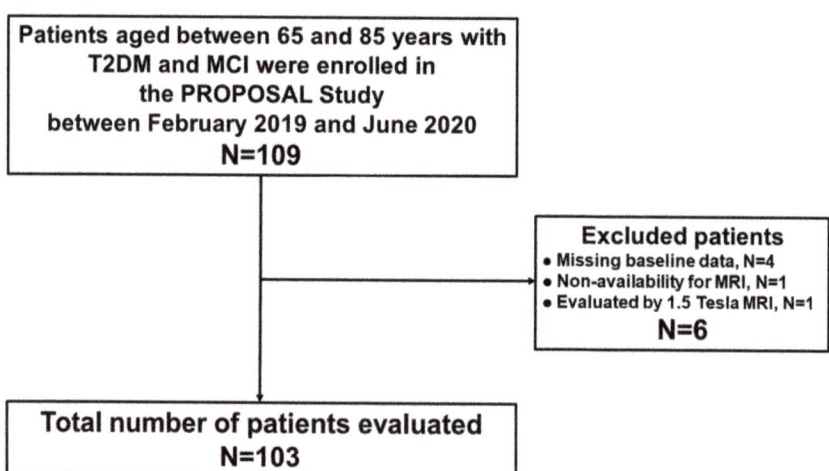

Figure 2. Patient inclusion flow chart. Blood glucose fluctuations were measured via CGM for at least 7 days in all patients. Abbreviations: CGM, continuous glucose monitoring; MCI, mild cognitive impairment; MRI, magnetic resonance imaging; T2DM, type 2 diabetes mellitus.

The patient's baseline characteristics stratified according to the WASID method are shown in Table 1.

Table 1. Baseline patient characteristics by degree of internal carotid artery siphon stenosis.

Variables	Intracranial Internal Carotid Artery Siphon Stenosis		
	Severe (n = 8)	Non-Severe (n = 95)	p Value
Baseline demographics			
Female (%)	6 (75)	26 (27)	0.01
Age, years	76 ± 5	76 ± 5	0.63
Cerebrovascular risk factors			
Hypertension (%)	6 (75)	88 (93)	0.14
Dyslipidemia (%)	8 (100)	83 (87)	0.59
Current or past smoking (%)	3 (38)	54 (57)	0.46
Atrial fibrillation (%)	1 (13)	16 (17)	1.00
Medical history of percutaneous coronary intervention or coronary artery bypass grafting (%)	4 (50)	41 (44)	0.73
Ischemic stroke episode (%)	3 (38)	42 (45)	1.00
Diabetes mellitus			
Duration, years	26 ± 10	23 ± 11	0.32
HbA1c at registration, %	7.8 ± 0.9	7.5 ± 0.9	0.47
Blood glucose at registration, mg/dL	136 ± 42	150 ± 42	0.54
Blood glucose (CGM average), mg/dL	148 ± 25	136 ± 28	0.19
SD, mg/dL	53 ± 12	39 ± 10	<0.01
%CV	36 ± 7	29 ± 6	<0.01
MAGE, mg/dL	114 ± 18	90 ± 23	<0.01

Continuous variables are shown as the mean (± SD), while categorical variables are shown as frequencies and percentages. Abbreviations: HbA1c, hemoglobin A1c; CGM, continuous glucose monitoring; SD, standard deviation; %CV, coefficient of variation; MAGE, mean amplitude of glycemic excursions.

3.2. Head Magnetic Resonance Angiography Findings

Of the 103 patients examined, 8 patients presented with severe (≥70%) ICA siphon stenosis (severe stenosis group: 8%), while 95 patients presented non-severe (<70%) ICA siphon stenosis (non-severe stenosis group: 92%). Among these 95 patients, 48 and 47 patients had moderate (50–70%) and mild (0–50%) ICA siphon stenosis, respectively. A representative case of severe stenosis of the left ICA siphon on MRA is shown in Figure 3.

Except ICA siphon, severe stenoses (≥70%) were not observed in any other intracranial arteries. In addition, moderate stenoses (50–70%) were only observed at the M1 portion of the MCA in 3 of the 103 patients. Regarding the consistency of intracranial artery stenosis evaluation, the inter-rater agreement of the quadratic weighted kappa statistic for the evaluation of the vessels constituting the intracranial artery was 0.952, indicating high consistency.

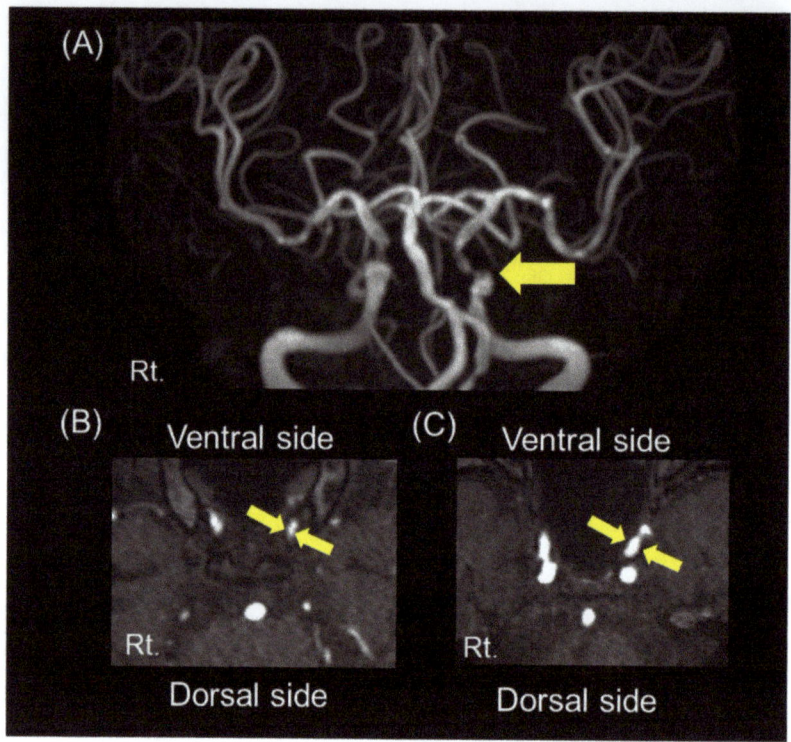

Figure 3. A representative case of severe internal carotid artery siphon stenosis. (**A**) Magnetic resonance angiography (MRA) showing the severe stenosis in the left internal carotid artery siphon (arrow). (**B,C**) MRA source images showing 74% stenosis of the internal carotid artery (ICA) siphon evaluated using the WASID method, with the narrowest portion (**B**, between arrows; 1.0 mm) of the siphon ICA and the widest portion (**C**, between arrows; 3.8 mm) of the petrous ICA.

3.3. Association between Glucose Fluctuation and Intracranial Artery Stenosis

Compared with the non-severe stenosis group ($n = 95$), the severe stenosis group ($n = 8$) showed significantly higher variability in the three indices of glucose fluctuation: SD (53 mg/dL vs. 39 mg/dL, $p < 0.01$), %CV (36 vs. 29, $p < 0.01$), and MAGE (114 mg/dL vs. 90 mg/dL, $p < 0.01$) (Table 1). Meanwhile, other vascular risk factors, such as smoking, hypertension, dyslipidemia, mean blood glucose, HbA1c, and duration years of T2DM, were not significantly different between the two groups (Table 1). Scatter plots showing the relationships between glucose fluctuation and ICA siphon stenosis are shown in Figure 4.

In univariable analysis, the severe stenosis group showed significantly higher SD (OR, 3.60; 95% CI, 1.60–8.08; $p < 0.01$), %CV (OR, 7.85; 95% CI, 1.90–32.5; $p < 0.01$), and MAGE (OR, 1.56; 95% CI, 1.11–2.20; $p = 0.01$). Multivariable logistic regression analysis showed that these factors remained significantly associated with severe ICA siphon stenosis after adjustment for sex (SD: OR, 3.00; 95% CI, 1.32–6.84; $p < 0.01$; %CV: OR, 5.55; 95% CI, 1.23–25.2; $p = 0.03$; and MAGE: OR, 1.52; 95% CI, 1.06–2.19; $p = 0.02$) (Table 2).

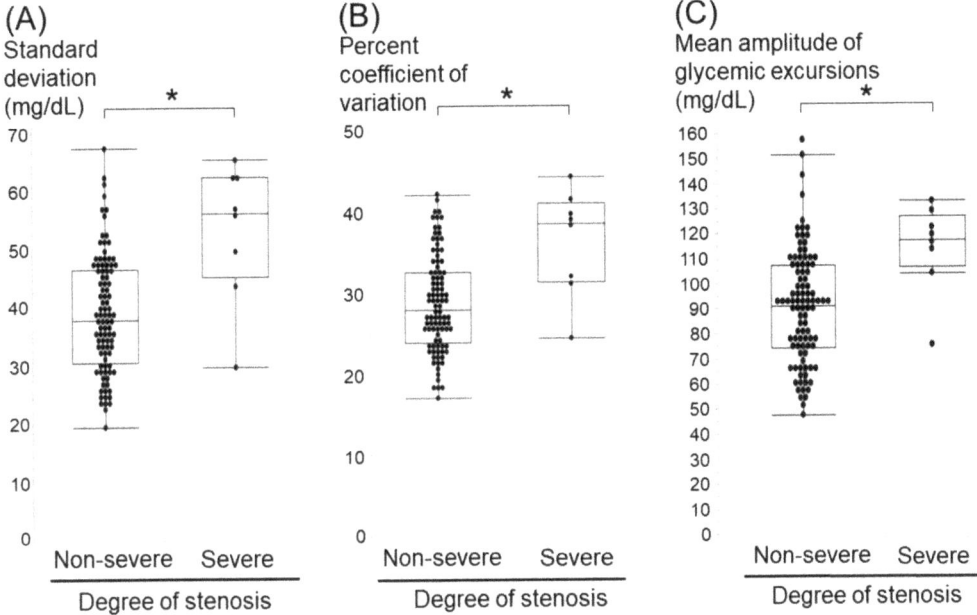

Figure 4. Scatter plots showing relationships between glucose fluctuation and internal carotid artery siphon stenosis. Glucose fluctuations assessed by standard deviation (SD) (**A**), coefficient of validation (%CV) (**B**), and mean amplitude of glycemic excursions (MAGE) (**C**) are significantly higher in the severe stenosis group than in the non-severe stenosis group (* $p < 0.01$).

Table 2. Multivariable analysis of influencing factors of stenosis adjusted for sex.

	SD (10 mg/dL)	p Value	%CV (/10)	p Value	MAGE (10 mg/dL)	p Value
Crude OR (95% CI)	3.60 (1.60–8.08)	<0.01	7.85 (1.90–32.5)	<0.01	1.56 (1.11–2.20)	0.01
Adjusted OR (95% CI)	3.00 (1.32–6.84)	<0.01	5.55 (1.23–25.2)	0.03	1.52 (1.06–2.19)	0.02

Abbreviations: SD, standard deviation; CV, coefficient of variation; MAGE, mean amplitude of glycemic excursions; OR, odds ratio; CI, confidence interval.

As for the cases with moderate (50–70%) and mild (0–50%) ICA siphon stenosis, there was no significant intergroup difference in all variables including SD, %CV, and MAGE (Table S1). There was also no significant intergroup difference in all variables including SD, %CV, and MAGE for the cases with moderate (50–70%) and mild (0–50%) MCA M1 stenosis (Table S2).

4. Discussion

The relationship between blood glucose fluctuation and intracranial artery stenosis in T2DM patients remains unclear. In this study, patients with severe ICA siphon stenosis had higher blood glucose fluctuations as assessed with SD, %CV, and MAGE. Meanwhile, there were no significant differences for other vascular risk factors, such as hypertension, dyslipidemia, mean blood glucose levels, HbA1c, and duration in years of T2DM. To our best knowledge, this is the first study to reveal the association between intracranial artery stenosis and glucose fluctuation.

There are several possible mechanisms by which blood glucose fluctuation causes the atherosclerotic stenosis of the major intracranial arteries. Atherosclerosis is a complex multifactorial disease and often causes diabetic macrovascular complications. Glucose fluctuation plays a key role in the development of atherosclerosis. One of the most common causative factors for atherosclerosis by glucose fluctuation is an increase in oxidative stress due to a rapid blood glucose change that causes vascular endothelial damage. Compared with chronic sustained hyperglycemia, glucose fluctuations induce a more specific effect on oxidative stress [8]. Severe blood glucose fluctuation is known to lower the number of vascular endothelial progenitor cells [28]. Blood glucose fluctuation is also correlated with carotid intima media thickness (IMT) [29], which is an indicator of subclinical atherosclerosis. Coronary plaque has been reported to be correlated with glucose fluctuation [30].

Additionally, glucose fluctuation usually includes hyperglycemia and hypoglycemia, and these are also associated with the presence and severity of cardiovascular disease in DM patients [31]. Hyperglycemia increases the advanced glycation endproducts (AGEs), and the binding of the AGEs to the receptor of AGEs induces oxidative stress and inflammation via the NF-kappa B pathway, leading to atherosclerosis [32]. Furthermore, a meta-analysis by Liang et al. showed that minimizing glucose fluctuation improved insulin resistance and carotid IMT thickness, thus lowering the risk of cardiovascular disease [33]. Reductions in glucose fluctuation by DPP-IV inhibitors can prevent atherosclerosis progression in T2DM patients by lowering inflammation and oxidative stress [34].

However, there is still limited evidence on the association between glucose fluctuations and cerebrovascular lesions. Glucose is the primary energy source for the brain, and severe glucose fluctuations have been associated with numerous types of central nervous system damage [35]. Several studies demonstrated that oxidative stress and inflammation due to blood glucose fluctuations impair the blood–brain barrier [36] or induce hypercoagulability and suppression of the fibrinolytic system [37]. Blood glucose fluctuations also worsen the progression of cerebral white matter lesions [38] and the prognosis of cerebral infarction [39,40]. Increasing evidence shows that glucose fluctuation significantly increases oxidative stress, leading to neuroinflammation and cognitive dysfunction [35]. However, the detailed mechanisms by which glucose fluctuation causes cerebrovascular lesions remain to be elucidated, highlighting the need for further studies.

With respect to the site of the intracranial artery stenosis, our study showed that intracranial artery stenosis particularly occurred at the siphon portion of the ICA. Few studies have examined the sites of intracranial artery stenosis. Atherosclerotic stenosis often occurs at sites with complex hemodynamics, such as arteries with high curvature or bifurcations. A study on fluid dynamics in morphology identified three preferred sites of stenoses along the carotid siphon with low and highly oscillatory wall shear stress [41]. Another review showed that low and oscillatory shear stress is closely associated with atherogenesis [42]. In our study, stenosis was also found along the carotid siphon area. As for the degree of the intracranial artery stenosis, Mo et al. [7] assessed the relationship between glucose fluctuation and degree of intracranial artery stenosis and found no significant relationship. However, stenosis was defined as more than 50% thickening of the arterial wall, and this could have affected the finding. A previous analysis of the predictors of ischemic stroke in symptomatic intracranial arterial stenosis showed that patients with $\geq 70\%$ intracranial stenosis have a ≥ 2 times higher risk of stroke than patients with <70% stenosis [3]. In this context, we compared patients with severe intracranial stenosis ($\geq 70\%$ stenosis) and non-severe intracranial stenosis (<70%), and found a significant difference in glucose fluctuation between them.

In this study, the proportion of female patients was higher in the severe ICA siphon stenosis group than in the non-severe group in the univariable analysis. A prospective multicenter study of 2864 consecutive acute ischemic stroke patients in China reported that women aged >63 years were more likely to have intracranial artery stenosis than men [43]. This sex difference in the risk of intracranial artery stenosis is complex and not easily explained. However, elderly women have more vascular risk factors, such as DM, hypertension and dyslipidemia, than elderly men [43]. Additionally, elderly females are more likely to have hormone imbalance. Low sex hormone–binding globulin levels and high free androgen index are strongly associated with cardiovascular risk factors (DM, dyslipidemia and inflammation) in multiethnic premenopausal and perimenopausal women [44]. This could explain the sex difference for intracranial artery stenosis. However, in this study, multivariable logistic regression analysis adjusted for sex showed that SD, %CV, and MAGE were independent factors associated with severe ICA siphon stenosis, although there was a possibility that sex difference could have affected the tolerance of vessel structural change.

Our findings support the idea that glucose fluctuation may help predict intracranial artery stenosis and accordingly direct preventive measures against ischemic stroke in T2DM patients. The rate of ischemic stroke episode was not significantly different between severe and non-severe ICA siphon stenosis. This may be due to the relatively small sample size of patients with severe stenosis or because patients with ≥80% carotid artery stenosis were excluded from the current study. However, identifying factors associated with severe intracranial artery stenosis is important because patients with severe intracranial stenosis have the highest rate of recurrent stroke [2,3]. Furthermore, glucose fluctuation is also associated with early neurological deterioration and poor functional outcome in patients with acute ischemic stroke [45]. Interventions for glucose fluctuation can prevent intracranial artery stenosis and ischemic stroke in T2DM patients.

This study has some limitations that need to be considered when interpreting the results. First, this was a cross-sectional study, and thus the causal association between glucose fluctuation and intracranial artery stenosis still needs to be clarified in studies with longer follow-up. Second, this study was conducted at a single center that was specialized for stroke and cardiovascular disease, and there was a relatively small number of patients with severe intracranial stenosis. Multicenter studies with a larger sample size are needed to further confirm the association between glucose fluctuation and ICA siphon stenosis. Third, patients with ≥80% carotid artery stenosis were excluded in this study because severe carotid artery stenosis is known to affect cognitive function [18]. This may lead to difficulty in interpretation of the results due to poor diabetes control of dementia patients. Glycemic variability is correlated with carotid IMT, which is an indicator of subclinical atherosclerosis [29]. Additionally, patients with intracranial artery stenosis tend to have carotid artery stenosis [46]. It is assumed that patients with ≥80% carotid artery stenosis have greater glycemic variability. It is therefore necessary to conduct future studies that include patients with carotid artery stenosis ≥80% along with a detailed neuropsychological assessment. Fourth, MRI may have lower accuracy than digital subtraction angiography (DSA) or computed tomography angiography (CTA) for evaluating stenosis. ICA siphon, where the stenosis was observed in this study, runs parallel to the axial images. Therefore, saturation of the blood signal may result in poor vessel delineation. However, some diabetes patients have chronic renal failure, which sometimes makes it difficult to perform DSA or CTA. Advances in vascular imaging technology are eagerly awaited.

5. Conclusions

Glucose fluctuation, as indicated by elevations in SD, %CV, and MAGE, is significantly associated with severe ICA siphon stenosis. Thus, glucose fluctuation can be a target of preventive therapies for intracranial artery stenosis and ischemic stroke.

Supplementary Materials: The following are available online at https://www.mdpi.com/article/10.3390/nu13072379/s1, Table S1. Baseline patient characteristics by degree of internal carotid artery siphon stenosis. Table S2. Baseline patient characteristics by degree of middle cerebral artery stenosis.

Author Contributions: Conceptualization, K.W.; methodology, F.E. and K.W.; software, F.E. and Y.N.; validation, F.E. and K.W.; formal analysis, F.E., K.N. (Kotaro Noda), Y.N. and K.N. (Kunihiro Nishimura); investigation, F.E. and A.T.; resources, F.E.; data curation, F.E., M.M. and A.T.; writing—

original draft preparation, F.E.; writing—review and editing, K.W., M.M., H.M., A.T., Y.H., Y.N., K.N. (Kunihiro Nishimura), K.H. and M.I.; visualization, F.E. and K.W.; supervision, M.I.; project administration, K.W.; funding acquisition, K.H. All authors have read and agreed to the published version of the manuscript.

Funding: This research was funded by Japan Agency for Medical Research and Development (AMED), grant number 18ek0210104h0001.

Institutional Review Board Statement: The study was conducted according to the guidelines of the Declaration of Helsinki, and registered part of the PROPOSAL study, University Hospital Medical Information Network clinical trials database (UMIN000038546). The study was approved by the Institutional Review Board of National Cerebral and Cardiovascular Center (approved number M30-110-3).

Informed Consent Statement: Informed consent was obtained from all subjects involved in the study. Written informed consent has been obtained from the patients to publish this paper.

Data Availability Statement: The data presented in this study are available on request from the corresponding author.

Acknowledgments: We are indebted to Yoko Ohashi and Sayaka Wada for their excellent secretarial assistance.

Conflicts of Interest: The authors declare no conflict of interest.

References

1. Cho, N.H.; Shaw, J.E.; Karuranga, S.; Huang, Y.; Fernandes, J.D.R.; Ohlrogge, A.W.; Malanda, B. IDF Diabetes Atlas: Global estimates of diabetes prevalence for 2017 and projections for 2045. *Diabetes Res. Clin. Pract.* **2018**, *138*, 271–281. [CrossRef] [PubMed]
2. Arenillas, J.F. Intracranial atherosclerosis: Current concepts. *Stroke* **2011**, *42*, S20–S23. [CrossRef]
3. Kasner, S.E.; Chimowitz, M.I.; Lynn, M.J.; Howlett-Smith, H.; Stern, B.J.; Hertzberg, V.S.; Frankel, M.R.; Levine, S.R.; Chaturvedi, S.; Benesch, C.G.; et al. Predictors of ischemic stroke in the territory of a symptomatic intracranial arterial stenosis. *Circulation* **2006**, *113*, 555–563. [CrossRef]
4. Shitara, S.; Fujiyoshi, A.; Hisamatsu, T.; Torii, S.; Suzuki, S.; Ito, T.; Arima, H.; Shiino, A.; Nozaki, K.; Miura, K.; et al. Intracranial artery stenosis and its association with conventional risk factors in a general population of Japanese men. *Stroke* **2019**, *50*, 2967–2969. [CrossRef] [PubMed]
5. Sun, Q.; Wang, Q.; Wang, X.; Ji, X.; Sang, S.; Shao, S.; Zhao, Y.; Xiang, Y.; Xue, Y.; Li, J.; et al. Prevalence and cardiovascular risk factors of asymptomatic intracranial arterial stenosis: The Kongcun town study in Shandong, China. *Eur. J. Neurol.* **2020**, *27*, 729–735. [CrossRef]
6. Wang, Y.-L.; Leng, X.-Y.; Dong, Y.; Hou, X.-H.; Tong, L.; Ma, Y.-H.; Xu, W.; Cui, M.; Dong, Q.; Tan, L.; et al. Fasting glucose and HbA1c levels as risk factors for the presence of intracranial atherosclerotic stenosis. *Ann. Transl. Med.* **2019**, *7*, 804. [CrossRef] [PubMed]
7. Mo, Y.; Zhou, J.; Li, M.; Wang, Y.; Bao, Y.; Ma, X.; Li, D.; Lu, W.; Hu, C.; Li, M.; et al. Glycemic variability is associated with subclinical atherosclerosis in Chinese type 2 diabetic patients. *Cardiovasc. Diabetol.* **2013**, *12*, 15. [CrossRef] [PubMed]
8. Monnier, L.; Mas, E.; Ginet, C.; Michel, F.; Villon, L.; Cristol, J.P.; Colette, C. Activation of oxidative stress by acute glucose fluctuations compared with sustained chronic hyperglycemia in patients with type 2 diabetes. *JAMA* **2006**, *295*, 1681–1687. [CrossRef]
9. Kaufman, F.R.; Gibson, L.C.; Halvorson, M.; Carpenter, S.; Fisher, L.K.; Pitukcheewanont, P. A pilot study of the continuous glucose monitoring system: Clinical decisions and glycemic control after its use in pediatric type 1 diabetic subjects. *Diabetes Care* **2001**, *24*, 2030–2034. [CrossRef] [PubMed]
10. Chen, X.M.; Zhang, Y.; Shen, X.P.; Huang, Q.; Ma, H.; Huang, Y.L.; Zhang, W.Q.; Wu, H.J. Correlation between glucose fluctuations and carotid intima-media thickness in type 2 diabetes. *Diabetes Res. Clin. Pract.* **2010**, *90*, 95–99. [CrossRef] [PubMed]
11. Gohbara, M.; Hibi, K.; Mitsuhashi, T.; Maejima, N.; Iwahashi, N.; Kataoka, S.; Akiyama, E.; Tsukahara, K.; Kosuge, M.; Ebina, T.; et al. Glycemic variability on continuous glucose monitoring system correlates with non-culprit vessel coronary plaque vulnerability in patients with first-episode acute coronary syndrome. *Circ. J.* **2016**, *80*, 202–210. [CrossRef]
12. Su, G.; Mi, S.; Tao, H.; Li, Z.; Yang, H.; Zheng, H.; Zhou, Y.; Ma, C. Association of glycemic variability and the presence and severity of coronary artery disease in patients with type 2 diabetes. *Cardiovasc. Diabetol.* **2011**, *10*, 19. [CrossRef]
13. Takahashi, H.; Iwahashi, N.; Kirigaya, J.; Kataoka, S.; Minamimoto, Y.; Gohbara, M.; Abe, T.; Okada, K.; Matsuzawa, Y.; Konishi, M.; et al. Glycemic variability determined with a continuous glucose monitoring system can predict prognosis after acute coronary syndrome. *Cardiovasc. Diabetol.* **2018**, *17*, 116. [CrossRef] [PubMed]

14. Matsubara, M.; Makino, H.; Washida, K.; Matsuo, M.; Koezuka, R.; Ohata, Y.; Tamanaha, T.; Honda-Kohmo, K.; Noguchi, M.; Tomita, T.; et al. A prospective longitudinal study on the relationship between glucose fluctuation and cognitive function in type 2 diabetes: PROPOSAL Study Protocol. *Diabetes Ther.* **2020**, *11*, 2729–2737. [CrossRef]
15. Fujiwara, Y.; Suzuki, H.; Yasunaga, M.; Sugiyama, H.; Ijuin, M.; Sakuma, N.; Inagaki, H.; Iwasa, H.; Ura, C.; Yatomi, N.; et al. Brief screening tool for mild cognitive impairment in older Japanese: Validation of the Japanese version of the Montreal Cognitive Assessment. *Geriatr. Gerontol. Int.* **2010**, *10*, 225–232. [CrossRef] [PubMed]
16. Trzepacz, P.T.; Hochstetler, H.; Wang, S.; Walker, B.; Saykin, A.J.; The Alzheimer's Disease Neuroimaging Initiative. Relationship between the Montreal Cognitive Assessment and Mini-mental State Examination for assessment of mild cognitive impairment in older adults. *BMC Geriatr.* **2015**, *15*, 107. [CrossRef] [PubMed]
17. North American Symptomatic Carotid Endarterectomy Trial Collaborators. Beneficial effect of carotid endarterectomy in symptomatic patients with high-grade carotid stenosis. *N. Engl. J. Med.* **1991**, *325*, 445–453. [CrossRef]
18. Marshall, R.S.; Pavol, M.A.; Cheung, Y.K.; Asllani, I.; Lazar, R.M. Cognitive impairment correlates linearly with mean flow velocity by transcranial doppler below a definable threshold. *Cerebrovasc. Dis. Extra* **2020**, *10*, 21–27. [CrossRef]
19. Zwieten, A.; Wong, G.; Ruospo, M.; Palmer, S.C.; Barulli, M.R.; Iurillo, A.; Saglimbene, V.; Natale, P.; Gargano, L.; Murgo, M.; et al. Prevalence and patterns of cognitive impairment in adult hemodialysis patients: The COGNITIVE-HD study. *Nephrol. Dial. Transplant.* **2018**, *33*, 1197–1206. [CrossRef] [PubMed]
20. Fischer, E. Die Lageabweichungen de vorderen hirnarterie im gefaessbild. *Zentralbl. Neurochir.* **1938**, *3*, 300–313.
21. Samuels, O.B.; Joseph, G.J.; Lynn, M.J.; Smith, H.A.; Chimowitz, M.I. A standardized method for measuring intracranial arterial stenosis. *AJNR* **2000**, *21*, 643–646.
22. Baradaran, H.; Patel, P.; Gialdini, G.; Al-Dasuqi, K.; Giambrone, A.; Kamel, H.; Gupta, A. Quantifying intracranial internal carotid artery stenosis on MR angiography. *AJNR* **2017**, *38*, 986–990. [CrossRef]
23. Turan, T.N.; Makki, A.A.; Tsappidi, S.; Cotsonis, G.; Lynn, M.J.; Cloft, H.J.; Chimowitz, M.I.; WASID investigators. Risk factors associated with severity and location of intracranial arterial stenosis. *Stroke* **2010**, *41*, 1636–1640. [CrossRef] [PubMed]
24. Bailey, T.; Bode, B.W.; Christiansen, M.P.; Klaff, L.J.; Alva, S. The performance and usability of a factory-calibrated flash glucose monitoring system. *Diabetes Technol. Ther.* **2015**, *17*, 787–794. [CrossRef] [PubMed]
25. Battelino, T.; Danne, T.; Bergenstal, R.M.; Amiel, S.A.; Beck, R.; Biester, T.; Bosi, E.; Buckingham, B.A.; Cefalu, W.T.; Close, K.L.; et al. Clinical targets for continuous glucose monitoring data interpretation: Recommendations from the international consensus on time in range. *Diabetes Care* **2019**, *42*, 1593–1603. [CrossRef] [PubMed]
26. Marics, G.; Lendvai, Z.; Lódi, C.; Koncz, L.; Zakariás, D.; Schuster, G.; Mikos, B.; Hermann, C.; Szabó, A.J.; Tóth-Heyn, P. Evaluation of an open access software for calculating glucose variability parameters of a continuous glucose monitoring system applied at pediatric intensive care unit. *Biomed. Eng. Online* **2015**, *14*, 37. [CrossRef] [PubMed]
27. Matsuoka, A.; Hirota, Y.; Takeda, A.; Kishi, M.; Hashimoto, N.; Ohara, T.; Higo, S.; Yamada, H.; Nakamura, T.; Hamaguchi, T.; et al. Relationship between glycated hemoglobin level and duration of hypoglycemia in type 2 diabetes patients treated with sulfonylureas: A multicenter cross-sectional study. *J. Diabetes Investig.* **2020**, *11*, 417–425. [CrossRef]
28. Inaba, Y.; Tsutsumi, C.; Haseda, F.; Fujisawa, R.; Mitsui, S.; Sano, H.; Terasaki, J.; Hanafusa, T.; Imagawa, A. Impact of glycemic variability on the levels of endothelial progenitor cells in patients with type 1 diabetes. *Diabetol. Int.* **2017**, *9*, 113–120. [CrossRef]
29. Di Flaviani, A.; Picconi, F.; Di Stefano, P.; Giordani, I.; Malandrucco, I.; Maggio, P.; Palazzo, P.; Sgreccia, F.; Peraldo, C.; Farina, F.; et al. Impact of glycemic and blood pressure variability on surrogate measures of cardiovascular outcomes in type 2 diabetic patients. *Diabetes Care* **2011**, *34*, 1605–1609. [CrossRef]
30. Otowa-Suematsu, N.; Sakaguchi, K.; Komada, H.; Nakamura, T.; Sou, A.; Hirota, Y.; Kuroda, M.; Shinke, T.; Hirata, K.-I.; Ogawa, W. Comparison of the relationship between multiple parameters of glycemic variability and coronary plaque vulnerability assessed by virtual histology-intravascular ultrasound. *J. Diabetes Investig.* **2017**, *9*, 610–615. [CrossRef]
31. Papachristoforou, E.; Lambadiari, V.; Maratou, E.; Makrilakis, K. Association of glycemic indices (Hyperglycemia, Glucose variability, and Hypoglycemia) with oxidative stress and diabetic complications. *J. Diabetes Res.* **2020**, 7489795. [CrossRef]
32. Katakami, N. Mechanism of development of atherosclerosis and cardiovascular disease in diabetes mellitus. *J. Atheroscler. Thromb.* **2018**, *25*, 27–39. [CrossRef]
33. Liang, S.; Yin, H.; Wei, C.; Xie, L.; He, H.; Liu, X. Glucose variability for cardiovascular risk factors in type 2 diabetes: A meta-analysis. *J. Diabetes Metab. Disord.* **2017**, *16*, 45. [CrossRef]
34. Barbieri, M.; Rizzo, M.R.; Marfella, R.; Boccardi, V.; Esposito, A.; Pansini, A.; Paolisso, G. Decreased carotid atherosclerotic process by control of daily acute glucose fluctuations in diabetic patients treated by DPP-IV inhibitors. *Atherosclerosis* **2013**, *227*, 349–354. [CrossRef] [PubMed]
35. Watt, C.; Sanchez-Rangel, E.; Hwang, J.J. Glycemic variability and CNS inflammation: Reviewing the connection. *Nutrients* **2020**, *12*, 3906. [CrossRef]
36. Sajja, R.K.; Cucullo, L. Altered glycaemia differentially modulates efflux transporter expression and activity in hCMEC/D3 cell line. *Neurosci. Lett.* **2015**, *598*, 59–65. [CrossRef] [PubMed]
37. Wada, S.; Yoshimura, S.; Inoue, M.; Matsuki, T.; Arihiro, S.; Koga, M.; Kitazono, T.; Makino, H.; Hosoda, K.; Ihara, M.; et al. Outcome prediction in acute stroke patients by continuous glucose monitoring. *J. Am. Heart Assoc.* **2018**, *7*, e008744. [CrossRef] [PubMed]

38. Livny, A.; Ravona-Springer, R.; Heymann, A.; Priess, R.; Kushnir, T.; Tsarfaty, G.; Rabinov, L.; Moran, R.; Hoffman, H.; Cooper, I.; et al. Long-term variability in glycemic control is associated with white matter hyperintensities in APOE4 genotype carriers with type 2 diabetes. *Diabetes Care* **2016**, *39*, 1056–1059. [CrossRef]
39. Hui, J.; Zhang, J.; Mao, X.; Li, Z.; Li, X.; Wang, F.; Wang, T.; Yuan, Q.; Wang, S.; Pu, M.; et al. The initial glycemic variability is associated with early neurological deterioration in diabetic patients with acute ischemic stroke. *Neurol. Sci.* **2018**, *39*, 1571–1577. [CrossRef]
40. Naess, H.; Thomassen, L.; Waje-Andreassen, U.; Glad, S.; Kvistad, C.E. High risk of neurological worsening of lacunar infarction. *Acta Neurol. Scand.* **2019**, *139*, 143–149. [CrossRef]
41. Zhang, C.; Xie, S.; Li, S.; Pu, F.; Deng, X.; Fan, Y.; Li, D. Flow patterns and wall shear stress distribution in human internal carotid arteries: The geometric effect on the risk for stenoses. *J. Biomech.* **2012**, *45*, 83–89. [CrossRef]
42. Cecchi, E.; Giglioli, C.; Valente, S.; Lazzeri, C.; Gensini, G.F.; Abbate, R.; Mannini, L. Role of hemodynamic shear stress in cardiovascular disease. *Atherosclerosis* **2011**, *214*, 249–256. [CrossRef]
43. Pu, Y.; Liu, L.; Wang, Y.; Zou, X.; Pan, Y.; Soo, Y.; Leung, T.; Zhao, X.; Wong, K.S.; Wang, Y.; et al. Geographic and sex difference in the distribution of intracranial atherosclerosis in China. *Stroke* **2013**, *44*, 2109–2114. [CrossRef] [PubMed]
44. Sutton-Tyrrell, K.; Wildman, R.P.; Matthews, K.A.; Chae, C.; Lasley, B.L.; Brockwell, S.; Pasternak, R.C.; Lloyd-Jones, D.; Sowers, M.F.; Torréns, J.I.; et al. Sex-hormone-binding globulin and the free androgen index are related to cardiovascular risk factors in multiethnic premenopausal and perimenopausal women enrolled in the Study of Woman across the Nation (SWAN). *Circulation* **2005**, *111*, 1242–1249. [CrossRef] [PubMed]
45. Lee, S.H.; Kim, Y.; Park, S.Y.; Kim, C.; Kim, Y.J.; Sohn, J.H. Pre-stroke glycemic variability estimated by glycated albumin is associated with early neurological deterioration and poor functional outcome in prediabetic patients with acute ischemic stroke. *Cerebrovasc. Dis.* **2021**, *50*, 26–33. [CrossRef] [PubMed]
46. Hoshino, T.; Sissani, L.; Labreuche, J.; Ducrocq, G.; Lavallée, P.C.; Meseguer, E.; Guidoux, C.; Cabrejo, L.; Hobeanu, C.; Gongora-Rivera, F.; et al. Prevalence of Systemic Atherosclerosis Burdens and Overlapping Stroke Etiologies and Their Associations with Long-term Vascular Prognosis in Stroke with Intracranial Atherosclerotic Disease. *JAMA Neurol.* **2018**, *75*, 203–211. [CrossRef]

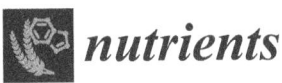

Article

Effects of Reducing L-Carnitine Supplementation on Carnitine Kinetics and Cardiac Function in Hemodialysis Patients: A Multicenter, Single-Blind, Placebo-Controlled, Randomized Clinical Trial

Miki Sugiyama [1,2], Takuma Hazama [1], Kaoru Nakano [1], Kengo Urae [1], Tomofumi Moriyama [1], Takuya Ariyoshi [1], Yuka Kurokawa [1], Goh Kodama [1], Yoshifumi Wada [3], Junko Yano [1,4], Yoshihiko Otsubo [5], Ryuji Iwatani [6], Yukie Kinoshita [7], Yusuke Kaida [1], Makoto Nasu [1], Ryo Shibata [1], Kyoko Tashiro [7] and Kei Fukami [1,*]

1. Division of Nephrology, Department of Medicine, Kurume University School of Medicine, Kurume, Fukuoka 830-0011, Japan; sugiyama_miki@med.kurume-u.ac.jp (M.S.); hazama_takuma@kurume-u.ac.jp (T.H.); nakano_kaoru@med.kurume-u.ac.jp (K.N.); urae_kengo@med.kurume-u.ac.jp (K.U.); moriyama_tomofumi@med.kurume-u.ac.jp (T.M.); ariyoshi_takuya@med.kurume-u.ac.jp (T.A.); kurokawa_yuka@med.kurume-u.ac.jp (Y.K.); kodama_gou@med.kurume-u.ac.jp (G.K.); akkun@med.kurume-u.ac.jp (J.Y.); kaida_yuusuke@kurume-u.ac.jp (Y.K.); nasusuma0210@med.kurume-u.ac.jp (M.N.); ryo0513@med.kurume-u.ac.jp (R.S.)
2. Sugi Hospital, Omuta, Fukuoka 837-0916, Japan
3. Wada Cardiovascular Clinic, Tosu, Saga 841-0071, Japan; houseikaiwada@outlook.jp
4. Kurume Ekimae Clinic, Kurume, Fukuoka 830-0023, Japan
5. Shin Koga Clinic, Kurume, Fukuoka 830-0033, Japan; y.otsubo@tenjinkai.or.jp
6. Koga 21 Hospital, Kurume, Fukuoka 839-0801, Japan; iwatani_ryuuji@kurume-u.ac.jp
7. Research Institute of Medical Mass Spectrometry, Kurume University School of Medicine, Kurume, Fukuoka 830-0011, Japan; kinoshita_yukie@med.kurume-u.ac.jp (Y.K.); k_tashiro23@med.kurume-u.ac.jp (K.T.)
* Correspondence: fukami@med.kurume-u.ac.jp; Tel.: +81-942317002

Abstract: L-carnitine (LC) supplementation improves cardiac function in hemodialysis (HD) patients. However, whether reducing LC supplementation affects carnitine kinetics and cardiac function in HD patients treated with LC remains unclear. Fifty-nine HD patients previously treated with intravenous LC 1000 mg per HD session (three times weekly) were allocated to three groups: LC injection three times weekly, once weekly, and placebo, and prospectively followed up for six months. Carnitine fractions were assessed by enzyme cycling methods. Plasma and red blood cell (RBC) acylcarnitines were profiled using tandem mass spectrometry. Cardiac function was evaluated using echocardiography and plasma B-type natriuretic peptide (BNP) levels. Reducing LC administration to once weekly significantly decreased plasma carnitine fractions and RBC-free carnitine levels during the study period, which were further decreased in the placebo group ($p < 0.001$). Plasma BNP levels were significantly elevated in the placebo group ($p = 0.03$). Furthermore, changes in RBC (C16 + C18:1)/C2 acylcarnitine ratio were positively correlated with changes in plasma BNP levels ($\beta = 0.389$, $p = 0.005$). Reducing LC administration for six months significantly decreased both plasma and RBC carnitine levels, while the full termination of LC increased plasma BNP levels; however, it did not influence cardiac function in HD patients.

Keywords: acylcarnitine; brain natriuretic peptide; cardiac function; cardiomyopathy; carnitine deficiency; CPT2; end-stage kidney disease; free fatty acid; heart failure; hemodialysis

1. Introduction

Heart failure (HF), as well as some of its complications, such as pulmonary edema, is a serious condition characterized by decreased myocardial contractility and abnormal hemodynamic state in patients with end-stage kidney disease (ESKD). The United States

Renal Data System revealed that an estimated 44% of patients on hemodialysis (HD) have chronic HF (CHF), and 5.4% of HD patients die of chronic HF [1] (https://render.usrds.org/2016/view/v2_09.aspx. Accessed date: 8 May 2021). The Japanese Society of Dialysis Transplantation has reported that HF is the most common cause of death in patients undergoing dialysis [2]. Furthermore, CHF is associated with impairments in activities of daily living and quality of life in HD patients [3]. Taken together, the prevention of HF development is a crucial therapeutic strategy for HD patients worldwide.

Carnitine is a natural substance that plays an important role in fatty acid β-oxidation and energy production in mitochondria [4]. Organic cation/carnitine transporter 2 (OCTN2) is capable of transporting free carnitine into the cytoplasm. In addition, carnitine palmitoyl-transferase 1 (CPT1) and CPT2 are the mitochondrial outer and inner membrane enzymes, respectively. These enzymes are responsible for delivering long-chain fatty acids into mitochondria, leading to β-oxidation and ATP synthesis. A lack of carnitine and dysfunction of OCTN2 and/or CPT2 results in the inability to produce energy from long-chain fatty acids, leading to the development of cardiomyopathy [5,6]. We, along with others, reported that serum carnitine levels are significantly decreased in HD patients due to the elimination of serum carnitine from the blood via HD [7,8]. Accordingly, HD-related carnitine deficiency may be one of the causative factors for the progression of HF in patients with ESKD. A meta-analysis demonstrated that L-carnitine (LC) supplementation may improve clinical symptoms and cardiac function and decrease serum levels of B-type natriuretic peptide (BNP) and NT-proBNP in patients with CHF [9]. Furthermore, LC supplementation for a year might improve cardiac function in HD patients [10], suggesting that LC treatment may have protective effects on HF in HD patients with carnitine deficiency.

In a recent study, we observed that plasma carnitine concentration is approximately ten-fold higher in HD patients treated with intravenous LC administration at a dose of 1000 mg three times weekly than in those receiving no LC treatment. This finding could be related to the fact that circulating carnitine cannot be excreted in urine and can only be eliminated by dialysis [11]. Furthermore, six months of intravenous LC treatment at a dose of 2000 mg per HD session increased muscle carnitine concentration by three-fold in HD patients [12]. However, the kinetics of serum carnitine fractions and changes in cardiac function after reducing or stopping LC treatment in HD patients remain unknown. Therefore, we prospectively examined the effects of reducing or stopping LC therapy on carnitine concentrations in plasma and red blood cells (RBCs) and cardiac function in HD patients treated with LC.

2. Materials and Methods

2.1. Patients and Study Protocol

This multicenter, single-blind, placebo-controlled, randomized clinical trial was conducted at Kurume University Hospital, Sugi Hospital, Wada Cardiovascular Clinic, Kurume Ekimae Clinic, Shin Koga Clinic, and Koga 21 Hospital. We recruited a total of 64 HD patients from December 2018 to June 2020. Patients over 20 years of age with ESKD undergoing HD who could provide written informed consent for study participation were enrolled in this study. All patients had already been diagnosed with dialysis-associated secondary carnitine deficiency and had been administered intravenous LC at a dose of 1000 mg per HD session three times weekly for at least three months. The exclusion criteria were as follows: under 20 years of age, unstable lower limb cramps and general fatigue, hemoglobin (Hb) levels below 10 g/dL, and patients deemed to have inadequate information by a physician.

Six months after the registration period, seven patients were excluded before randomization. Among these seven patients, one had Hb levels below 10 g/dL, one did not receive LC, one was referred to another clinic, and four had been administered LC once weekly (Figure 1). The remaining 57 patients were finally included and randomly assigned using simple randomization procedures (computer-generated list of random numbers) by the clinical research coordinator (CRC). They were allocated to LC 1000 mg (5 mL) three times weekly (LC-3) (*n* = 19), LC 1000 mg once and placebo (saline 5 mL) twice weekly (LC-1) (*n* = 18), or placebo three times weekly (LC-0) (*n* = 20) groups (Figure 1).

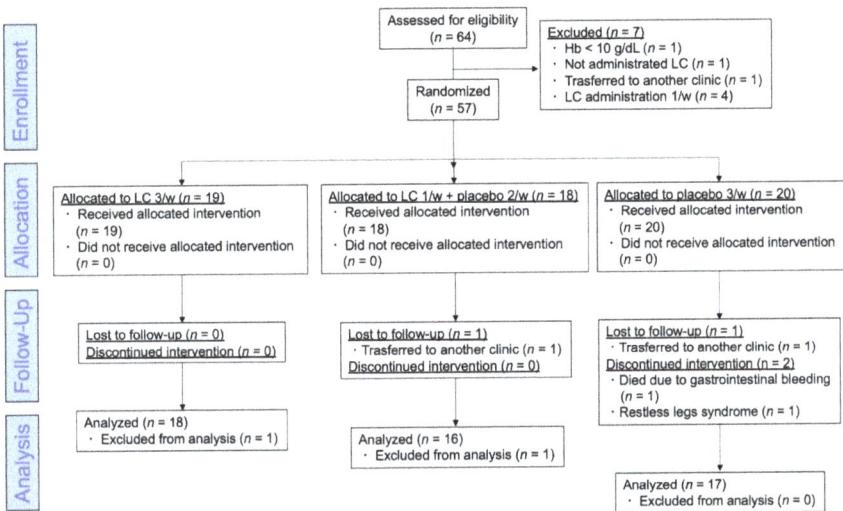

Figure 1. CONSORT flow diagram of this trial. Sixty-four hemodialysis patients were assessed for eligibility, and 57 were randomized and allocated to LC 3/week, LC 1/week + placebo 2/week, and placebo 3/week groups and followed up for six months. Hb: hemoglobin; LC: L-carnitine.

The participants were blinded to the intervention after the assignment. At baseline, 30 days, 90 days, and 176 days of the study period, patients provided a complete history and underwent physical examination, including blood pressure (BP) and blood chemistry test, just before HD sessions at two-day intervals. The study protocol is shown in Figure 2. All data and samples were collected by the CRC at Kurume University Hospital. The patients were dialyzed for 4–5 h with high-flux dialyzers three times weekly. All patients received 1000 mg of LC intravenously immediately after HD sessions. The primary endpoint was the effects of dose reduction or discontinuation of LC on the kinetics of plasma and RBC carnitine concentration and cardiac function. Additional analyses were performed to evaluate changes in plasma BNP levels before and after the study period.

2.2. Clinical, Demographic, and Anthropometric Measurements

The patients' medical histories were ascertained using a questionnaire. Vigorous physical activity and smoking were avoided for at least 30 min before HD sessions. Blood was drawn from an arteriovenous shunt just before starting the HD sessions to determine Hb, total protein, serum albumin, total cholesterol, low-density lipoprotein cholesterol, blood urea nitrogen, calcium, and phosphate levels. These parameters were analyzed by commercially available laboratories (Daiichi Pure Chemicals, Tokyo, Japan, and Wako Pure Chemical Industries, Osaka, Japan). Plasma BNP was measured using a chemiluminescent immunoassay (CRC Corporation, Fukuoka, Japan). Plasma carnitine fraction (total carnitine, free carnitine, and acylcarnitine) levels were determined by an enzymatic cycling method, as previously described [13]. Free carnitine and acylcarnitines in plasma and RBC were profiled using tandem mass spectrometry at baseline, 30 days, 90 days, and 176 days after beginning the study, according to a previously described method [14,15]. Changes in plasma BNP and acylcarnitine ratio were defined as the differences between the baseline values (pre-data) and those at 176 days (post-data). Changes in these data were calculated using the following formula: (post-data−pre-data)/pre-data × 100 (%).

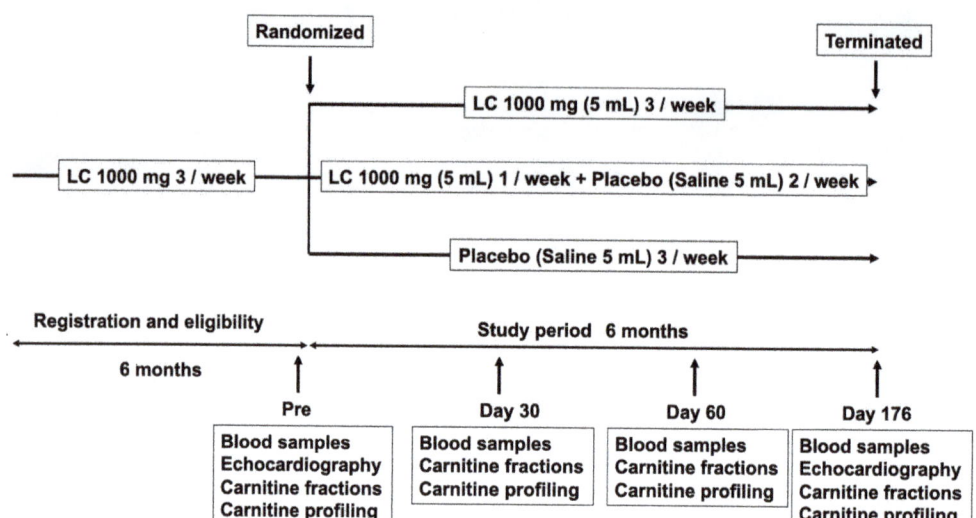

Figure 2. Trial design. Patients were randomized to LC 1000 mg 3/week, LC 1000 mg 1/week + placebo 2/week, and placebo 3/week groups and followed up for six months. Blood samples, including carnitine fractions and profiling, were examined before the study period, day 30, day 60, and day 176 of the study period. Echocardiography was evaluated before and on day 176 of the study period. LC: L-carnitine.

2.3. Evaluation of Cardiac Function

Systolic and diastolic cardiac functions were evaluated using transthoracic echocardiography by professional technicians at each hospital who were unaware of the participants' clinical data. Left ventricular (LV) mass index (LVMI) was determined using the standard formula as follows: Devereux formula = 1.04 × ((LV end-diastolic diameter + interventricular septal thickness at end-diastole + posterior wall thickness at end-diastole)^3 − (LV end-diastolic diameter)^3) − 13.6 [16]. LV ejection fraction (LVEF) was calculated to determine systolic myocardial function using the standard biplane Simpson's method from the formula: LVEF = ((end-diastolic volume) − (end-systolic volume))/end-diastolic volume. LV filling index (E/e') was calculated as the ratio of the transmitral flow velocity to the annular velocity as a marker of diastolic cardiac function.

2.4. Statistical Analysis

To compare clinical variables at baseline and on day 176 of the study period, the paired t-test was used. Non-parametric analysis (Wilcoxon signed-rank test) was used to determine differences between baseline plasma and RBC-free carnitine because the data did not follow a normal distribution using the Shapiro–Wilk test. One-way ANOVA with post-hoc Tukey HSD test was used to compare the data among the three groups. For exploratory data analysis, univariate and multiple regression analyses were performed to determine correlations between changes in BNP levels and clinical variables, including acylcarnitine ratios. Natural logarithmic transformation was used due to the skewness of the BNP distribution. Data are presented as mean ± standard deviation. Statistical significance was set at $p < 0.05$, and all statistical analyses were performed using the JMP Pro version.15 software (SAS Institute Inc., Cary, NC, USA).

3. Results

3.1. Demographic Data at Baseline

During the study period, two patients were referred to another clinic, one died due to gastrointestinal bleeding, and one patient discontinued treatment due to restless legs syndrome. Two patients were excluded from the study because RBC acylcarnitine levels were not measured. Finally, a total of 51 patients completed the treatment in the groups: LC-3 group (n = 18), LC-1 group (n = 16), and LC-0 group (n = 17) (Figure 1). No significant adverse events related to LC treatment stoppage were observed during the study period. No significant differences in age, HD duration, duration of previous LC treatment, or other clinical parameters, except for phosphate, were observed among the groups. The baseline phosphate level was higher in the LC-0 group than in the LC-1 group (p = 0.038) (Table 1). The baseline plasma total and free carnitines, acylcarnitine, and RBC-free carnitine levels were extremely high in all groups and were not different among the groups. The baseline free carnitine levels in RBCs were significantly higher than those in plasma in patients assessed by tandem mass spectrometry (462 ± 215, 293 ± 66 µmol/L, p < 0.0001). The baseline cardiac function and BNP levels were not different among the study groups.

Table 1. Clinical characteristics at baseline.

	LC 3 Times/w (LC-3)	LC 1 Time/w + Placebo 2 Times/w (LC-1)	Placebo 3 Times/w (LC-0)	p (LC-3 vs. LC-1)	p (LC-3 vs. LC-0)	p (LC-1 vs. LC-0)
Number	18	16	17	N/A		
Age (years)	64.5 ± 13.3	69.4 ± 12.7	69.5 ± 9.8	0.471	0.438	0.999
Sex (no.) (male/female)	12/6	10/6	10/7	N/A		
HD duration (months)	178 ± 91	150 ± 95	164 ± 120	0.721	0.916	0.926
Duration of LC treatment (months)	40 ± 21	35 ± 21	44 ± 27	0.788	0.860	0.484
Body weight (kg)	61.0 ± 13.2	57.4 ± 11.0	54.6 ± 10.7	0.656	0.249	0.765
Systolic BP (mmHg)	151 ± 27	141 ± 31	145 ± 24	0.516	0.792	0.892
Hemoglobin (g/dL)	11.2 ± 0.9	11.4 ± 0.7	11.7 ± 0.9	0.853	0.263	0.577
Total protein (g/dL)	6.26 ± 0.46	6.30 ± 0.51	6.45 ± 0.39	0.967	0.427	0.598
Serum albumin (g/dL)	3.57 ± 0.36	3.49 ± 0.27	3.54 ± 0.27	0.701	0.952	0.870
Total cholesterol (mg/dL)	164 ± 31	155 ± 28	159 ± 29	0.699	0.901	0.925
LDL-cholesterol (mg/dL)	89 ± 21	81 ± 20	88 ± 22	0.445	0.967	0.602
BUN (mg/dL)	56.6 ± 11.8	52.2 ± 14.0	61.5 ± 16.1	0.633	0.554	0.145
Corrected Ca (mg/dL)	8.73 ± 0.65	8.63 ± 0.39	8.49 ± 0.45	0.849	0.362	0.707
Phosphate (mg/dL)	4.64 ± 0.86	4.05 ± 0.90	4.97 ± 1.30	0.236	0.616	0.038
Plasma total carnitine (µmol/L)	454 ± 128	424 ± 119	466 ± 117	0.761	0.948	0.580
Plasma free carnitine (µmol/L)	270 ± 44	264 ± 40	284 ± 43	0.901	0.601	0.365
Plasma acylcarnitine (µmol/L)	183 ± 91	160 ± 83	182 ± 81	0.712	0.999	0.742
Acyl/free ratio	0.66 ± 0.24	0.59 ± 0.21	0.62 ± 0.21	0.633	0.909	0.872
RBC-free carnitine (µmol/L)	407 ± 203	456 ± 215	525 ± 224	0.781	0.242	0.629
LVEF (%)	65.3 ± 13.9	65.5 ± 10.1	65.8 ± 7.3	0.999	0.990	0.996
E/e'	13.9 ± 6.0	14.2 ± 7.1	13.2 ± 5.7	0.990	0.942	0.894
LVMI (g/m^2)	122 ± 26	108 ± 23	115 ± 44	0.420	0.786	0.817
BNP [†] (pg/mL)	317 (34–1150)	424 (15–1380)	460 (44–1440)	0.866	0.541	0.858

Acyl/free: acylcarnitine/free carnitine; BNP: B-type natriuretic peptide; BUN: blood urea nitrogen; Ca: calcium; E/e': ratio of early transmitral velocity E to mitral annular early diastolic velocity e'; HD: hemodialysis; LC: L-carnitine; LVMI: left ventricular mass index; LDL: low-density lipoprotein; RBC: red blood cell. [†] Because of the skewness of the BNP distribution, a natural logarithmic transformation was used for analysis.

3.2. Effects of Reducing or Stopping LC Administration on Clinical Variables and Carnitine Fractions

In Table 2, the comparison of clinical variables and carnitine fractions between baseline and day 176 of the study period is represented by the *p*-value. After the study period, body weight significantly decreased and the total protein, albumin, and total and LDL-cholesterol levels in the serum increased in the LC-3 group rather than the LC-1 and LC-0 groups (Table 2).

Table 2. Clinical characteristics at baseline and day 176 of the study period.

	LC 3 Times/w			LC 1 Time/w + Placebo 2 Times/w			Placebo 3 Times/w		
	Pre	Day 176	*p*	Pre	Day 176	*p*	Pre	Day 176	*p*
Body weight (kg)	61.0 ± 13.2	60.0 ± 13.0	0.036	57.4 ± 11.0	56.8 ± 10.4	0.063	54.6 ± 10.7	54.4 ± 11.2	0.555
Systolic BP (mmHg)	151 ± 27	154 ± 25	0.613	141 ± 31	149 ± 30	0.149	145 ± 24	140 ± 24	0.416
Hemoglobin (g/dL)	11.2 ± 0.9	11.0 ± 0.8	0.472	11.4 ± 0.7	11.2 ± 0.8	0.455	11.7 ± 0.9	11.4 ± 1.2	0.274
Total protein (g/dL)	6.26 ± 0.46	6.38 ± 0.43	0.043	6.30 ± 0.51	6.40 ± 0.40	0.377	6.45 ± 0.39	6.31 ± 0.40	0.079
Serum albumin (g/dL)	3.57 ± 0.36	3.67 ± 0.37	0.012	3.49 ± 0.27	3.50 ± 0.26	0.849	3.54 ± 0.27	3.50 ± 0.30	0.311
Total cholesterol (mg/dL)	164 ± 31	169 ± 30	0.044	155 ± 28	157 ± 24	0.765	159 ± 29	157 ± 30	0.573
LDL-cholesterol (mg/dL)	89 ± 21	96 ± 20	0.002	81 ± 20	83 ± 18	0.522	88 ± 22	87 ± 22	0.908
BUN (mg/dL)	56.6 ± 11.8	60.1 ± 12.6	0.052	52.2 ± 14.0	57.8 ± 16.5	0.065	61.5 ± 16.1	65.4 ± 19.0	0.211
Corrected Ca (mg/dL)	8.73 ± 0.65	8.78 ± 0.56	0.655	8.63 ± 0.39	8.73 ± 0.40	0.426	8.49 ± 0.45	8.48 ± 0.51	0.961
Phosphate (mg/dL)	4.64 ± 0.86	4.99 ± 0.76	0.180	4.05 ± 0.90	4.32 ± 1.21	0.373	4.97 ± 1.30	4.93 ± 1.36	0.910
Plasma total carnitine (μmol/L)	454 ± 128	431 ± 117	0.318	424 ± 119	143 ± 37	<0.0001	466 ± 117	66 ± 20	<0.0001
Plasma free carnitine (μmol/L)	270 ± 44	260 ± 44	0.383	264 ± 40	93 ± 28	<0.0001	284 ± 43	41 ± 14	<0.0001
Plasma acylcarnitine (μmol/L)	183 ± 91	171 ± 87	0.348	160 ± 83	50 ± 12	<0.0001	182 ± 81	25 ± 8	<0.0001
Acyl/free ratio	0.66 ± 0.24	0.65 ± 0.26	0.955	0.59 ± 0.21	0.56 ± 0.15	0.631	0.62 ± 0.21	0.62 ± 0.14	0.963
RBC-free carnitine (μmol/L)	407 ± 203	418 ± 157	0.717	456 ± 215	179 ± 80	<0.0001	525 ± 224	50 ± 21	<0.0001

Acyl/free: acylcarnitine/free carnitine; BP: blood pressure; BUN: blood urea nitrogen; Ca: calcium; LC: L-carnitine; LDL: low-density lipoprotein; RBC: red blood cell.

Significant decreases in the plasma total carnitine, free carnitine, and acylcarnitine levels assessed by enzyme cycling methods were observed at 30 days after reducing or stopping LC administration. In addition, all carnitine fraction levels were further reduced at 90 and 176 days in the LC-1 and LC-0 groups ($p < 0.0001$) (Figure 3A–C). Significant differences in plasma carnitine fraction levels between the LC-1 and LC-0 groups were similarly observed in this study (Figure 3A–C). The acyl/free carnitine ratio was not affected by the reduction or cessation of LC therapy during the study (Figure 3D).

In addition, we examined free carnitine levels in RBCs, reflecting tissue carnitine levels. Free carnitine levels in RBCs were decreased in the LC-1 and LC-0 groups compared with those in the LC-3 group during the study ($p < 0.0001$) (Figure 4). Similarly, there was a significant difference in free carnitine levels in RBCs between the LC-1 and LC-0 groups during the study (Figure 4).

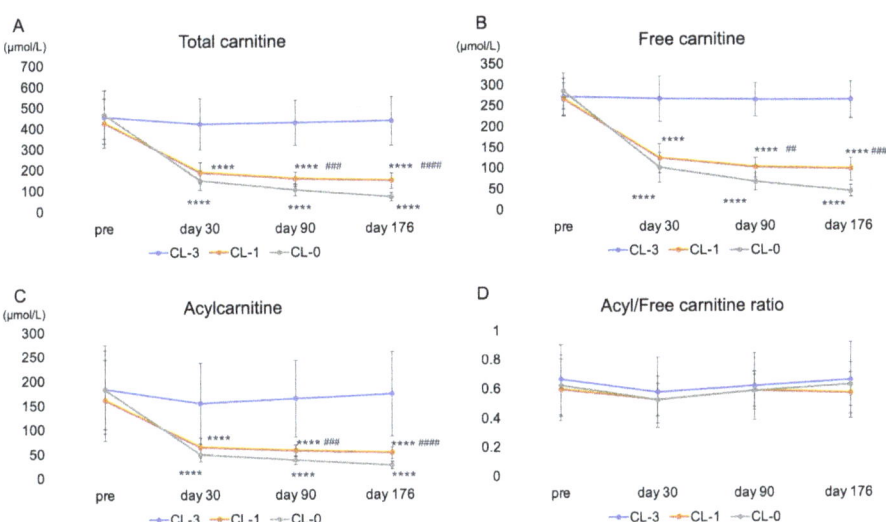

Figure 3. Kinetics of plasma total carnitine, free carnitine, acylcarnitine levels, and acyl/free carnitine ratio during the study. (**A**) plasma total carnitine levels; (**B**) plasma free carnitine levels; (**C**) plasma acylcarnitine levels; (**D**) acyl/free carnitine ratio. LC-3: LC 1000 mg three times weekly; LC-1: LC 1000 mg once and placebo (saline 5 mL) twice weekly; LC-0: placebo three times weekly (LC-0). **** $p < 0.0001$ vs. LC-3; ## $p < 0.01$; ### $p < 0.001$; #### $p < 0.0001$ vs. LC-0.

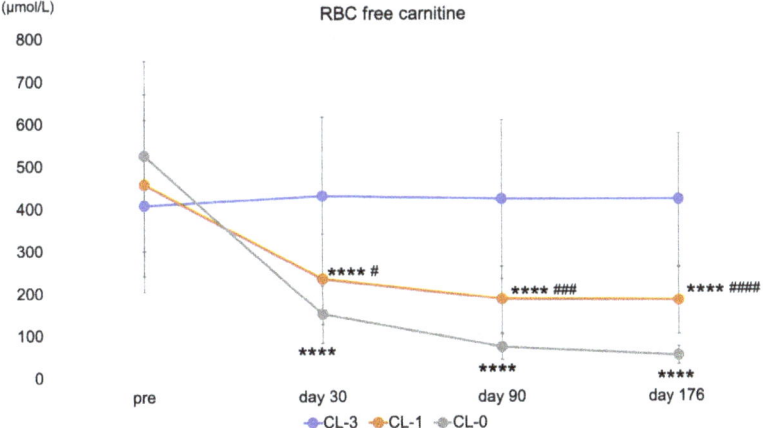

Figure 4. Kinetics of RBC-free carnitine level during the study. LC-3: LC 1000 mg three times weekly; LC-1: LC 1000 mg once and placebo (saline 5 mL) twice weekly; LC-0: placebo three times weekly (LC-0). **** $p < 0.0001$ vs. LC-3; # $p < 0.05$; ### $p < 0.001$; #### $p < 0.0001$ vs. LC-0.

3.3. Effects of Reducing or Stopping LC Administration on Cardiac Function and Plasma BNP Levels

Reducing or stopping LC administration did not change systolic and diastolic cardiac functions assessed by LVEF and E/e', respectively. There was no difference in LVMI before and after the study period in any of the groups. However, only stopping LC treatment for six months significantly increased BNP levels ($p = 0.03$) (Table 3).

Table 3. Effects of reducing or stopping LC treatment on LV function, LVMI, and BNP levels.

	LC 3 Times/w			LC 1 Time/w + Placebo 2 Times/w			Placebo 3 Times/w		
	Pre	Day 176	p	Pre	Day 176	p	Pre	Day 176	p
LVEF (%)	65.3 ± 13.9	63.7 ± 10.8	0.446	65.5 ± 10.1	65.4 ± 7.6	0.967	65.8 ± 7.3	65.3 ± 7.4	0.774
E/e'	13.9 ± 6.0	14.1 ± 7.0	0.737	14.2 ± 7.1	14.0 ± 6.2	0.893	13.2 ± 5.7	15.1 ± 8.9	0.224
LVMI (g/m^2)	122 ± 26	129 ± 33	0.330	108 ± 23	107 ± 39	0.873	115 ± 44	120 ± 44	0.207
BNP [†] (pg/mL)	317 (34–1150)	396 (51–1270)	0.255	424 (15–1380)	433 (57–1580)	0.422	460 (44–1440)	631 (44–1450)	0.030

BNP: B-type natriuretic peptide; E/e': ratio of early transmitral velocity E to mitral annular early diastolic velocity e'; LC: L-carnitine; LV: left ventricular; LVMI: left ventricular mass index. [†] Because of the skewness of the BNP distribution, a natural logarithmic transformation was used for analysis.

3.4. Correlations between Changes in BNP Levels and Clinical Variables and Acylcarnitine Ratios

To further explore which variables could be independently associated with BNP levels, we assessed correlations between changes in BNP and clinical variables and acylcarnitine ratios, such as (C16 + C18:1)/C2, a marker of CPT2 deficiency; C0/(C16 + C18), a marker of CPT1 deficiency; C8/C10, a marker of medium-chain acyl-CoA dehydrogenase deficiency; and C14/C3, another marker of CPT2 deficiency, by univariate and multiple regression analyses in all HD patients. We speculated that independent determinants of the changes in BNP might be involved in the pathogenesis of carnitine deficiency-associated HF. Changes in systolic BP were positively associated with changes in BNP levels (β = 0.373, SE = 0.152, p = 0.007) (Table 4). Changes in plasma (C16 + C18:1)/C2, C0/(C16 + C18), C8/C10, and C14/C3 were not associated with changes in BNP levels (Table 4) (Figure 5A). Although changes in RBC C0/(C16 + C18), C8/C10, and C14/C3 were not associated with BNP, changes in RBC (C16 + C18:1)/C2 were positively correlated with changes in BNP levels (β = 0.398, SE = 0.283, p = 0.005) (Table 4) (Figure 5B). Both changes in systolic BP and RBC (C16 + C18:1)/C2 were the sole independent determinants of changes in BNP levels in these patients (R^2 = 0.259) (Table 4).

Table 4. Univariate and multiple regression analyses for the covariates of changes in BNP.

	Univariate Regression			Multiple Regression		
	β	SE	p	β	SE	p
ΔBody weight	0.069	0.024	0.630			
ΔSystolic blood pressure	0.373	0.152	0.007	0.331	0.109	0.011
ΔHemoglobin	−0.077	0.097	0.590			
ΔTotal protein	−0.038	0.051	0.789			
ΔAlbumin	−0.032	0.052	0.826			
ΔTotal cholesterol	0.000	0.095	0.999			
ΔLDL-cholesterol	−0.106	0.145	0.461			
ΔBlood urea nitrogen	−0.220	0.180	0.121			
ΔCorrected Ca	0.011	0.051	0.441			
ΔPhosphate	−0.144	0.285	0.312			
ΔPlasma total carnitine	−0.114	0.349	0.427			
ΔPlasma free carnitine	−0.135	0.344	0.345			
ΔPlasma acylcarnitine	−0.063	0.352	0.661			
ΔAcyl/Free ratio	0.229	0.233	0.110			
ΔPlasma (C16 + C18:1)/C2	0.219	1.191	0.123			
ΔPlasma C0/(C16 + C18)	−0.156	1458.7	0.273			
ΔPlasma C8/C10	−0.206	0.160	0.147			
ΔPlasma C14/C3	0.016	2.451	0.912			
ΔRBC (C16 + C18:1)/C2	0.389	0.283	0.005	0.350	0.058	0.007
ΔRBC C0/(C16 + C18)	−0.131	0.282	0.359			
ΔRBC C8/C10	−0.154	0.218	0.281			
ΔRBC C14/C3	0.160	0.923	0.160			

R^2 = 0.259. Acyl/free: acylcarnitine/free carnitine; BNP: B-type natriuretic peptide; Ca: calcium; Δ: delta; LDL: low-density lipoprotein; RBC: red blood cell.

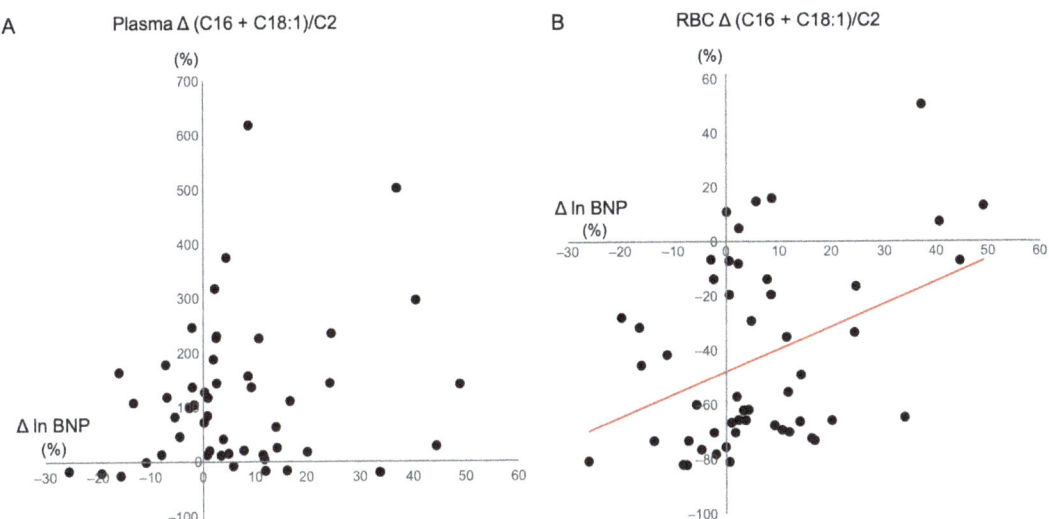

Figure 5. Correlation between changes in BNP with (C16 + C18:1)/C2 in (**A**) plasma; and (**B**) RBCs. BNP: B-type natriuretic peptide; RBC: red blood cell.

4. Discussion

In this study, we demonstrated that reducing or stopping LC administration for six months significantly decreased all plasma carnitine fractions and RBC-free carnitine levels. In addition, stopping LC treatment significantly increased plasma BNP levels. Moreover, changes in systolic BP and RBC (C16 + C18:1)/C2 values were the sole independent determinants of changes in BNP levels. To the best of our knowledge, this is the first report to demonstrate that stopping LC administration increased BNP levels in HD patients treated with LC.

Translocation of long-chain free fatty acids into mitochondria by carnitine shuttle plays a pivotal role in energy production via β-oxidation [17]. Therefore, carnitine deficiency induces cardiac dysfunction and muscle atrophy in HD patients. We previously reported a significant decrease in plasma carnitine fraction levels in HD patients [8]. Higuchi et al. reported the beneficial effects of LC on cardiac function and LVMI assessed by echocardiography and NT-proBNP in carnitine-deficient HD patients [10]. However, the effects of reducing or stopping LC on cardiac function have not yet been reported. In this study, we demonstrated that reducing or stopping LC administration for six months significantly reduced plasma and RBC carnitine fraction levels. Furthermore, plasma BNP levels significantly increased only in patients who stopped LC treatment, suggesting that stopping LC for six months may contribute to the future progression of cardiac dysfunction in HD patients. Indeed, suspension of LC therapy has been reported to result in signs and symptoms of recurrence (muscular weakness, fatigue, cardiac enlargement, and low cardiac function) in patients with primary carnitine deficiency treated with LC [18]. However, regardless of the increase in BNP levels, LV function assessed by EF and E/e', markers of systolic and diastolic cardiac function, respectively, and LVMI did not change before or after reduction or discontinuation of LC therapy. This result might be explained by the concentration of carnitine fractions during the study. At the end of the study, free carnitine levels in the plasma were still within the normal range, even after stopping the LC therapy for six months. These findings suggest that the inadequate deficiency of carnitine by stopping LC therapy might not have influenced cardiac function in these patients. Taken together, long-term studies are needed to clarify the deleterious effects of stopping LC administration on cardiac function in carnitine-deficient HD patients.

In our study, changes in systolic BP and RBC (C16 + C18:1)/C2 ratio, a marker of CPT2 deficiency, were only positively correlated with changes in plasma BNP levels. CPT2 deficiency in humans is diagnosed by abnormal acylcarnitine profile obtained from blood spotted on filter paper with an increased (C16 + C18:1)/C2 ratio [19]. CPT2 plays a central role in ATP synthesis in cardiomyocytes mitochondria. Genetic deletion of mouse CPT2 induces cardiac hypertrophic remodeling, which activates the mammalian target of the rapamycin complex, thereby reducing protein acetylation and accumulating lipid droplets [20]. Furthermore, LC supplementation is effective in severe CPT2 deficiency [21], indicating that stopping LC supplementation may influence the activity of CPT2 in cardiomyocytes, leading to an increase in BNP levels in HD patients. Furthermore, we found that changes in the (C16 + C18:1)/C2 ratio in RBC, not in plasma, were associated with changes in plasma BNP levels. Acylcarnitine levels in RBCs are higher than those in plasma [22]. In addition, elevated RBC carnitine levels by LC administration decreased very slowly even after irrigation suggesting a low carnitine turnover in RBCs [22]. These findings indicate that the acylcarnitine ratio in RBC, rather than that in plasma, appears to be an accurate tissue acylcarnitine profile in HD patients.

This study has several limitations. First, the sample size of the patients was small; thus, the statistical power was weak. Second, the short study duration might have affected the efficacy of reducing or stopping LC in cardiac function. Therefore, further large and long-term clinical studies are warranted to verify the effect of reduction in LC treatment on the cardiac function of HD patients.

Carnitine deficiency induces mitochondrial damages through the impairment of β-oxidation and ATP production. However, the exact mechanism underlying the exacerbation of cardiomyocyte injury by hemodialysis-induced carnitine deficiency through the manipulation of carnitine-related mitochondrial enzymes, such as CPT1 and CPT2, is not fully understood. Hence, future research using a carnitine-deficient experimental model might be required to examine the mediating mechanism underlying carnitine deficiency-associated myocardial injury.

5. Conclusions

In conclusion, reducing LC administration for six months significantly decreased both plasma and RBC carnitine levels. Moreover, stopping LC increased plasma BNP levels; however, this stoppage did not influence cardiac function in HD patients.

Author Contributions: J.Y. and K.F.; Methodology, K.F.; Software, K.F.; Validation, Y.K. (Yusuke Kaida) and K.F.; Formal Analysis, K.F.; Investigation, Y.K. (Yusuke Kaida), R.S., and K.F.; Resources, Y.K. (Yukie Kinoshita) and K.T.; Data Curation, M.S., T.H., K.N., K.U., T.M., T.A., Y.K. (Yuka Kurokawa), G.K., Y.W., Y.O., R.I., and M.N.; Writing—Original Draft Preparation, K.F.; Visualization, K.F.; Supervision, K.F.; Project Administration, K.F.; Funding Acquisition, K.F. All authors have read and agreed to the published version of the manuscript.

Funding: This research was funded in part by a Grant-in-Aid for Welfare and Scientific Research (C) (no. 19K08693) from the Ministry of Education, Culture, Sports, Science, and Technology of Japan (K.F.).

Institutional Review Board Statement: The study was conducted according to the guidelines of the Declaration of Helsinki and registered with the University Hospital Medical Information Network clinical trials database (UMIN000037330). The study protocol was approved by the Institutional Ethics Committees of Kurume University School of Medicine (Approval Number: 18179).

Informed Consent Statement: Informed consent was obtained from all patients as specified in the recommendations set by the International Committee of Medical Journal Editors.

Data Availability Statement: The data presented in this study are available on request from the corresponding author.

Acknowledgments: We would like to thank all of investigators.

Conflicts of Interest: K.F. has received honoraria, including lecture fees, from Otsuka Pharmaceutical Co., Ltd. All other authors declare no conflict of interest.

References

1. House, A.A.; Wanner, C.; Sarnak, M.J.; Piña, I.L.; McIntyre, C.W.; Komenda, P.; Kasiske, B.L.; Deswal, A.; de Filippi, C.R.; Cleland, J.G.F.; et al. Heart Failure in Chronic Kidney Disease: Conclusions From a Kidney Disease: Improving Global Outcomes (KDIGO) Controversies Conference. *Kidney Int.* **2019**, *95*, 1304–1317. [CrossRef] [PubMed]
2. Nitta, K.; Abe, M.; Masakane, I.; Hanafusa, N.; Taniguchi, M.; Hasegawa, T.; Nakai, S.; Wada, A.; Hamano, T.; Hoshino, J.; et al. Annual dialysis data report 2018, JSDT Renal Data Registry: Dialysis fluid quality, hemodialysis and hemodiafiltration, peritoneal dialysis, and diabetes. *Ren. Replace Ther.* **2020**, *6*, 51. [CrossRef]
3. Liang, K.V.; Pike, F.; Argyropoulos, C.; Weissfeld, L.; Teuteberg, J.; Dew, M.A.; Unruh, M.L. Heart Failure Severity Scoring System and Medical- and Health-Related Quality-of-Life Outcomes: The HEMO Study. *Am. J. Kidney Dis.* **2011**, *58*, 84–92. [CrossRef] [PubMed]
4. Evans, A.M.; Fornasini, G. Pharmacokinetics of L-Carnitine. *Clin. Pharmacokinet.* **2003**, *42*, 941–967. [CrossRef]
5. Chapoy, P.R.; Angelini, C.; Brown, W.J.; Stiff, J.E.; Shug, A.L.; Cederbaum, S.D. Systemic Carnitine Deficiency–A Treatable Inherited Lipid-Storage Disease Presenting as Reye's Syndrome. *N. Engl. J. Med.* **1980**, *303*, 1389–1394. [CrossRef]
6. Semba, S.; Yasujima, H.; Takano, T.; Yokozaki, H. Autopsy Case of the Neonatal Form of Carnitine Palmitoyltransferase-II Deficiency Triggered by a Novel Disease-Causing Mutation del1737C. *Pathol. Int.* **2008**, *58*, 436–441. [CrossRef]
7. Evans, A. Dialysis-Related Carnitine Disorder and Levocarnitine Pharmacology. *Am. J. Kidney Dis.* **2003**, *41* (Suppl. 4), S13–S26. [CrossRef]
8. Adachi, T.; Fukami, K.; Yamagishi, S.; Kaida, Y.; Ando, R.; Sakai, K.; Adachi, H.; Otsuka, A.; Ueda, S.; Sugi, K.; et al. Decreased Serum Carnitine Is Independently Correlated With Increased Tissue Accumulation Levels of Advanced Glycation End Products in Haemodialysis Patients. *Nephrology (Carlton)* **2012**, *17*, 689–694. [CrossRef]
9. Song, X.; Qu, H.; Yang, Z.; Rong, J.; Cai, W.; Zhou, H. Efficacy and Safety of L-Carnitine Treatment for Chronic Heart Failure: A Meta-Analysis of Randomized Controlled Trials. *BioMed Res. Int.* **2017**, *2017*, 6274854. [CrossRef]
10. Higuchi, T.; Abe, M.; Yamazaki, T.; Okawa, E.; Ando, H.; Hotta, S.; Oikawa, O.; Kikuchi, F.; Okada, K.; Soma, M. Levocarnitine Improves Cardiac Function in Hemodialysis Patients With Left Ventricular Hypertrophy: A Randomized Controlled Trial. *Am. J. Kidney Dis.* **2016**, *67*, 260–270. [CrossRef]
11. Yano, J.; Kaida, Y.; Maeda, T.; Hashida, R.; Tonan, T.; Nagata, S.; Hazama, T.; Nakayama, Y.; Ito, S.; Kurokawa, Y.; et al. l-Carnitine Supplementation vs. Cycle Ergometer Exercise for Physical Activity and Muscle Status in Hemodialysis Patients: A Randomized Clinical Trial. *Ther. Apher. Dial.* **2020**. [CrossRef]
12. Siami, G.; Clinton, M.E.; Mrak, R.; Griffis, J.; Stone, W. Evaluation of the Effect of Intravenous L-Carnitine Therapy on Function, Structure and Fatty Acid Metabolism of Skeletal Muscle in Patients Receiving Chronic Hemodialysis. *Nephron* **1991**, *57*, 306–313. [CrossRef]
13. Takahashi, M.; Ueda, S.; Misaki, H.; Sugiyama, N.; Matsumoto, K.; Matsuo, N.; Murao, S. Carnitine Determination by an Enzymatic Cycling Method With Carnitine Dehydrogenase. *Clin. Chem.* **1994**, *40*, 817–821. [CrossRef]
14. Shigematsu, Y.; Hirano, S.; Hata, I.; Tanaka, Y.; Sudo, M.; Sakura, N.; Tajima, T.; Yamaguchi, S. Newborn Mass Screening and Selective Screening Using Electrospray Tandem Mass Spectrometry in Japan. *J. Chromatogr. B Analyt. Technol. Biomed. Life Sci.* **2002**, *776*, 39–48. [CrossRef]
15. Chace, D.H.; Kalas, T.A.; Naylor, E.W. Use of Tandem Mass Spectrometry for Multianalyte Screening of Dried Blood Specimens From Newborns. *Clin. Chem.* **2003**, *49*, 1797–1817. [CrossRef]
16. Devereux, R.B.; Reichek, N. Echocardiographic Determination of Left Ventricular Mass in Man. Anatomic Validation of the Method. *Circulation* **1977**, *55*, 613–618. [CrossRef]
17. Longo, N.; Frigeni, M.; Pasquali, M. Carnitine Transport and Fatty Acid Oxidation. *Biochim. Biophys. Acta* **2016**, *1863*, 2422–2435. [CrossRef]
18. Agnetti, A.; Bitton, L.; Tchana, B.; Raymond, A.; Carano, N. Primary Carnitine Deficiency Dilated Cardiomyopathy: 28 Years Follow-Up. *Int. J. Cardiol.* **2013**, *162*, e34–e35. [CrossRef]
19. Gempel, K.; Kiechl, S.; Hofmann, S.; Lochmüller, H.; Kiechl-Kohlendorfer, U.; Willeit, J.; Sperl, W.; Rettinger, A.; Bieger, I.; Pongratz, D.; et al. Screening for Carnitine Palmitoyltransferase II Deficiency by Tandem Mass Spectrometry. *J. Inherit. Metab. Dis.* **2002**, *25*, 17–27. [CrossRef]
20. Pereyra, A.S.; Hasek, L.Y.; Harris, K.L.; Berman, A.G.; Damen, F.W.; Goergen, C.J.; Ellis, J.M. Loss of Cardiac Carnitine Palmitoyltransferase 2 Results in Rapamycin-Resistant, Acetylation-Independent Hypertrophy. *J. Biol. Chem.* **2017**, *292*, 18443–18456. [CrossRef]
21. Bonnefont, J.P.; Djouadi, F.; Prip-Buus, C.; Gobin, S.; Munnich, A.; Bastin, J. Carnitine Palmitoyltransferases 1 and 2: Biochemical, Molecular and Medical Aspects. *Mol. Aspects Med.* **2004**, *25*, 495–520. [CrossRef]
22. Wanner, C.; Wäckerle, B.; Boeckle, H.; Schollmeyer, P.; Hörl, W.H. Plasma and Red Blood Cell Carnitine and Carnitine Esters During L-Carnitine Therapy in Hemodialysis Patients. *Am. J. Clin. Nutr.* **1990**, *51*, 407–410. [CrossRef]

Article

The Effects of Long-Term Nutrition Counseling According to the Behavioral Modification Stages in Patients with Cardiovascular Disease

Keiko Matsuzaki [1,*], Nobuko Fukushima [2], Yutaka Saito [3], Naoya Matsumoto [4], Mayu Nagaoka [5], Yousuke Katsuda [6] and Shin-ichiro Miura [6]

1. Department of Nutrition, Fukuoka University Nishijin Hospital, Fukuoka 814-8522, Japan
2. Fukuoka Women's Junior College Health and Nutrition, Fukuoka 818-0193, Japan; fuku.c.fukushima@gmail.com
3. Department of Cardiovascular Medicine, Public Yame General Hospital, Fukuoka 834-0033, Japan; ymhp2388@yamehp.jp
4. Department of Rehabilitation, Fukuoka University Nishijin Hospital, Fukuoka 814-8522, Japan; nmatsumoto@fukuoka-u.ac.jp
5. Department of Pharmacy, Fukuoka University Nishijin Hospital, Fukuoka 814-8522, Japan; mnagaoka@fukuoka-u.ac.jp
6. Department of Cardiovascular Medicine, Fukuoka University Nishijin Hospital, Fukuoka 814-8522, Japan; katsuda@fukuoka-u.ac.jp (Y.K.); miuras@cis.fukuoka-u.ac.jp (S.-i.M.)
* Correspondence: eiyoukeiko@fukuoka-u.ac.jp; Tel.: +81-92-831-1211

Abstract: Background: the behavioral modification stages (BMS) are widely used; however, there are no reports on long-term nutrition counseling for cardiovascular disease (CVD) according to BMS. Aim: to study the effects of long-term nutrition counseling based on the BMS in patients with CVD. Methods: fifteen patients with CVD who participated in nutrition counseling were enrolled between June 2012 and December 2016. We provided BMS and dietary questionnaires to estimate the stage score (SS), salt intake, and drinking habits (non-drinking group ($n = 7$)/drinking group ($n = 8$)), and measured the blood pressure (BP), body mass index (BMI), and biochemical markers before and after hospitalization at 6 months, 1 year, and 1.5 years after leaving the outpatient department (OPD). Results: a significant decreased salt intake and increase in SS were found at 1.5 years. It significantly decreased the BP and salt intake in the non-drinking group at 1.5 years. Conclusions: long-term nutrition counseling according to BMS improved salt intake and BP in the non-drinking group. However, in the drinking group, increased salt intake might weaken the BP improvement. Temperance and low-sodium intake are essential factors that control BP, especially in drinkers.

Keywords: behavioral modification stages; nutrition counseling; patient education

1. Introduction

Currently, cardiovascular disease (CVD) is the second leading cause of death along with malignant neoplasm in Japan [1]. In Japan, in particular, where the population aged >65 years exceeds 27.3% of the total population [2], increased mortality from cardiovascular disease has become a social problem. However, the implementation of guideline-based medical therapy in elderly patients with CVD was insufficient to prevent the recurrence of CVD [3].

Lifestyle-related diseases, such as hypertension, are strongly involved in the development of CVD or congestive heart disease (CHF). Therefore, to prevent CVD, daily habits should be improved from early in the day, such as implementing nutritional and exercise therapies and quitting smoking [4,5]. Furthermore, it is reported that recurrence of CHF in elderly patients is caused by their refusal to incorporate behavioral changes—and they continue to consume excessive amounts of salt [6]. Behavioral changes, such as decreased salt intake, are important factors in patients with CVD or CHF. Recently, the trans-theoretical model (TTM) has been used to improve the lifestyle and provide specific guidance to patients with type 2 diabetes [7–11]. TTM theorizes behavioral modification of dietary habits; it suggests behavioral modification by estimating personal readiness to changes and performs specific, individual intervention programs. Behavioral modification stages (BMS) have been indicated in one of the concepts, as well as the preparatory state of psychology, and its practice situations, of five stages: 1) precontemplation (participants have no intention of changing their behavior within the next 6 months); 2) contemplation (they are aware a problem exists and intend to change their behavior within the next 6 months, but not within 1 month); 3) preparation (they are ready for the change within the next 1 month); 4) action (they actively modified their behavior within the last 6 months); and 5) maintenance (they sustained their behavioral changes for >6 months) [12,13].

However, no reports on nutrition counseling using the TTM and long-term follow-up in patients with CVD have been described. We evaluated the effects of long-term nutrition counseling based on the BMS in patients with CVD. Therefore, we hypothesized that long-term nutrition counseling, according to the BMS, should induce lifestyle modification, in particular improvement of high blood pressure and decreased salt intake.

2. Materials and Methods

2.1. Investigation Period

This study was conducted from June 2012 to December 2016.

2.2. Inclusion Criteria

The participants were patients who had no coronary restenosis after percutaneous coronary intervention at Fukuoka University Nishijin Hospital. The study protocol is indicated in Figure 1. Finally, 15 patients with CVD participated in nutrition counseling. We provided BMS and dietary questionnaires to estimate the stage score (SS), salt intake, and drinking habits, and measured the BP, body mass index (BMI), and biochemical markers at hospitalization to 6 months, 1 year, and 1.5 years after leaving the outpatient department (OPD). Nine, four, and two patients had angina, heart failure (with ischemic heart disease history), and acute myocardial infarction, respectively.

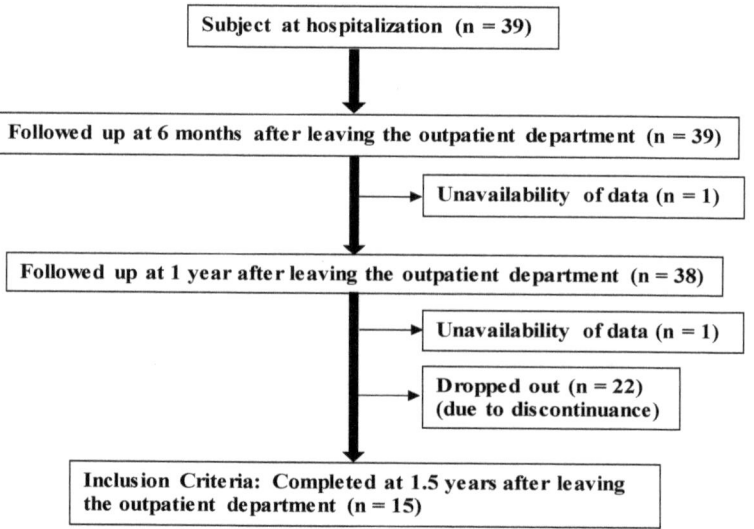

Figure 1. Study protocol.

2.3. Methods

2.3.1. Research Ethics and Patient Consent

Informed consent was obtained from all patients via consent confirm. The investigation conforms to the principles outlined in the Declaration of Helsinki. The present study was approved by the ethics committee of Fukuoka Medical Association Hospital (Fukuoka University Nishijin Hospital at present) (approval number: N19-03-001) and was prospectively performed form June 2012 to December 2016.

2.3.2. BMS Questionnaire

Prior to individual nutrition counseling, patients were provided with self-administered BMS questionnaires about dietary intake [8]. Dietary intake in BMS was assessed using five stages of the first described BMS. Furthermore, we performed the scores as follows: precontemplation, 0; contemplation, 1; preparation, 2; action, 3; and maintenance, 4.

2.3.3. Dietary Survey Questionnaire

Patients were provided with three-day food record questionnaires [14], with self-reports regarding their standard dietary intakes (in OPD, 3 days before nutrition counseling) for 3 days before hospitalization. An interview survey on dietary intake was conducted by a managerial dietician during nutrition counseling. To investigate the amount of drinking per day, and the drinking frequency for 1 week, we conducted interview surveys. The calculation of alcohol intake was based on the Standard Tables of Food Composition in Japan, 2015 (Seventh Revised Version) [15]. Furthermore, we calculated the alcohol intake on an average day.

2.3.4. Nutrition Counseling

Nutrition counseling involved making appropriate improvement suggestions in dietary habits and behavior. Cardiologists provided counseling and nutritional intake directions (energy, protein, fat, and salt intake). Counseling to promote a diet focused on increased consumption of, vegetables, mushrooms, seaweed, and fish and decreased consumption of foods that are high in salt (sodium), deep-fried food, and food with added sugar. Recommendations applied to risk factors for CVD, such as high blood pressure and high cholesterol [4,5]. Long-term nutrition counseling included counseling done during hospitalization, and 6 months, 1 year, and then 1.5 years after leaving the OPD. We determined BMS on dietary intake and dietary survey contents, and then nutrition counseling (30-min individual interview) was performed according to the preparatory state (BMS) at each time. The same managerial dietician set a target along BMS with patients at each time point.

Counseling was guided by referring to the Ministry of Health, Labor, and Welfare, Japan Safety, and Health Council (2018): the standard medical checkup and health guidance program (definitive) [10]. There are five stages, as follows.

The precontemplation stage: the managerial dietician confirmed the many benefits of changing dietary habits. We explained that, without changing dietary habits, it is much easier for the recrudescence of CVD.

The contemplation stage: the managerial dietician proposed a behavior change on the dietary habits. High blood pressure and high cholesterol can be improved by increasing consumption of vegetables, mushrooms, seaweed, and fish, while reducing the consumption of food high in salt (sodium), deep-fried food, and added sugars. We explained that such behavior changes could assist in reducing the risk of CVD.

The preparation stage: when patients seemed to have a problem regarding dietary intake, the managerial dietician could assist to establish some behavioral objectives on how to improve. We proposed increasing the consumption of vegetables, mushrooms, seaweed, and fish while reducing consumption of high salt (sodium), deep-fried food, and food with added sugar.

The action stage: the managerial dietician identified the behavior problem then provided appropriate correction actions. We suggested continuing consumption of vegetables, mushrooms, seaweed, and fish, while decreasing consumption of food high in salt (sodium), deep-fried food, and food with added sugar.

The maintenance stage: the managerial dietician identified the plan that prevented interruptions in behavioral modifications, concerning dietary habits with patients. We insisted on the continued increase of consumption of vegetables, mushrooms, seaweed, and fish, and reduced consumption of food high in salt (sodium), deep-fried foods, and food with added sugar. We asked patients with concerns about dietary habits.

We assumed a deviation from and retractability in BMS beforehand and established a target [10,11]. Moreover, we investigated factors such as dining out, usage of prepared food, snacking, and exercise habits.

2.3.5. Dietary Intake

Dietary intake investigated energy, carbohydrate, protein, fat, dietary fiber, potassium, and sodium from a three-day food record questionnaire. The calculation of the salt intake was based on the Microsoft Excel software—Excel Eiyoukun version 8.0 (kenpakusha, Tokyo, Japan) [16] from "Sodium (mg)/1000 × 2.54" [15].

2.4. Investigation Item

The data from the medical records were collected—that is, age, weight, BMI (weight (kg)/height (m) × height (m)), total cholesterol (T-Cho), high-density lipoprotein cholesterol (HDL-Cho), low-density lipoprotein cholesterol (LDL-Cho), hemoglobin A1c (HbA1c), uric acid (UA), estimated glomerular filtration rate (eGFR), BP. Regarding alcohol consumption, the patients were divided into the drinking ($n = 8$) and non-drinking groups ($n = 7$). The data on SS, salt intake, and alcohol intake at hospitalization, 6 months, 1 year, and 1.5 years after leaving the OPD, were compared.

The relation between salt intake and each factor (sex, age, snacking, drinking habit) after 1.5 years of leaving was also determined. Regarding alcohol consumption (1.5 years after leaving, the non-drinking group ($n = 7$), the drinking group < thrice a week ($n = 3$), the drinking group > four times a week ($n = 5$)) and salt intake, the drinking habit and the respective compared with salt intake and BP were considered.

2.5. Measuring Method of Blood Pressure

We normally inform our patients to come to the hospital at 11:00 a.m., and a clinical nurse measures the patient's BP. BP was collected using a double cuff electronic sphygmomanometer (Terumo ES-H55).

2.6. Calculating Dietary Intake

The calculation of the dietary intake was based on the Microsoft Excel software—Excel Eiyoukun version 8.0 (kenpakusha, Tokyo, Japan) [16], from the standard table of food composition in Japan 2015 (Seventh Revised Version) [15].

2.7. Statistical Analysis

All analyses were performed using SPSS Statistics Version 22 (IBM, Tokyo, Japan). The weight, BMI, T-Cho, HDL-Cho, LDL-Cho, neutral lipid, HbA1c, UA, eGFR, energy, carbohydrate, protein, fat, dietary fiber, and potassium, with their means expressed as mean (standard deviation), were compared with salt intake, alcohol intake, BP, SS about dietary intake, drinking habits (the non-drinking group ($n = 7$)/the drinking group ($n = 8$)), and the respective SS and salt intake, BP were performed by statistical analysis of one-way analysis of variance, subjected to the general linear model with replicate.

Using the multiple regression analysis, the relation between salt intake (dependent variable) and each factor (sex, age, snacking, the drinking habit; independent variable) 1.5 years after leaving was identified. Then, a stepwise method was used. Furthermore, multiple comparisons regarding the drinking habits (after 1.5 years, non-drinking group ($n = 7$), drinking group < thrice a week ($n = 3$), drinking group > four times a week ($n = 5$)) and salt intake were done using the Bonferroni correction. The correlation between alcohol intake and salt intake were calculated using the Spearman's rank correlation coefficient. Student's t-test was used to between the non-drinking and drinking groups (The weight, BMI, T-Cho, HDL-Cho, LDL-Cho, neutral lipid, HbA1c, UA, and eGFR). Chi-squared test was used for the daily habits, and the medications between the non-drinking and drinking groups. Student's t-test was used to compare SS and salt intake, BP between the non-drinking and drinking groups, with the two-way analysis of variance (without repetitions). p values < 0.05 were considered statistically significant (two-tailed test).

3. Results

3.1. Changes in Anthropometry and Blood Biochemical Examination

Table 1 presents the changes in patients' body. The patients' respective BMIs shows (mean (SD)): 26.1 (3.2), 25.7 (3.3), 25.7 (3.3), and 26.2 (3.8) kg/m^2. BMI was significantly lower at 6 months after leaving than that at hospitalization ($p < 0.05$).

Table 1. Changes in anthropometry and blood biochemical examination ($n = 15$).

	Hospitalization	6 Months	1 Year	1.5 Years	p Value		
Male		$n = 11$			Hospitalization vs		
Female		$n = 4$					
Age (years old)		71.3 (8.4)					
HT (%)		93.3			6 months	1 year	1.5 years
DM (%)		53.3					
HL (%)		80.0					
Weight (kg)	69.8 (14.9)	68.7 (14.8)	68.8 (14.8)	70.0 (15.9)	n.s.	n.s.	n.s.
BMI (kg/m^2)	26.1 (3.2)	25.7 (3.3)	25.7 (3.3)	26.2 (3.8)	0.040 *	n.s.	n.s.
T-Cho (mg/dl)	169.8 (37.0)	174.3 (32.2)	171.8 (31.6)	160.4 (30.2)	n.s.	n.s.	n.s.
HDL-Cho (mg/dl)	50.0 (11.1)	50.6 (13.2)	47.6 (10.3)	47.3 (10.5)	n.s.	n.s.	n.s.
LDL-Cho (mg/dl)	93.1 (34.1)	95.7 (29.6)	94.6 (29.3)	85.3 (29.1)	n.s.	n.s.	n.s.
Neutral lipid (mg/dl)	133.8 (65.4)	140.3 (54.8)	148.1 (71.3)	139.1 (53.2)	n.s.	n.s.	n.s.
HbA1c (%)	6.6 (1.1)	6.5 (0.7)	6.5 (0.7)	6.5 (0.7)	n.s.	n.s.	n.s.
UA (mg/dl)	6.6 (1.0)	6.7 (1.1)	6.6 (0.9)	6.6 (0.8)	n.s.	n.s.	n.s.
eGFR (ml/min/1.73m^2)	55.8 (17.6)	56.2 (18.8)	53.7 (20.8)	53.8 (21.5)	n.s.	n.s.	n.s.

Mean (SD) * $p < 0$. Abbreviations: HT, hypertension; DM, diabetes mellitus; HL, hyperlipidemia; BMI, body mass index; T-Cho, total cholesterol; HDL-Cho, high-density lipoprotein cholesterol; LDL-Cho, low-density lipoprotein cholesterol; HbA1c, hemoglobin A1c; UA, uric acid; eGFR, estimated glomerular filtration rate; n.s., not significant. BMI was significantly lower at 6 months after leaving than that at hospitalization ($p < 0.05$).

3.2. Changes in Daily Habits

Changes in daily habits are indicated in Table 2. Dining out, snacking, prepared food, and exercise habits almost remained unchanged.

Table 2. Changes in the daily ($n = 15$).

		Admission Time	$1\frac{1}{2}$ Years after Leaving	p Value
Dining out habits	Yes	11	12	0.307
	No	4	3	
Usage of prepared food	Yes	12	10	0.494
	No	3	5	
Snacking	Yes	14	13	1.000
	No	1	2	
Exercise habits	Yes	10	13	1.000
	No	5	2	

3.3. Cardiovascular Disease and Medications

Table 3 presents cardiovascular disease and medication information. Medications for the treatment of diabetes accounted for 11.4%. Alpha-blocker was addition one patient 1 year later about antihypertensive drug. Calcium channel blocker was addition one patient 1.5 years later, and Angiotensin II receptor blocker dose reduction one patient. Antiplatelet aggregation drug come off three patients 1.5 years later. HMG-CoA reductase inhibitor and anticlotting drug were addition respectively one patient 1.5 years later.

Table 3. Cardiovascular disease and medications (at the time of hospitalization) ($n = 15$).

Drug	Number	(%)
Antiplatelet aggregation drug	23	21.9
HMG-CoA reductase inhibitor	10	9.5
Beta-blocking drug	9	8.6
Vasodilating drug	9	8.6
Calcium channel blocker	9	8.6
Angiotensin II receptor blocker	7	6.7
Diuretic drug	6	5.7
DPP-4 inhibitor	6	5.7
Diuretic antihypertensive drug	5	4.8
Environmental Protection Agency drug	4	3.8
Angiotensin-converting enzyme inhibitor	3	2.9
Non-pudding type selective xanthine oxidase inhibitor	3	2.9
Anticlotting drug	3	2.9
Anti-arrhythmic drug	2	1.9
Sulphonyl urea drug	2	1.9
α—glucosidase inhibitor	1	1.0
Biguanide	1	1.0
Long acting insulin	1	1.0
Fast acting insulin	1	1.0

3.4. Changes in SS Regarding Dietary Intake

Score results of the BMS questionnaire were indicated. Changes in SS regarding dietary intake are indicated in Figure 2a. SS after nutrition counseling were significantly higher than those at hospitalization and 1.5 years after leaving ($p < 0.01$); SS at hospitalization, 6 months, 1 year, and 1.5 years after leaving were 2.7 (0.9), 3.3 (0.7), 3.8 (0.4), and 3.9 (0.3) points, respectively.

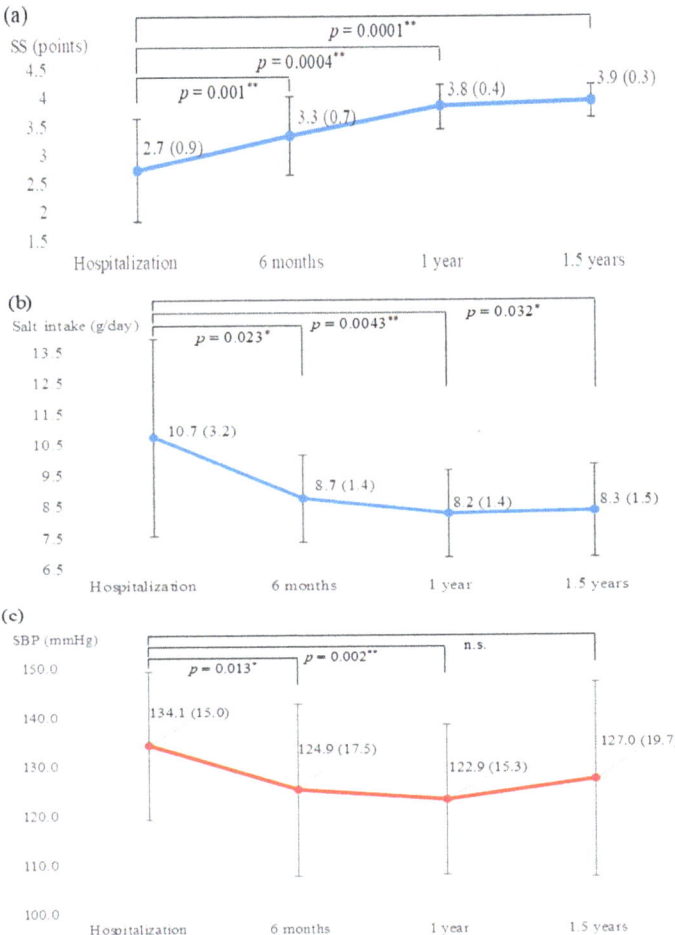

Figure 2. Change in SS regarding dietary intake, salt intake, and BP. Mean (SD). * $p < 0.05$, ** $p < 0.01$, $n = 15$. Abbreviations: SS, stage scores; SBP, systolic blood pressure; n.s., not significant. (**a**) A significant increase in SS was found 1.5 years after leaving compared with that at hospitalization ($p < 0.01$). (**b**) ESI decreased in 1.5 years after leaving compared with that at hospitalization ($p < 0.05$). (**c**) SBPs significantly decreased at 6 months and 1 year compared with hospitalization ($p < 0.05$), however an upward trend in 1.5 years from 1 year after leaving.

3.5. Changes in the Salt Intake

The salt intake in patients at the time of hospitalization and 6 months, 1 year, and 1.5 years after leaving were 10.7 (3.2), 8.7 (1.4), 8.2 (1.4), and 8.3 (1.5) g/day, respectively. It decreased in 1 year as well as 1.5 years after leaving, compared with that at hospitalization (at 1 year $p = 0.0043$, at 1.5 years $p = 0.032$) (Figure 2b).

3.6. Changes in the Nutrient Intake

Changes in the nutrient intake are indicated in Table 4. Energy, carbohydrate, protein, fat, dietary fiber, and potassium were almost unchanged. Dietary fiber was of low value over this time period.

Table 4. Changes in the nutrient intake ($n = 15$).

	Hospitalization	6 Months	1 Year	1.5 Years	*p* Value		
					Hospitalization vs		
					6 Months	1 Year	1.5 years
Energy (kcal)	2042.0 (376.9)	1823.2 (284.3)	1789.7 (285.2)	1828.9 (362.4)	n.s.	n.s.	n.s.
Carbohydrate (g)	315.7 (64.2)	283.4 (52.6)	277.8 (51.1)	277.1 (56.7)	n.s.	n.s.	n.s.
Protein (g)	80.3 (13.3)	72.4 (10.5)	72.0 (10.9)	79.3 (25.2)	n.s.	n.s.	n.s.
Fat (g)	50.9 (17.5)	44.5 (13.4)	43.4 (13.4)	44.8 (17.3)	n.s.	n.s.	n.s.
Dietary fiber (g)	16.7 (3.4)	17.0 (2.7)	17.0 (4.7)	15.2 (4.3)	n.s.	n.s.	n.s.
Potassium (mg)	3094.5 (567.7)	2969.3 (553.7)	2976.8 (756.3)	2914.9 (606.5)	n.s.	n.s.	n.s.

3.7. Changes in the BP

Systolic BPs (SBPs) of patients at hospitalization and 6 months, 1 year, and 1.5 years after leaving were 134.1 (15.0), 124.9 (17.5), 122.9 (15.3), and 127.0 (19.7) mmHg, respectively (Figure 2c). SBPs significantly decreased at 6 months and 1 year compared with that at hospitalization (at 6 months $p = 0.013$, at 1 year $p = 0.002$); however, an upward trend was seen in 1.5 years from 1 year after leaving.

3.8. Relation between the Salt Intake of Patients 1.5 Years after Leaving and Each Factor

Concerning the relation with salt intake at 1.5 years after leaving, each factor (sex, age, snacking, the drinking habit) was compared. A significant positive correlation coefficient of 0.515 was noted between the salt intake and drinking habit ($p = 0.049$).

3.9. Changes in Anthropometry and Blood Biochemical Examination (the Drinking Group and Non-Drinking Group)

Changes in the patient bodies in the non-drinking group were compared with the drinking group, as seen in Table 5. The eGFR of the non-drinking group was significantly lower than that of the drinking group at 1 year and 1.5 years after leaving (at 1 year $p = 0.023$, at 1.5 years $p = 0.045$).

Table 5. Changes in anthropometry and blood biochemical examination (the drinking group and non-drinking group).

	The Drinking Group ($n = 8$)				The Non-Drinking Group ($n = 7$)				The Drinking Group vs The Non-Drinking Group			
	Hospitalization	6 Months	1 Year	1.5 Years	Hospitalization	6 Months	1 Year	1.5 Years	Hospitalization	6 Months	1 Year	1.5 Years
									p Value			
Weight (kg)	72.4 (18.9)	70.8 (18.5)	70.8 (18.5)	72.1 (20.0)	66.9 (9.0)	66.3 (10.0)	66.6 (9.9)	67.6 (10.5)	n.s.	n.s.	n.s.	n.s.
BMI (kg/m²)	26.4 (3.6)	25.9 (3.6)	25.9 (3.7)	26.3 (4.3)	25.7 (2.8)	25.5 (3.1)	25.6 (3.1)	26.0 (3.5)	n.s.	n.s.	n.s.	n.s.
T-Cho (mg/dl)	174.8 (38.1)	173.6 (39.7)	169.8 (41.6)	149.1 (34.7)	164.0 (37.9)	175.1 (24.0)	174.1 (17.1)	173.3 (19.2)	n.s.	n.s.	n.s.	n.s.
HDL-Cho (mg/dl)	52.0 (10.3)	50.9 (13.2)	46.9 (8.4)	49.0 (8.4)	47.6 (12.4)	50.3 (14.3)	48.3 (12.8)	45.3 (12.9)	n.s.	n.s.	n.s.	n.s.
LDL-Cho (mg/dl)	98.7 (41.0)	95.6 (39.4)	95.1 (40.2)	75.3 (36.6)	86.7 (26.3)	95.7 (15.2)	94.0 (11.0)	96.7 (11.2)	n.s.	n.s.	n.s.	n.s.
Neutral lipid (mg/dl)	120.3 (23.5)	135.5 (48.3)	138.8 (63.2)	123.9 (33.8)	149.3 (93.9)	145.7 (65.1)	158.9 (83.4)	156.4 (68.0)	n.s.	n.s.	n.s.	n.s.
HbA1c (%)	6.5 (0.8)	6.5 (0.8)	6.5 (0.8)	6.4 (0.5)	6.7 (1.5)	6.5 (0.7)	6.5 (0.7)	6.6 (0.8)	n.s.	n.s.	n.s.	n.s.
UA (mg/dl)	6.5 (1.1)	6.3 (0.9)	6.4 (1.1)	6.7 (0.9)	6.7 (0.9)	7.2 (1.1)	6.8 (0.4)	6.5 (0.7)	n.s.	n.s.	n.s.	n.s.
eGFR (ml/min/1.73 m²)	62.8 (13.9)	63.3 (13.6)	64.6 (19.9)	63.9 (20.7)	48.0 (19.1)	48.2 (21.6)	41.2 (14.3)	42.1 (16.8)	n.s.	n.s.	0.023 *	0.045 *

Mean (SD) * $p < 0.05$ Abbreviations: BMI, body mass index; T-Cho, total cholesterol; HDL-Cho, high-density lipoprotein cholesterol; LDL-Cho, low-density lipoprotein cholesterol; HbA1c, hemoglobin A1c; UA, uric acid; eGFR, estimated glomerular filtration rate; n.s., not significant.

3.10. Cardiovascular Disease and Medications (the Drinking Group and Non-Drinking Group)

There was no significant difference between the drinking and non-drinking groups at the time of hospitalization.

3.11. Drinking Habit and SS

SS in the non-drinking ($n = 7$) and drinking ($n = 8$) groups were compared (Figure 3a). In both groups, SS at hospitalization and 6 months, 1 year, and 1.5 years after leaving had significantly increased (the non-drinking group: 2.9 (0.9), 3.4 (0.5), 3.9 (0.4), and 4.0 (0.0) points, respectively; all, $p < 0.05$, the drinking group: 2.6 (0.9), 3.1 (0.8), 3.8 (0.5), and 3.8 (0.5) points, respectively; all, $p < 0.05$). SS of the drinking group tended to be lower than that of the non-drinking group.

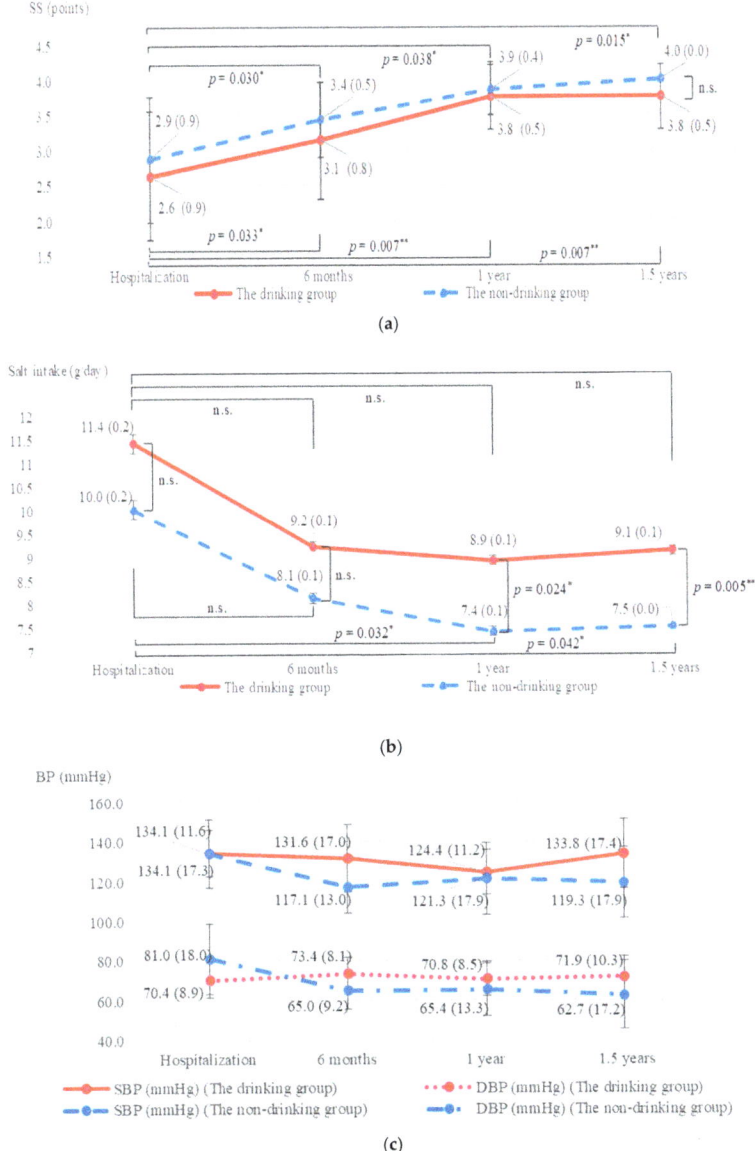

Figure 3. *Cont.*

		p value					
		Hospitalization vs			1 y vs	The drinking group vs The non-drinking group (Hospitalization – 1.5 years)	
		6 months	1 year	1.5 years	1.5 years	SBP	DBP
SBP (mmHg)	The drinking group (n = 8)	n.s.	0.036 *	n.s.	0.049 *	n.s.	n.s.
DBP (mmHg)		n.s.	n.s.	n.s.	n.s.		
SBP (mmHg)	The non-drinking group (n = 7)	0.004 **	0.041 *	0.046 *	n.s.		
DBP (mmHg)		0.019 *	0.034 *	0.031 *	n.s.		

Mean (SD) * p < 0.05, ** p < 0.01   n = 15

Figure 3. Change in the drinking habit and SS, salt intake and BP. (**a**) In both groups, SS at hospitalization and 1.5 years after leaving had significantly increased ($p < 0.05$). SS of the drinking group tended to be lower than that of the non-drinking group. (**b**) The salt intake in the non-drinking group, 1 year, and 1.5 years after leaving were lower than hospitalization ($p < 0.05$). From hospitalization to 1.5 years after leaving, salt intake was lower in the non-drinking group than that in the drinking group ($p < 0.01$). (**c**) In the non-drinking group, SBPs at hospitalization and 1.5 years after leaving, which showed a decrease ($p < 0.05$).

3.12. Drinking Habit and Salt Intake

Alcohol intake showed an upward trend in the drinking group at the time of hospitalization and 6 months, 1 year, and 1.5 years after leaving were 20.3 (26.7), 19.6 (27.1), 14.9 (20.3), and 24.6 (31.1) g/day, respectively ($p = 0.254$). At 1.5 years after leaving, salt intake in the non-drinking group ($n = 7$), drinking group < thrice a week ($n = 3$), and drinking group > four times a week ($n = 5$) were 7.5 (0.7), 8.0 (0.6), and 9.7 (1.8) g/day, respectively. The non-drinking group had significantly lower salt intake than the drinking group >four times a week ($p = 0.041$). A significant positive correlation coefficient of 0.628 was noted between alcohol intake and salt intake ($p = 0.012$). Salt intake in the non-drinking ($n = 7$) and drinking ($n = 8$) groups were compared (Figure 3b). At hospitalization and 6 months and 1 year after leaving, in the drinking group, it tended to decrease (11.4 (0.2), 9.2 (0.1), and 8.9 (0.1) g/day, respectively). However, 1.5 years after leaving, it was 9.1 (0.1) g/day, which notably increased (not significant). Salt intake in the non-drinking group, at hospitalization and 6 months, 1 year, and 1.5 years after leaving, were 10.0 (0.2), 8.1 (0.1), 7.4 (0.1), and 7.5 (0.0) g/day, respectively. Furthermore, it significantly decreased at 1 year and 1.5 years compared with hospitalization ($p < 0.05$). From hospitalization to 1.5 years after leaving, salt intake was lower in the non-drinking group than that in the drinking group ($p < 0.01$).

3.13. Changes in the Drinking Habit and BP

Changes in the drinking habit and BP are indicated in Figure 3c. A comparison of these between the non-drinking ($n = 7$) and drinking ($n = 8$) groups was determined. In the drinking group, SBPs tended to decrease at hospitalization, 6 months, and 1 year after leaving: 134.1 (11.6), 131.6 (17.0), and 124.4 (11.2) mmHg, respectively (hospitalization vs. 1 year after leaving, $p < 0.05$). However, 1.5 years after, it was 133.8 (17.4) mmHg, which was higher than that in 1 year after leaving ($p < 0.05$).

In the non-drinking group, SBPs significantly decreased at hospitalization and 6 months, 1 year, and 1.5 years after leaving: 134.1 (17.3), 117.1 (13.0), 121.3 (17.9), and 119.3 (17.9) mmHg, respectively ($p < 0.05$). In the non-drinking group, DBPs at hospitalization and 6 months, 1 year, and 1.5 years after leaving had significantly decreased (81.0 (18.0), 65.0 (9.2), 65.4 (13.3), and 62.7 (17.2) mmHg, respectively; all, $p < 0.05$).

4. Discussion

This is the first report assessing the effects of long-term nutrition counseling according to behavioral modification stages for patients with CVD. We discussed on what kind of help we can assist. The decision-making and execution power are all left to the patient's own initiative, and medical staff have no way to interfere. However, diet therapy can allow patients to be treated in their daily lives. In conjunction with changes in behavior, the long-term nutrition counseling is reflected in the reduction of salt intake and the improvement of blood pressure.

This strategy improved long-term behavioral modification, salt intake, and hypertension, and its effectiveness was significant in non-drinking patients with CVD. It is well known that excessive salt intake increases BP [17–20]. In this study, a significant long-term decrease in salt intake and SBP was observed in the non-drinking group, but not in the drinking-group. Thus, long-term decreased salt intake might have resulted in decreased BP in the non-drinking group. Studies have shown that single or repetitive nutrition counseling alone could lead to decreased salt intake and BP, but the long-term effects were unknown [21,22]. In this study, effective behavioral changed and long-term BP reduction could be obtained by repeating nutrition counseling based on TTM. Thus, it was suggested that behavioral change was an important factor to keep long-term BP reduction.

In the drinking group, SBPs had significantly decreased in the short term, but the effects of BP disappeared after 1.5 years. Long-term nutrition counseling with behavioral modification stages went wrong in the drinking group. It is necessary to grope the planning of temperance and abstinence as a target of behavioral modification in social concerns. Yoshimura et al. reported that alcohol consumption is associated with salt intake and BP, and salt sensitivity improved by reducing alcohol intake [23]. Salt intake was also excessive for the drinking group at hospitalization in this study. Salt intake and SBPs had significantly decreased after 1 year in the drinking group. However, the salt intake and BP tended to increase 1.5 years after hospitalization in the drinking group. Moreover, in this study, 1.5 years after hospitalization, due to intake, beef jerky, salted nuts, and pickle (salt intake >2 g) consumption increased in the drinking group (data not shown) [15]. These were regarded as factors of the salt intake and BP tended to increase. Thus, in the long-term drinkers, increased salt intake during alcohol intake might weaken the effect for BP. Therefore, temperance and stricter sodium reduction [24,25] in drinkers [20,26,27] are essential.

Most of the patients in this study were elderly with an average age of 71 years old. Akita et al. reported that guideline-based drug therapy alone for elderly cardiovascular patients was insufficient to prevent recurrence of CHF [3], and Tsuchihashi et al. also reported that one-third of the triggers for relapse of CHF in elderly patients are because of excess salt intake [6]. Therefore, repetitive nutrition counseling based on TTM was effective in preventing recurrence in elderly patients with CVD. Furthermore, there is no significant improvement about lipid profile and dietary fiber intake. It will be problematic in target setting of nutrition counseling in the future. In this study, target setting to the drinkers of temperance, and stricter sodium reduction, with behavioral modification stages are important. To prevent the development or recurrence of CVD, we should also support the acquisition of self-management skills [28], as well as long-term improvement of dietary intake and daily lifestyle habits. This is crucial because absence of effective behavior changes may exacerbate the symptoms, resulting in long-term consequences.

The findings of this study have to be seen in light of some limitations. The small sample of patients with CVD. Since this study is small, a large-scale, prospective study is necessary to obtain a final conclusion. Moreover, we were not considering the change of medication in this study, but that was a number of minor changes.

In conclusion, this study suggests that acquisition of effective behavior modifications by long-term nutrition counseling, according to behavioral modification stages, is important for patients with CVD.

Author Contributions: K.M. designed the study, and wrote the initial draft of the manuscript. Y.K. and S.-i.M. contributed to data analysis and interpretation, and assisted in manuscript preparation. All other authors have contributed to data collection and interpretation, and critically reviewed the manuscript. All authors agreed to be accountable for all aspects of the work in ensuring that questions related to the accuracy or integrity of any part of the work are appropriately investigated and resolved. All authors have read and agreed to the published version of the manuscript.

Funding: This study has not received funding.

Institutional Review Board Statement: The study was conducted according to the guidelines of the Declaration of Helsinki, and approved by the ethics committee of Fukuoka Medical Association Hospital (Fukuoka University Nishijin Hospital at present) (approval number: N19-03-001, 1 March 2019 of approval).

Informed Consent Statement: Informed consent was obtained from all subjects involved in the study.

Data Availability Statement: The data that support the findings of this study are available from the corresponding author upon reasonable request.

Conflicts of Interest: The Authors declare that there is no conflict of interest.

References

1. Ministry of Health Japan, Labour and Welfare. Source: A Population Movement Investigation in 2018. Available online: http://www.mhlw.go.jp/toukei/saikin/hw/jinkou/kakutei18 (accessed on 28 November 2019).
2. Ministry of Internal Affairs and Communications Department of Statistics Japan. Source: Demographic Forecast. 2019. Available online: http://www.stat.go.jp/data/jinsui/new.html (accessed on 20 June 2019).
3. Akita, K.; Kohno, T.; Kohsaka, S.; Shiraishi, Y.; Nagatomo, Y.; Izumi, Y.; Goda, A.; Mizuno, A.; Sawano, M.; Inohara, T.; et al. Current use of guideline-based medical therapy in elderly patients admitted with acute heart failure with reduced ejection fraction and its impact on event-free survival. *Int. J. Cardiol.* **2017**, *235*, 162–168. [CrossRef] [PubMed]
4. Iestra, J.A.; Kromhout, D.; van der Schouw, Y.T.; Grobbee, D.E.; Boshuizen, H.C.; van Staveren, W.A. Effect size estimates of lifestyle and dietary change on all-cause mortality in coronary artery disease patients. *Circulation* **2005**, *112*, 924–934. [CrossRef] [PubMed]
5. The American College of Cardiology Foundation; The American Heart Association. ACC/AHA Guideline on the Primary Prevention of Cardiovascular Disease. *J. Am. Coll. Cardiol.* **2019**, *74*, 177–232. [CrossRef]
6. Tsuchihashi, M.; Tsutsui, H.; Kodama, K.; Kasagi, F.; Takeshita, A. Clinical characteristics and prognosis of hospitalized patients with congestive heart failure—A study in Fukuoka, Japan. *Jpn. Circ. J.* **2000**, *64*, 953–959. [CrossRef]
7. Jones, H.; Edwards, L.; Vallis, T.M.; Ruggiero, L.; Rossi, S.R.; Rossi, J.S.; Greene, G.; Prochaska, J.O. Changes in diabetes self–care behaviors make a difference in glycemic control: The diabetes stages of change (DiSC) study. *Diabetes Care* **2003**, *26*, 732–737. [CrossRef]
8. Ministry of Health Japan, Labour and Welfare Safety and Health Council. Source: Standard Medical Checkup and Health Guidance Program (Definitive). Available online: https://www.mhlw.go.jp/file/06-seisakujouhou-10900000-kenkoukyoku/0000_3.pdf (accessed on 16 February 2018).
9. Prochaska, J.O.; Redding, C.A.; Evers, K.E. *The Transtheoretical Model and Stages of Change, Health Behavior and Health Education*, 3rd ed.; Glanz, K., Rimer, B.K., Lewis, F.M., Eds.; Jossey-Bass: San Francisco, CA, USA, 2002; pp. 97–121.
10. Prochaska, J.O.; Velicer, W.F. The transtheoretical model of health behavior change. *Am. J. Health Promot.* **1997**, *12*, 38–48. [CrossRef] [PubMed]
11. Johnson, S.S.; Paiva, A.L.; Cummins, C.O.; Johnson, J.L.; Dyment, S.J.; Wright, J.A.; Prochaska, J.O.; Prochaska, J.M.; Sherman, K. Transtheoretical model based multiple behavior intervention for weight management: Effectiveness on a population basis. *Prev. Med.* **2008**, *46*, 238–246. [CrossRef]
12. Prochaska, J.O.; DiClemente, C.C.; Norcross, J.C. In search of how people change. Applications to addictive behavior. *Am. Psychol.* **1992**, *47*, 1102–1114. [CrossRef]
13. Rosen, C.S. Is the sequencing of change processes by stage consistent across health problems? A meta-analysis. *Health Psychol.* **2000**, *19*, 593–604. [CrossRef]
14. Thompson, F.E.; Byers, T. Dietary Assessment Resource Manual. *J. Nutr.* **1994**, *124*, 2245–2317.
15. Ministry of Education Japan, Culture, Sports, Science and Technology; Office for Resources; Policy Division Science; Technology Policy Bureau. Source: Standard Table of Food Composition in Japan 2015 (Seventh Revised Version). Available online: http://www.mext.go.jp/a_menu/syokuhinseibun/1365295.htm (accessed on 25 December 2015).
16. Excel Eiyoukun Ver. 8.0. Available online: https://www.kenpakusha.co.jp/np/code/600821-01/ (accessed on 1 May 2016).
17. Intersalt Cooperative Research Group. Intersalt: An international study of electrolyte excretion and blood pressure. Results for 24-hour urinary sodium and potassium excretion. *Br. Med. J.* **1988**, *297*, 319–328. [CrossRef] [PubMed]
18. Salonen, J.T.; Tuomilehto, J.; Tanskanen, A. Relation of blood pressure to reported intake of salt, saturated fats, and alcohol in healthy middle-aged population. *J. Epidemiol. Community Health* **1983**, *37*, 32–37. [CrossRef] [PubMed]
19. Morgan, T.; Adam, W.; Gillies, A.; Wilson, M.; Morgan, G.; Carney, S. Hypertension treated by salt restriction. *Lancet* **1978**, *1*, 227–230. [CrossRef]
20. Meneely, G.R.; Dahl, L.K. Electrolytes in hypertension: The effects of sodium chloride. The evidence from animal and human studies. *Med. Clin. N. Am.* **1961**, *45*, 271–283. [CrossRef]

21. Asai, K.; Kobayashi, T.; Miyata, H.; Tanaka, Y.; Okada, Y.; Sakai, K.; Negoro, H.; Kamba, T.; Tsuji, H.; Shide, K.; et al. The short-term impact of dietary counseling on sodium intake and blood pressure in renal allograft recipients. *Prog. Transpl.* **2006**, *26*, 365–371. [CrossRef] [PubMed]
22. Kim, E.J.; Cho, S.W.; Kang, J.Y.; Choi, T.I.; Park, Y. Effects of a 12-week lifestyle intervention on health outcome and serum adipokines in middle-aged Korean men with borderline high blood pressure. *J. Am. Coll. Nutr.* **2012**, *31*, 352–360. [CrossRef]
23. Yoshimura, R.; Yamamoto, R.; Shinzawa, M.; Tomi, R.; Ozaki, S.; Fujii, Y.; Ito, T.; Tanabe, K.; Moriguchi, Y.; Isaka, Y.; et al. Drinking frequency modifies an association between salt intake and blood pressure: A cohort study. *J. Clin. Hypertens.* **2020**, *22*, 649–655. [CrossRef]
24. Pimenta, E.; Gaddam, K.K.; Oparil, S.; Aban, I.; Husain, S.; Dell'Italia, L.J.; Calhoun, D.A. Effects of dietary sodium reduction on blood pressure in subjects with resistant hypertension: Results from a randomized trial. *Hypertension* **2009**, *54*, 475–481. [CrossRef]
25. Sacks, F.M.; Svetkey, L.P.; Vollmer, W.M.; Appel, L.J.; Bray, G.A.; Harsha, D.; Obarzanek, E.; Conlin, P.R.; Miller, E.R.; Simons-Morton, D.G.; et al. Effects on blood pressure of reduced dietary sodium and the Dietary Approaches to Stop Hypertension (DASH) diet. DASH-Sodium Collaborative Research Group. *N. Engl. J. Med.* **2001**, *344*, 3–10. [CrossRef]
26. Nakamura, K.; Okamura, T.; Hayakawa, T.; Hozawa, A.; Kadowaki, T.; Murakami, Y.; Kita, Y.; Okayama, A.; Ueshima, H. The proportion of individuals with alcohol-induced hypertension among total hypertensives in a general Japanese population: NIPPON DATA90. *Hypertens. Res.* **2007**, *30*, 663–668. [CrossRef]
27. Xue, X.; Jiang, H.; Maria, G.; Motsamai, O.I.; Whelton, P.K. Effects of alcohol reduction on blood pressure: A meta-analysis of randomized controlled trials. *Hypertension* **2001**, *38*, 1112–1117.
28. Anderson, R.M.; Funnell, M.M.; Butler, P.M.; Arnold, M.S.; Fitzgerald, J.T.; Feste, C.C. Patient empowerment. Results of a randomized controlled trial. *Diabetes Care* **1995**, *18*, 943–949. [CrossRef] [PubMed]

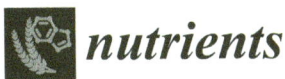

Article

Secular Decreasing Trend in Plasma Eicosapentaenoic and Docosahexaenoic Acids among Patients with Acute Coronary Syndrome from 2011 to 2019: A Single Center Descriptive Study

Tomoaki Okada [1], Toru Miyoshi [2,*], Masayuki Doi [1], Kosuke Seiyama [1], Wataru Takagi [1], Masahiro Sogo [1], Kazumasa Nosaka [1], Masahiko Takahashi [1], Keisuke Okawa [1] and Hiroshi Ito [2]

1. Department of Cardiology, Kagawa Prefectural Central Hospital, 1-2-1 Asahi-machi, Takamatsu City 760-8557, Japan; ju_10monomoto0622@yahoo.co.jp (T.O.); mdoimd@gmail.com (M.D.); k.seiyama9543@gmail.com (K.S.); t_wataru1206@yahoo.co.jp (W.T.); msogo0517@gmail.com (M.S.); kn_orch@yahoo.co.jp (K.N.); masahiko0707@infoseek.jp (M.T.); drop-in-bigriver@hotmail.co.jp (K.O.)
2. Department of Cardiovascular Medicine, Okayama University Graduate School of Medicine, Dentistry and Pharmaceutical Sciences, 2-5-1 Shikata-cho, Okayama City 700-8558, Japan; itomd@md.okayama-u.ac.jp
* Correspondence: miyoshit@cc.okayama-u.ac.jp; Tel.: +81-86-235-7351

Abstract: Despite intensive lipid-lowering interventions, patients treated with statins develop atherosclerotic cardiovascular disease (ASCVD), and these patients have an increased risk of developing recurrent cardiovascular events during follow-up. Therefore, there is a need to focus on the residual risks in patients in statin therapy to further reduce ASCVD. The aim of this study was to retrospectively investigate the 10-year trend (2011–2019) regarding changes in polyunsaturated fatty acids (PUFAs) in patients with acute coronary syndrome (ACS) in a single center. We included 686 men and 203 women with ACS admitted to Kagawa Prefectural Central Hospital. Plasma PUFAs, including eicosapentaenoic acid (EPA), docosahexaenoic acid (DHA), arachidonic acid (AA), and dihomo-γ-linolenic acid (DGLA), were measured at admission for suspected ACS. A secular decreasing trend in the levels of EPA and DHA and the EPA/AA ratio, but not of AA and DGLA, was observed. The analyses based on age (>70 or <70 years) and sex showed that the decreasing trend in the levels of EPA and DHA did not depend on age and remained significant only in men. Further studies are needed to obtain robust evidence to justify that the administration of n-3 PUFA contributes to the secondary prevention of ACS.

Keywords: atherosclerotic cardiovascular disease; polyunsaturated fatty acids; eicosapentaenoic acid; docosahexaenoic acid; arachidonic acid; descriptive study

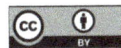

1. Introduction

Atherosclerotic cardiovascular disease (ASCVD) is the leading cause of mortality, accounting for 30% of all global deaths [1]. There are several methods to prevent ASCVD, including smoking cessation, increased physical activity, and weight loss [2]. The recent guidelines for the prevention of ASCVD recommend lipid-lowering agents, particularly statins, as the essence of primary and secondary prevention of ASCVD [3–5]. However, despite intensive lipid-lowering interventions, patients treated with statins develop ASCVD, and these patients have an increased recurrent risk of cardiovascular events [6–8]. Therefore, the residual risks in patients on statin therapy need to be the focus to further reduce ASCVD. An observational study showed that lower n-3 polyunsaturated fatty acids (PUFAs), especially eicosapentaenoic acid (EPA) and docosahexaenoic acid (DHA), were associated with the incidence of ASCVD [9]. Other studies have demonstrated that a low ratio of EPA to arachidonic acid (AA) is associated with a greater risk of cardiovascular disease [10–12]. Therefore, active screening of PUFAs is beneficial in identifying patients at high risk for ASCVD. A survey of a community-dwelling middle-aged and elderly Japanese population over 13 years from 1997 to 2012 showed that EPA and DHA concentrations increased in those aged over 60 years [13]. However, there is no data on the secular trend of PUFAs in patients with ASCVD. To establish appropriate intervention for secondary prevention, more recent data, especially in patients with ASCVD, is needed.

Therefore, we investigated the 10-year trend regarding changes in PUFAs in patients with acute coronary syndrome (ACS) based on data from a single center.

2. Materials and Methods

This was a single-center, retrospective, observational study. We enrolled 889 patients who were treated for ACS at the Kagawa Prefectural Central Hospital between January 2011 and December 2019. All these patients were evaluated for plasma EPA, DHA, AA, and dihomo-γ-linolenic acid (DGLA) on the day of admission for suspected ACS. ACS was diagnosed according to the American College of Cardiology/American Heart Association 2007 guideline; recent-onset chest pain, associated with ST segment and/or negative T wave electrocardiogram (ECG) changes and/or positive cardiac enzymes (creatine kinase or troponin T) [14]. Patients were excluded if they were administered pure EPA formulations.

This study was approved by the ethics committee of Kagawa Prefectural Central Hospital. The requirement for informed consent was waived because of the low-risk nature of the study and the inability to obtain consent directly from all the study subjects. Instead, we announced this study protocol extensively at Kagawa Prefectural Central Hospital and on the hospital website (http://www.chp-kagawa.jp/) and provided patients with the opportunity to withdraw from the study. The study was conducted in accordance with the principles of the Declaration of Helsinki.

2.1. Blood Sampling

Blood samples were obtained in the emergency room, and plasma levels of EPA, DHA, AA, and DGLA were measured at an external laboratory (SRL Inc., Tokyo, Japan). Routine laboratory tests, including total cholesterol, fasting triglycerides, low-density lipoprotein cholesterol (LDL-C), high-density lipoprotein cholesterol (HDL-C), hemoglobin A1c, and serum creatinine, were performed using an automated analyzer at Kagawa Prefectural Central Hospital. LDL concentration was assayed directly.

2.2. Assessment of Additional Risk Factors

Hypertension was confirmed according to the Japanese Society of Hypertension Guidelines for the Management of Hypertension 2014 [15]. Diabetes mellitus was defined as having a previous diagnosis of diabetes mellitus in the medical records, having a hemoglobin A1c (national glycohemoglobin standardization program calculation) level $\geq$ 6.5%, or receiving treatment with oral antidiabetic agents or insulin. Dyslipidemia was defined according to the Japan Atherosclerosis Society Guidelines for Prevention of Atherosclerotic Cardiovascular Diseases 2017 [16]. Smoking status was defined as currently smoking.

2.3. Statistical Analysis

Continuous variables are presented as mean ± standard deviation or mean ± 95% confidence interval (CI). Categorical variables are presented as frequency and proportion (%). The observation period was divided into three terms: the first term (2011–2013), second term (2014–2016), and third term (2017–2019). Differences among groups were evaluated using the chi-square test for categorical variables, and differences in continuous variables were compared by analysis of variance. Analysis of covariance allowed the comparison of PUFAs among groups while taking into account age and sex. For multiple comparisons, the Bonferroni post-hoc test was applied. A 2-tailed p-value of <0.05 was considered statistically significant. All statistical analyses were performed using SPSS 27.0 for Windows (IBM, Armonk, NY, USA).

3. Results

Analysis of the patient characteristics and lipid profile of the study population according to the terms as shown in Table 1, patients in the third term were significantly older than those in the second term. The prevalence of dyslipidemia in the third term was significantly lower than that in the second term. There was a higher prevalence of patients with current smoking habit and statin use in the second term than in the first and third terms, respectively. The level of hemoglobin A1c in the second term was significantly lower than that in the first term. The level of triglyceride in the third term was significantly lower than that in the first term, whereas the levels of LDL-C and HDL-C did not differ among the three terms.

Table 1. Patient characteristics in the first, second and third terms.

	First Term (2011–2013), $n = 238$	Second Term (2014–2016), $n = 285$	Third Term (2017–2019), $n = 366$	p Value
Age, years	70.3 ± 11.4	68.5 ± 12.1	71.7 ± 12.7 #	0.003
Male/female	181 (76)/57 (24)	227 (80)/58 (20)	278 (76)/88 (24)	0.480
Body mass index, kg/m^2	23.7 ± 3.8	23.9 ± 3.4	23.8 ± 3.8	0.765
Hypertension	165 (69)	211 (74)	264 (72)	0.489
Diabetes mellitus	92 (39)	95 (33)	140 (38)	0.340
Dyslipidemia	159 (67)	199 (70)	219 (60) #	0.023
Current smoker	69 (29)	124 (43.8) *	107 (29) #	<0.001
AMI/UAP	160 (67)/78 (33)	194 (68)/91 (32)	245 (67)/121 (33)	0.097
History of CAD	37 (16)	32 (11)	47 (13)	0.34
Statin	39 (16)	74 (26) *	67 (18) #	0.012
Ezetimibe	N/A	5 (2)	7 (2)	0.710
ACEI/ARB	65 (28)	108 (37)	106 (28)	0.770
β-blocker	22 (9)	28 (10)	31 (8)	0.995
Serum creatinine, mg/dL	1.00 ± 0.91	0.98 ± 0.88	1.18 ± 1.49	0.057
Hemoglobin A1c, %	6.4 ± 1.3	6.0 ± 0.9 *	6.2 ± 1.1	0.005
Total cholesterol, mg/dL	181 ± 39	185 ± 44	180 ± 40	0.223
LDL-C, mg/dL	114 ± 33	116 ± 36	113 ± 34	0.692
Triglyceride, mg/dL	110 ± 131	114 ± 99	94 ± 77 #	0.037
HDL-C, mg/dL	42 ± 10	44 ± 12	44 ± 12	0.257
EPA, μg/mL	63.0 ± 42.2	60.2 ± 38.3	51.6 ± 33.2 *#	<0.001
DHA, μg/mL	138.1 ± 51.7	130.2 ± 51.0	116.0 ± 43.8 *#	<0.001
AA, μg/mL	169.6 ± 45.6	178.3 ± 53.2	180.8 ± 55.7 *	0.032
DGLA, μg/mL	36.0 ± 14.7	39.3 ± 15.2 *	36.0 ± 14.8 #	0.010
EPA/AA	0.37 ± 0.22	0.35 ± 0.22	0.29 ± 0.18 *#	<0.001

Categorical variables are presented as number of patients (%). Continuous variables are presented as mean ± standard deviation. AMI, acute myocardial infarction; UAP, unstable angina pectoris; CAD, coronary artery disease; N/A, not available; ACEI/ARB, angiotensin-converting-enzyme inhibitor/angiotensin II Receptor Blocker; HDL-C, high-density lipoprotein cholesterol; LDL-C, low-density lipoprotein cholesterol; EPA, eicosapentaenoic acid; DHA, docosahexaenoic acid; DGLA, dihomo-γ-linolenic acid; AA, arachidonic acid. * $p < 0.05$ versus first term and # $p < 0.05$ versus second term. For multiple comparisons, the Bonferroni post-hoc test was applied.

On analyzing the secular trend of EPA, AA, DGLA, AA, and EPA/AA levels in all patients, and according to age (>70 or < 70years) and sex (Table 2), the levels of EPA and DHA in the third term were significantly lower than those in the first and second terms, respectively. The AA level in the third term was significantly higher than that in the first term. The DGLA level in the second term was significantly higher than that in the first and third terms. Regarding the influence of age on the trend, the levels of EPA and DHA in the third term remained significantly lower than those in the first term in both patients aged <70 years and >70 years. Regarding the influence of sex on the trend, the levels of EPA and DHA in the third term remained significantly lower than those in the first term in men, but not in women. The levels of AA and DGLA did not differ among the three terms regardless of age and sex. The EPA/AA ratio in the third term was significantly lower than that in the first term regardless of age, and this difference remained significant in men, but not in women.

Table 2. Secular trend in polyunsaturated fatty acids in all patients.

	First Term (2011–2013)	Second Term (2014–2016)	Third Term (2017–2019)	p Value
EPA, µg/mL				
All patients	63.0 ± 42.2	60.2 ± 38.3	51.6 ± 33.2 *#	<0.001
Age ≤ 70 years	62.8 ± 40.1	57.9 ± 37.4	49.5 ± 31.2 *	0.010
Age > 70 years	65.9 ± 50.4	62.6 ± 36.6	53.4 ± 34.9 *	0.018
Men	64.5 ± 43.9	58.8 ± 36.7	51.7 ± 31.7 *	0.002
Women	63.8 ± 50.3	64.8 ± 38.3	51.3 ± 37.8	0.080
DHA, µg/mL				
All patients	138.1 ± 51.7	130.2 ± 51.0	116.0 ± 43.8 *#	<0.001
Age ≤ 70 years	142.9 ± 62.5	128.6 ± 49.0	110.9 ± 41.9 *	<0.001
Age > 70 years	139.0 ± 48.1	131.6 ± 48.4	120.2 ± 45.1 *	0.004
Men	140.5 ± 59.1	126.3 ± 46.0 *	111.7 ± 38.9 *,#	<0.001
Women	142.2 ± 44.4	143.9 ± 56.0	129.4 ± 54.7	0.183
AA, µg/mL				
All patients	169.6 ± 45.6	178.3 ± 53.2	180.8 ± 55.7 *	0.032
Age ≤ 70 years	179.4 ± 53.1	185.7 ± 53.2	192.0 ± 61.7	0.225
Age > 70 years	161.9 ± 39.4	164.7 ± 46.4	171.5 ± 48.4	0.186
Men	169.7 ± 48.1	171.3 ± 50.5	179.4 ± 53.3	0.093
Women	174.1 ± 45.8	194.8 ± 50.3	185.5 ± 63.1	0.150
DGLA, µg/mL				
All patients	36.0 ± 14.7	39.3 ± 15.2 *	36.0 ± 14.8 #	0.010
Age ≤ 70 years	40.1 ± 17.2	42.8 ± 16.0	39.6 ± 14.3	0.124
Age > 70 years	32.4 ±12.7	33.5 ± 11.1	33.1 ± 14.6	0.813
Men	36.6 ± 15.6	38.2 ± 15.0	36.2 ± 15.6	0.298
Women	35.2 ± 15.5	40.1 ± 13.4	35.6 ± 12.2	0.066
EPA/AA				
All patients	0.37 ± 0.22	0.35 ± 0.22	0.29 ± 0.18 *,#	<0.001
Age ≤ 70 years	0.35 ± 0.19	0.32 ± 0.20	0.27 ± 0.17 *	0.002
Age > 70 years	0.40 ± 0.28	0.439 ± 0.23	0.31 ± 0.19 *	0.001
Men	0.38 ± 0.24	0.36 ± 0.21	0.30 ± 0.21 *	<0.001
Women	0.35 ± 0.22	0.35 ± 0.23	0.27 ± 0.17	0.035

Continuous variables are presented as mean ± standard deviation. EPA, eicosapentaenoic acid; DHA, docosahexaenoic acid; DGLA, dihomo-γ-linolenic acid; AA, arachidonic acid. * $p < 0.05$ versus first term and # $p < 0.05$ versus second term. For multiple comparisons, the Bonferroni post-hoc test was applied.

Next, the secular trends of EPA, AA, DGLA, and EPA/AA levels in patients with and without diabetes were analyzed separately (Tables 3 and 4). The trend in patients with diabetes was similar to that in all patients. However, in patients without diabetes, the levels of EPA in the third term were significantly lower than those in the second term in women >70 years; the levels of DHA in the third term were significantly lower than those in the second term regardless age and sex; and the EPA/AA ratio in the third term was significantly lower than that in the first and the second terms in women >70 years.

Based on Figure 1, which shows the secular trend in the age- and sex-adjusted EPA, AA, DGLA, and EPA/AA levels, the adjusted levels of PUFAs [mean (95% CI)] in the first, second, and third terms were 62.4 (55.5–69.2), 57.6 (52.4–62.8), and 47.7 (42.6–52.8) of EPA (µg/mL, $p = 0.001$); 142.4 (133.9–150.6), 128.7 (122.3–13.5.1), and 116.6 (110.3–122.9) of DHA (µg/mL, $p < 0.001$); 174.9 (165.7–14.0), 182.7 (175.8–189.6), 186.8 (180.1–193.6) of AA ($p = 0.102$); 39.2 (36.8–41.7), 40.2 (38.4–42.0), and 37.0 (35.2–38.8) of DGLA (µg/mL, $p = 0.045$), 0.63 (0.32–0.40), 0.33 (0.30–0.36), and 0.26 (0.23–0.29) of EPA/AA ($p < 0.001$), respectively.

Table 3. Secular trend in polyunsaturated fatty acids in patients with diabetes.

	First Term (2011–2013), n = 92	Second Term (2014–2016), n = 95	Third Term (2017–2019), n = 139	p Value
EPA, μg/mL				
Age ≤ 70 years	71.2 ± 44.3	58.1 ± 32.2	46.3 ± 28.2 *,#	0.001
Age > 70 years	71.4 ± 50.5	62.5 ± 40.8	54.3 ± 41.4 *	0.125
Men	71.6 ± 49.3	59.9 ± 37.8	48.2 ± 28.5 *,#	<0.001
Women	70.2 ± 37.1	61.4 ± 31.8	60.0 ± 56.1	0.732
DHA, μg/mL				
Age ≤ 70 years	145.4 ± 67.4	127.7 ± 46.8	106.2 ± 43.7 *,#	0.001
Age > 70 years	146.3 ± 51.1	131.4 ± 58.3	120.6 ± 54.7 *	0.055
Men	144.6 ± 65.0	125.9 ± 47.8 *	106.6 ± 37.1 *,#	<0.001
Women	150.4 ± 38.8	142.9 ± 66.4	142.1 ± 77.6	0.903
AA, μg/mL				
Age ≤ 70 years	183.0 ± 58.8	239.4 ± 331.6	194.8 ± 70.9	0.297
Age > 70 years	162.6 ± 36.6	173.0 ± 38.6	170.4 ± 42.5	0.455
Men	173.0 ± 52.6	210.2 ± 272.1	178.3 ± 50.9	0.266
Women	177.1 ± 45.1	199.6 ± 64.4	191.2 ± 78.1	0.569
DGLA, μg/mL				
Age ≤ 70 years	42.6 ± 19.2	44.5 ± 16.4	39.9 ± 14.4	0.348
Age > 70 years	32.5 ± 12.2	34.7 ± 12.8	31.2 ± 11.0	0.280
Men	38.2 ± 17.7	39.8 ± 15.1	34.7 ± 13.1 #	0.063
Women	37.8 ± 15.3	40.1 ± 17.5	36.2 ± 13.9	0.694
EPA/AA				
Age ≤ 70 years	0.38 ± 0.20	0.31 ± 0.19	0.25 ± 0.14 *,#	<0.001
Age > 70 years	0.45 ± 0.33	0.36 ± 0.24	0.31 ± 0.19 *	0.016
Men	0.42 ± 0.27	0.34 ± 0.23	0.28 ± 0.16 *,#	<0.001
Women	0.40 ± 0.23	0.31 ± 0.14	0.30 ± 0.23	0.220

Continuous variables are presented as mean ± standard deviation. EPA, eicosapentaenoic acid; DHA, docosahexaenoic acid; DGLA, dihomo-γ-linolenic acid; AA, arachidonic acid. * $p < 0.05$ versus first term and # $p < 0.05$ versus second term. For multiple comparisons, the Bonferroni post-hoc test was applied.

Table 4. Secular trend in polyunsaturated fatty acids in patients without diabetes.

	First Term (2011–2013), n = 146	Second Term (2014–2016), n = 190	Third Term (2017–2019), n = 227	p Value
EPA, μg/mL				
Age ≤ 70 years	54.9 ± 29.5	57.7 ± 42.6	51.3 ± 32.8	0.434
Age > 70 years	60.9 ± 45.4	63.2 ± 35.2	52.8 ± 30.0 #	0.096
Men	56.8 ± 32.1	58.6 ± 38.6	53.9 ± 33.6	0.491
Women	60.7 ± 52.0	66.7 ± 42.2	46.8 ± 22.7 #	0.036
DHA, μg/mL				
Age ≤ 70 years	134.7 ± 47.5	129.0 ± 54.2	113.7 ± 40.8 *,#	0.009
Age > 70 years	131.7 ± 42.3	132.3 ± 46.0	119.9 ± 37.8 *,#	0.057
Men	131.1 ± 45.1	127.1 ± 48.4	115.0 ± 39.9 *,#	0.006
Women	139.1 ± 44.3	144.3 ± 56.8	122.9 ± 37.1 #	0.057
AA, μg/mL				
Age ≤ 70 years	175.0 ± 41.2	185.0 ± 53.1	190.3 ± 56.1 *	0.146
Age > 70 years	158.5 ± 41.0	163.7 ± 51.3	172.2 ± 52.0	0.151
Men	164.0 ± 40.1	169.8 ± 54.1	180.1 ± 54.8 *	0.031
Women	174.9 ± 45.9	197.1 ± 43.8 *	182.5 ± 54.3	0.137
DGLA, μg/mL				
Age ≤ 70 years	37.6 ± 13.1	43.4 ± 16.7 *	39.4 ± 14.3	0.027
Age > 70 years	31.6 ± 11.9	33.7 ± 10.7	34.3 ± 16.5	0.420
Men	34.7 ± 12.4	38.4 ± 15.7 *	37.2 ± 16.9	0.177
Women	34.4 ± 14.1	41.4 ± 11.8 *	35.3 ± 11.4 #	0.024

Table 4. Cont.

	First Term (2011–2013), n = 146	Second Term (2014–2016), n = 190	Third Term (2017–2019), n = 227	p Value
EPA/AA				
Age ≤ 70 years	0.31 ±0.16	0.32 ± 0.22	0.28 ± 0.18	0.312
Age > 70 years	0.37 ± 0.22	0.40 ± 0.22	0.31± 0.18 *,#	0.006
Men	0.35 ± 0.18	0.35 ± 0.22	0.31 ± 0.20	0.101
Women	0.33 ± 0.22	0.36 ± 0.26	0.26 ± 0.12 #	0.038

Continuous variables are presented as mean ± standard deviation. EPA, eicosapentaenoic acid; DHA, docosahexaenoic acid; DGLA, dihomo-γ-linolenic acid; AA, arachidonic acid. * $p < 0.05$ versus first term and # $p < 0.05$ versus second term. For multiple comparisons, the Bonferroni post-hoc test was applied.

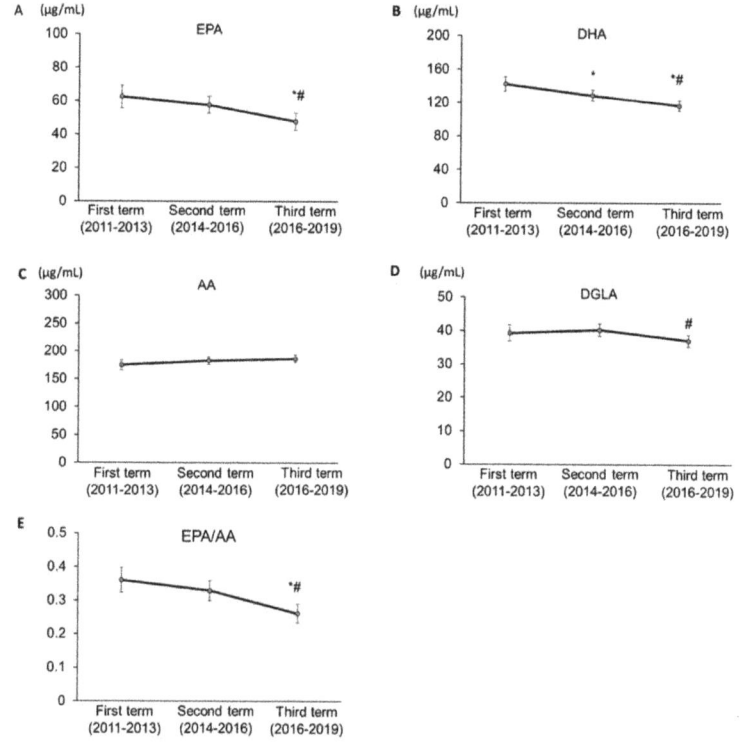

Figure 1. Secular trend in age- and sex- adjusted polyunsaturated fatty acids and EPA/AA. (**A**) EPA, (**B**) DHA, (**C**) AA, (**D**) DGLA, and (**E**) EPA/AA Data are presented as mean ± 95% confidence interval. EPA, eicosapentaenoic acid; DHA, docosahexaenoic acid; DGLA, dihomo-γ-linolenic acid; AA, arachidonic acid. * $p < 0.05$ versus first term and # $p < 0.05$ versus second term. Analysis of covariance allowed the comparison of PUFAs among groups while taking into account age and sex. For multiple comparisons, the Bonferroni post-hoc test was applied.

4. Discussion

This study demonstrated a decreasing trend in the levels of EPA, DHA, and EPA/AA, but not of AA and DGLA. Analyses based on age (<70 and >70 years) and sex showed that this decreasing trend in the levels of EPA and DHA did not depend on age and was significant only in men. To our knowledge, this is the first study to describe changes in PUFAs over a decade in patients with ACS.

A previous study from 1997 to 2012 in a contemporary healthy Japanese population living in an urban area showed a secular increasing trend in the serum levels of EPA and DHA in the population aged over 60 years [17]. The present study evaluated subsequent changes in PUFAs from 2011 to 2019 in patients with ACS and demonstrated a decreasing trend in plasma EPA and DHA. After 2010, a substantial reduction in the fish intake in the Japanese elderly population was reported [18], which could be an explanation of this decreasing trend of n-3 PUFAs in the present study, as fish intake is closely correlated with circulating n-3 PUFAs level [19]. Another explanation is the difference in participant characteristics between the general population and patients with ACS. A previous study in patients with ACS showed that the mean levels of EPA and DHA during 2004 and 2011 were 73.4 µg/mL and 146.9 µg/mL, respectively, which were slightly higher than those in the first term (2011–2013) in our study (63.0 µg/mL and 138.1 µg/mL, respectively). Furthermore, the level of AA during 2004 and 2011 in patients with ACS was reported to be 159.9 µg/mL, which was moderately lower than that in the first term in the present study of 169.6 µg/mL. Thus, in patients with ACS, a decreasing trend in the levels of EPA, DHA, and EPA/AA may have continued before 2011. However, further larger studies are needed to confirm this decreasing trend in patients with ACS.

The mechanisms underlying the favorable effects of n-3 PUFAs remain partly unknown [20], whereas previous experimental studies showed that n-3 PUFAs have multiple actions towards prevention of ASCVD, including anti-inflammatory effect [21], inhibition of platelet aggregation [22], and improvement of endothelial function [23]. Several studies using intra-coronary imaging showed that circulating EPA levels were associated with lipid plaque volume, [24] and fibrous-cap thickness of the plaque [25]. A randomized control study evaluating coronary plaque change by multidetector computed tomography showed that treatment with n-3 PUFA formulation for 18 months significantly reduced the accumulation of low-attenuation plaque, which is a component of vulnerable plaque, compared to placebo [26]. Furthermore, a recent study showed that the proportion of EPA in serum phosphatidylcholine at the time of ACS was associated with further clinical adverse events [27]. Thus, clinical trials and basic experiments suggest an important association between n-3 PUFAs and the development of ASCVD.

The Japanese Registry of All Cardiac and Vascular Disease showed that the number of patients with ACS is slightly increasing in Japan (http://www.j-circ.or.jp/jittai_chosa/). Furthermore, despite significant improvement in cardiovascular events by intensive statin treatment, up to 40% of statin-treated patients continue to experience recurrent cardiovascular events [8]. Thus, the control of risk factors beyond LDL-C and residual risk is an emerging problem for preventing ASCVD. In this context, n-3 PUFA has been evaluated as a residual cardiovascular risk factor. Our study demonstrated the secular decreasing trend in the levels of EPA, DHA, and EPA/AA without significant changes in LDL-C and HDL-C. Although our study did not evaluate the association between the secular decreasing trend and the incidence of ASCVD, it highlights the importance of n-3 PUFAs in the development of ACS.

Previous studies have shown that triglyceride-rich lipoproteins, the main carriers of triglycerides, are associated with foam cell formation via macrophage uptake directly at the arterial wall, which results in the development of atherosclerosis [28]. In addition, recent genetic studies have provided robust evidence of the role of triglycerides in the causal pathway for ASCVD [29]. Thus, supplemental n-3 PUFA lower triglyceride can be used as a treatment in patients with hypertriglyceridemia. However, the clinical benefit of the treatment of hypertriglyceridemia for the prevention of ASCVD has not been established. Future clinical trials are needed to determine whether triglyceride-lowering therapies reduce the risk of ASCVD in patients with hypertriglyceridemia. In addition, lipoprotein(a), which is composed of an LDL-like particle and characteristic glycoprotein apolipoprotein(a) connected by a disulfide bond, has been recognized as a residual risk of ASCVD [30]. Thus, the control of residual risks is an emerging issue to prevent ASCVD after the achievement of substantial reduction of LDL-C.

Although a few clinical studies have shown the effectiveness of n-3 PUFAs in high-risk patients, the benefit of n-3 PUFAs in the prevention of ASCVD remains controversial [31–42]. For primary prevention, a study of cardiovascular events in diabetes (ASCEND) [43] and a long-term outcomes study to assess STatin Residual Risk Reduction With EpaNova in HiGh Cardiovascular Risk PatienTs With Hypertriglyceridemia (STRENGTH) [44] failed to show a significant reduction in ASCVD by n-3 PUFA formulation in high risk patients. The Vitamin D and Omega-3 Trial (VITAL) showed that supplemental n-3 PUFAs did not significantly reduce the primary cardiovascular end point of major cardiovascular events (composite of myocardial infarction, stroke, and cardiovascular mortality), but were associated with significant reductions in total myocardial infarction, percutaneous coronary intervention, and fatal myocardial infarction [45]. On the other hand, for secondary prevention, Reduction of Cardiovascular Events With EPA—Intervention Trial (REDUCE-IT) [46] showed a significant reduction in ASCVD. There were several differences among the studies. One issue is the formulation of n-3 PUFAs. The ASCEND, the VITAL, and the STRENGTH tested mixed formulations of EPA and DHA, whereas the REDUCE-IT evaluated pure EPA formulation. Another issue is the dose of n-3 PUFA. Participants in the ASCEND and the VITAL received 1 g/day of n-3 PUFA, whereas participants in the STRENGTH and the REDUCE-IT received 4 g/day. A high dose of n-3 PUFA formulation may be preferable because circulating EPA levels were shown to be tightly linked with ASCVD outcomes in the REDUCE-IT trial [46]. Furthermore, it is possible that the specific formulation of n-3 PUFAs makes a difference because the biological roles of EPA and DHA in tissue are different [18]. Further large-scale, carefully planned, and controlled clinical studies are needed to provide solid evidence that n-3 PUFAs can prevent ASCVD.

There are several limitations in this study. This study was retrospectively performed at a single center located in a costal provincial city. Therefore, the study results cannot be applied directly to patients living in urban areas. Second, this study did not aim to analyze the causal relationship between the decrease in the levels of EPA and DHA, EPA/AA, and the incidence of ACS. Further investigation is needed to achieve robust evidence on the role of n-3 PUFAs in preventing ASCVD.

5. Conclusions

This study demonstrated a decreasing trend in the levels of EPA and DHA, and EPA/AA in men from 2011 to 2019 without significant changes in the levels of LDL-C and HDL-C. This decreasing trend in the levels of EPA and DHA did not depend on age and was significant only in men. Considering the results of recent large-scale trials, administration of a sufficient dose of n-3 PUFAs may contribute to the secondary prevention of ACS, but further studies are needed to obtain robust evidence.

Author Contributions: Conceptualization, M.D.; formal analysis, M.D. and T.M.; investigation, T.O., K.S., W.T., M.S., K.N., M.T. and K.O.; writing—original draft preparation, T.O. and T.M.; writing—review and editing, H.I. All authors have read and agreed to the published version of the manuscript.

Funding: This research received no external funding.

Institutional Review Board Statement: The study was conducted according to the guidelines of the Declaration of Helsinki and approved by the Ethics Committee of Kagawa Prefectural Central Hospital.

Informed Consent Statement: Patient consent was waived due to the low-risk nature of the study and the inability to obtain consent directly from all the study subjects.

Data Availability Statement: The data presented in this study are available on request from the corresponding author.

Conflicts of Interest: The authors declare no conflict of interest.

References

1. Roth, G.A.; Abate, D.; Abate, K.H.; Abay, S.M.; Abbafati, C.; Abbasi, N.; Abbastabar, H.; Abd-Allah, F.; Abdela, J.; Abdelalim, A.; et al. Global, regional, and national age-sex-specific mortality for 282 causes of death in 195 countries and territories, 1980–2017: A systematic analysis for the global burden of disease study 2017. *Lancet* **2018**, *392*, 1736–1788. [CrossRef]
2. Piepoli, M.F.; Hoes, A.W.; Agewall, S.; Albus, C.; Brotons, C.; Catapano, A.L.; Cooney, M.T.; Corrà, U.; Cosyns, B.; Deaton, C.; et al. 2016 European Guidelines on cardiovascular disease prevention in clinical practice: The Sixth Joint Task Force of the European Society of Cardiology and Other Societies on Cardiovascular Disease Prevention in Clinical Practice (constituted by representatives of 10 societies and by invited experts) Developed with the special contribution of the European Association for Cardiovascular Prevention & Rehabilitation (EACPR). *Eur. Heart J.* **2016**, *37*, 2315–2381. [PubMed]
3. Arnett, D.K.; Blumenthal, R.S.; Albert, M.A.; Buroker, A.B.; Goldberger, Z.D.; Hahn, E.J.; Himmelfarb, C.D.; Khera, A.; Lloyd-Jones, D.; McEvoy, J.W.; et al. 2019 ACC/AHA guideline on the primary prevention of cardiovascular disease: A report of the American College of Cardiology/American Heart Association Task Force on Clinical Practice Guidelines. *J. Am. Coll. Cardiol.* **2019**, *74*, e177–e232. [CrossRef] [PubMed]
4. Mach, F.; Baigent, C.; Catapano, A.L.; Koskinas, K.C.; Casula, M.; Badimon, L.; Chapman, M.J.; De Backer, G.G.; Delgado, V.; Ference, B.A.; et al. 2019 ESC/EAS Guidelines for the management of dyslipidaemias: Lipid modification to reduce cardiovascular risk. *Atherosclerosis* **2019**, *290*, 140–205. [CrossRef] [PubMed]
5. Kimura, K.; Kimura, T.; Ishihara, M.; Nakagawa, Y.; Nakao, K.; Miyauchi, K.; Sakamoto, T.; Tsujita, K.; Hagiwara, N.; Miyazaki, S.; et al. JCS 2018 Guideline on diagnosis and treatment of acute coronary syndrome. *Circ. J.* **2019**, *83*, 1085–1196. [CrossRef] [PubMed]
6. Stone, S.G.; Serrao, G.W.; Mehran, R.; Tomey, M.I.; Witzenbichler, B.; Guagliumi, G.; Peruga, J.Z.; Brodie, B.R.; Dudek, D.; Möckel, M.; et al. Incidence, predictors, and implications of reinfarction after primary percutaneous coronary intervention in ST-segment-elevation myocardial infarction: The harmonizing outcomes with revascularization and stents in acute myocardial infarction trial. *Circ. Cardiovasc. Interv.* **2014**, *7*, 543–551. [CrossRef]
7. Motivala, A.A.; Tamhane, U.; Ramanath, V.S.; Saab, F.; Montgomery, D.G.; Fang, J.; Kline-Rogers, E.; May, N.; Ng, G.; Froehlich, J.; et al. A prior myocardial infarction: How does it affect management and outcomes in recurrent acute coronary syndromes? *Clin. Cardiol.* **2008**, *31*, 590–596. [CrossRef]
8. Sachdeva, A.; Cannon, C.P.; Deedwania, P.C.; Labresh, K.A.; Smith, S.C., Jr.; Dai, D.; Hernandez, A.; Fonarow, G.C. Lipid levels in patients hospitalized with coronary artery disease: An analysis of 136,905 hospitalizations in Get with the Guidelines. *Am. Heart J.* **2009**, *157*, 111–117. [CrossRef]
9. Iso, H.; Kobayashi, M.; Ishihara, J.; Sasaki, S.; Okada, K.; Kita, Y.; Kokubo, Y.; Tsugane, S.; JPHC Study Group. Intake of fish and n3 fatty acids and risk of coronary heart disease among Japanese: The Japan Public Health Center-Based (JPHC) Study Cohort I. *Circulation* **2006**, *113*, 195–202. [CrossRef]
10. Domei, T.; Yokoi, H.; Kuramitsu, S.; Soga, Y.; Arita, T.; Ando, K.; Shirai, S.; Kondo, K.; Sakai, K.; Goya, M.; et al. Ratio of serum n-3 to n-6 polyunsaturated fatty acids and the incidence of major adverse cardiac events in patients undergoing percutaneous coronary intervention. *Circ. J.* **2012**, *76*, 423–429. [CrossRef]
11. Ueeda, M.; Doumei, T.; Takaya, Y.; Ohnishi, N.; Takaishi, A.; Hirohata, S.; Miyoshi, T.; Shinohata, R.; Usui, S.; Kusachi, S. Association of serum levels of arachidonic acid and eicosapentaenoic acid with prevalence of major adverse cardiac events after acute myocardial infarction. *Heart Vessel.* **2011**, *26*, 145–152. [CrossRef] [PubMed]
12. Ninomiya, T.; Nagata, M.; Hata, J.; Hirakawa, Y.; Ozawa, M.; Yoshida, D.; Ohara, T.; Kishimoto, H.; Mukai, N.; Fukuhara, M.; et al. Association between ratio of serum eicosapentaenoic acid to arachidonic acid and risk of cardiovascular disease: The Hisayama Study. *Atherosclerosis* **2013**, *231*, 261–267. [CrossRef] [PubMed]
13. Otsuka, R.; Kato, Y.; Imai, T.; Ando, F.; Shimokata, H. Secular trend of serum docosahexaenoic acid, eicosapentaenoic acid, and arachidonic acid concentrations among Japanese-a 4- and 13-year descriptive epidemiologic study. *Prostaglandins Leukot. Essent. Fatty Acids* **2015**, *94*, 35–42. [CrossRef] [PubMed]
14. King, S.B., 3rd; Smith, S.C., Jr.; Hirshfeld, J.W., Jr.; Jacobs, A.K.; Morrison, D.A.; Williams, D.O.; Feldman, T.E.; Kern, M.J.; O'Neill, W.W.; Schaff, H.V.; et al. 2007 focused update of the ACC/AHA/SCAI 2005 guideline update for percutaneous coronary intervention: A report of the American College of Cardiology/American Heart Association Task Force on Practice guidelines. *J. Am. Coll. Cardiol.* **2008**, 172–209. [CrossRef] [PubMed]
15. Shimamoto, K.; Ando, K.; Fujita, T.; Hasebe, N.; Higaki, J.; Horiuchi, M.; Imai, Y.; Imaizumi, T.; Ishimitsu, T.; Ito, M.; et al. The Japanese Society of Hypertension Guidelines for the Management of Hypertension (JSH 2014). *Hypertens. Res.* **2014**, *37*, 253–390. [PubMed]
16. Kinoshita, M.; Yokote, K.; Arai, H.; Iida, M.; Ishigaki, Y.; Ishibashi, S.; Umemoto, S.; Egusa, G.; Ohmura, H.; Okamura, T.; et al. Japan Atherosclerosis Society (JAS) Guidelines for Prevention of Atherosclerotic Cardiovascular Diseases 2017. *J. Atheroscler. Thromb.* **2018**, *25*, 846–984. [CrossRef] [PubMed]
17. Yanagisawa, N.; Shimada, K.; Miyazaki, T.; Kume, A.; Kitamura, Y.; Ichikawa, R.; Ohmura, H.; Kiyanagi, T.; Hiki, M.; Fukao, K.; et al. Polyunsaturated fatty acid levels of serum and red blood cells in apparently healthy Japanese subjects living in an urban area. *J. Atheroscler. Thromb.* **2010**, *17*, 285–294. [CrossRef] [PubMed]
18. Yokoyama, S. Beneficial effect of retuning to "Japan Diet" for the Japanese. *J. Atheroscler. Thromb.* **2019**, *26*, 1–2. [CrossRef]

19. Shijo, Y.; Maruyama, C.; Nakamura, E.; Nakano, R.; Shima, M.; Mae, A.; Okabe, Y.; Park, S.; Kameyama, N.; Hirai, S. Japan diet intake changes serum phospholipid fatty acid compositions in middle-aged men: A pilot study. *J. Atheroscler. Thromb.* **2019**, *26*, 3–13. [CrossRef]
20. Mason, R.P.; Libby, P.; Bhatt, D.L. Emerging mechanisms of cardiovascular protection for the omega-3 fatty acid eicosapentaenoic acid. *Arterioscler. Thromb. Vasc. Biol.* **2020**, *40*, 1135–1147. [CrossRef]
21. Bäck, M.; Hansson, G.K. Omega-3 fatty acids, cardiovascular risk, and the resolution of inflammation. *FASEB J.* **2019**, *33*, 1536–1539. [CrossRef] [PubMed]
22. Krämer, H.J.; Stevens, J.; Grimminger, F.; Seeger, W. Fish oil fatty acids and human platelets: Dose-dependent decrease in dienoic and increase in trienoic thromboxane generation. *Biochem. Pharmacol.* **1996**, *52*, 1211–1217. [CrossRef]
23. Mason, R.P.; Dawoud, H.; Jacob, R.F.; Sherratt, S.C.R.; Malinski, T. Eicosapentaenoic acid improves endothelial function and nitric oxide bioavailability in a manner that is enhanced in combination with a statin. *Biomed. Pharmacother.* **2018**, *103*, 1231–1237. [CrossRef] [PubMed]
24. Niki, T.; Wakatsuki, T.; Yamaguchi, K.; Taketani, Y.; Oeduka, H.; Kusunose, K.; Ise, T.; Iwase, T.; Yamada, H.; Soeki, T.; et al. Effects of the addition of eicosapentaenoic acid to strong statin therapy on inflammatory cytokines and coronary plaque components assessed by integrated backscatter intravascular ultrasound. *Circ. J.* **2016**, *80*, 450–460. [CrossRef] [PubMed]
25. Nishio, R.; Shinke, T.; Otake, H.; Nakagawa, M.; Nagoshi, R.; Inoue, T.; Kozuki, A.; Hariki, H.; Osue, T.; Taniguchi, Y.; et al. Stabilizing effect of combined eicosapentaenoic acid and statin therapy on coronary thin-cap fibroatheroma. *Atherosclerosis* **2014**, *234*, 114–119. [CrossRef]
26. Budoff, M.J.; Bhatt, D.L.; Kinninger, A.; Lakshmanan, S.; Muhlestein, J.B.; Le, V.T.; May, H.T.; Shaikh, K.; Shekar, C.; Roy, S.K.; et al. Effect of icosapent ethyl on progression of coronary atherosclerosis in patients with elevated triglycerides on statin therapy: Final results of the EVAPORATE trial. *Eur. Heart J.* **2020**, *41*, 3925–3932. [CrossRef]
27. Lázaro, I.; Rueda, F.; Cediel, G.; Ortega, E.; García-García, C.; Sala-Vila, A.; Bayés-Genís, A. Circulating omega-3 fatty acids and incident adverse events in patients with acute myocardial infarction. *J. Am. Coll. Cardiol.* **2020**, *76*, 2089–2097. [CrossRef]
28. Nordestgaard, B.G.; Varbo, A. Triglycerides and cardiovascular disease. *Lancet* **2014**, *384*, 626–635. [CrossRef]
29. Nordestgaard, B.G. Triglyceride-rich lipoproteins and atherosclerotic cardiovascular disease: New insights from epidemiology, genetics, and biology. *Circ. Res.* **2016**, *118*, 547–563. [CrossRef]
30. Cesaro, A.; Schiavo, A.; Moscarella, E.; Coletta, S.; Conte, M.; Gragnano, F.; Fimiani, F.; Monda, E.; Caiazza, M.; Limongelli, G.; et al. Lipoprotein(a): A genetic marker for cardiovascular disease and target for emerging therapies. *J. Cardiovasc. Med. (Hagerstown)* **2020**. [CrossRef]
31. Abdelhamid, A.S.; Brown, T.J.; Brainard, J.S.; Biswas, P.; Thorpe, G.C.; Moore, H.J.; Deane, K.H.; Summerbell, C.D.; Worthington, H.V.; Song, F.; et al. Omega-3 fatty acids for the primary and secondary prevention of cardiovascular disease. *Cochrane Database Syst. Rev.* **2020**, CD003177. [CrossRef] [PubMed]
32. Alexander, D.D.; Miller, P.E.; Van Elswyk, M.E.; Kuratko, C.N.; Bylsma, L.C. A Meta-Analysis of Randomized Controlled Trials and Prospective Cohort Studies of Eicosapentaenoic and Docosahexaenoic Long-Chain Omega-3 Fatty Acids and Coronary Heart Disease Risk. *Mayo Clin. Proc.* **2017**, *92*, 15–29. [CrossRef] [PubMed]
33. Aung, T.; Halsey, J.; Kromhout, D.; Gerstein, H.C.; Marchioli, R.; Tavazzi, L.; Geleijnse, J.M.; Rauch, B.; Ness, A.; Galan, P.; et al. Associations of Omega-3 Fatty Acid Supplement Use with Cardiovascular Disease Risks: Meta-analysis of 10 Trials Involving 77917 Individuals. *JAMA Cardiol.* **2018**, *3*, 225–234. [CrossRef] [PubMed]
34. Bernasconi, A.A.; Wiest, M.M.; Lavie, C.J.; Milani, R.V.; Laukkanen, J.A. Effect of Omega-3 Dosage on Cardiovascular Outcomes: An Updated Meta-Analysis and Meta-Regression of Interventional Trials. *Mayo Clin. Proc.* **2020**. [CrossRef]
35. Cabiddu, M.F.; Russi, A.; Appolloni, L.; Mengato, D.; Chiumente, M. Omega-3 for the prevention of cardiovascular diseases: Meta-analysis and trial-sequential analysis. *Eur. J. Hosp. Pharm.* **2020**. [CrossRef]
36. Casula, M.; Olmastroni, E.; Gazzotti, M.; Galimberti, F.; Zambon, A.; Catapano, A.L. Omega-3 polyunsaturated fatty acids supplementation and cardiovascular outcomes: Do formulation, dosage, and baseline cardiovascular risk matter? An updated meta-analysis of randomized controlled trials. *Pharmacol. Res.* **2020**, *160*, 105060. [CrossRef]
37. Doshi, R.; Kumar, A.; Thakkar, S.; Shariff, M.; Adalja, D.; Doshi, A.; Taha, M.; Gupta, R.; Desai, R.; Shah, J.; et al. Meta-analysis Comparing Combined Use of Eicosapentaenoic Acid and Statin to Statin Alone. *Am. J. Cardiol.* **2020**, *125*, 198–204. [CrossRef]
38. Hoang, T.; Kim, J. Comparative Effect of Statins and Omega-3 Supplementation on Cardiovascular Events: Meta-Analysis and Network Meta-Analysis of 63 Randomized Controlled Trials Including 264,516 Participants. *Nutrients* **2020**, *12*, 2218. [CrossRef]
39. Hu, Y.; Hu, F.B.; Manson, J.E. Marine Omega-3 Supplementation and Cardiovascular Disease: An Updated Meta-Analysis of 13 Randomized Controlled Trials Involving 127 477 Participants. *J. Am. Heart Assoc.* **2019**, *8*, e013543. [CrossRef]
40. Lombardi, M.; Chiabrando, J.G.; Vescovo, G.M.; Bressi, E.; Del Buono, M.G.; Carbone, S.; Koenig, R.A.; Van Tassell, B.W.; Abbate, A.; Biondi-Zoccai, et al. Impact of Different Doses of Omega-3 Fatty Acids on Cardiovascular Outcomes: A Pairwise and Network Meta-analysis. *Curr. Atheroscler. Rep.* **2020**, *22*, 45. [CrossRef]
41. Maki, K.C.; Palacios, O.M.; Bell, M.; Toth, P.P. Use of supplemental long-chain omega-3 fatty acids and risk for cardiac death: An updated meta-analysis and review of research gaps. *J. Clin. Lipidol.* **2017**, *11*, 1152–1160. [CrossRef] [PubMed]
42. Popoff, F.; Balaciano, G.; Bardach, A.; Comande, D.; Irazola, V.; Catalano, H.N.; Izcovich, A. Omega 3 fatty acid supplementation after myocardial infarction: A systematic review and meta-analysis. *BMC Cardiovasc. Disord.* **2019**, *19*, 136. [CrossRef] [PubMed]

43. Bhatt, D.L.; Steg, P.G.; Miller, M.; Brinton, E.A.; Jacobson, T.A.; Ketchum, S.B.; Doyle, R.T.; Juliano, R.A.; Jiao, L.; Granowitz, C.; et al. Cardiovascular risk reduction with icosapent ethyl for hypertriglyceridemia. *N. Engl. J. Med.* **2019**, *380*, 11–22. [CrossRef] [PubMed]
44. ASCEND Study Collaborative Group; Bowman, L.; Mafham, M.; Wallendszus, K.; Stevens, W.; Buck, G.; Barton, J.; Murphy, K.; Aung, T.; Haynes, R.; et al. Effects of n-3 fatty acid supplements in diabetes mellitus. *N. Engl. J. Med.* **2018**, *379*, 1540–1550. [PubMed]
45. Manson, J.E.; Cook, N.R.; Lee, I.M.; Christen, W.; Bassuk, S.S.; Mora, S.; Gibson, H.; Albert, C.M.; Gordon, D.; Copeland, T.; et al. Marine n-3 fatty acids and prevention of cardiovascular disease and cancer. *N. Engl. J. Med.* **2019**, *380*, 23–32. [CrossRef] [PubMed]
46. Nicholls, S.J.; Lincoff, A.M.; Garcia, M.; Bash, D.; Ballantyne, C.M.; Barter, P.J.; Davidson, M.H.; Kastelein, J.J.P.; Koenig, W.; McGuire, D.K.; et al. Effect of high-dose omega-3 fatty acids vs corn oil on major adverse cardiovascular events in patients at high cardiovascular risk: The STRENGTH randomized clinical trial. *JAMA* **2020**, *324*, 2268–2280. [CrossRef] [PubMed]

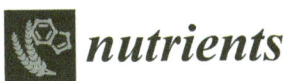

Article

Protein Intake and Physical Activity in Newly Diagnosed Patients with Acute Coronary Syndrome: A 5-Year Longitudinal Study

Andrea Greco [1,*], Agostino Brugnera [1], Roberta Adorni [2], Marco D'Addario [2], Francesco Fattirolli [3,4], Cristina Franzelli [5], Cristina Giannattasio [6,7], Alessandro Maloberti [6,7], Francesco Zanatta [2] and Patrizia Steca [2]

1. Department of Human and Social Sciences, University of Bergamo, 24129 Bergamo, Italy; agostino.brugnera@unibg.it
2. Department of Psychology, University of Milano-Bicocca, 20126 Milan, Italy; roberta.adorni1@unimib.it (R.A.); marco.daddario@unimib.it (M.D.); francesco.zanatta@unimib.it (F.Z.); patrizia.steca@unimib.it (P.S.)
3. Department of Medical and Surgical Critical Care, Cardiac Rehabilitation Unit, University of Florence, 50139 Florence, Italy; francesco.fattirolli@unifi.it
4. Azienda Ospedaliero-Universitaria Careggi, 50134 Florence, Italy
5. Cardiac Rehabilitation Centre-CTO Hospital, 20126 Milan, Italy; cristina.franzelli@asst-pini-cto.it
6. School of Medicine, Surgery University of Milano-Bicocca, 20126 Milan, Italy; cristina.giannattasio@unimib.it (C.G.); alessandro.maloberti@ospedaleniguarda.it (A.M.)
7. Cardiology IV, "A. De Gasperis" Department, Ospedale Niguarda Ca' Granda, 20162 Milan, Italy
* Correspondence: andrea.greco@unibg.it

Abstract: Cardiovascular disease is one of the most common causes of hospitalization and is associated with high morbidity and mortality rates. Among the most important modifiable and well-known risk factors are an unhealthy diet and sedentary lifestyle. Nevertheless, adherence to healthy lifestyle regimes is poor. The present study examined longitudinal trajectories (pre-event, 6-, 12-, 24-, 36-, and 60-month follow-ups) of protein intake (fish, legumes, red/processed meat) and physical activity in 275 newly-diagnosed patients with acute coronary syndrome. Hierarchical Generalized Linear Models were performed, controlling for demographic and clinical variables, the season in which each assessment was made, and the presence of anxiety and depressive symptoms. Significant changes in protein intake and physical activity were found from pre-event to the six-month follow-up, suggesting the adoption of healthier behaviors. However, soon after the six-month follow-up, patients experienced significant declines in their healthy behaviors. Both physical activity and red/processed meat intake were modulated by the season in which the assessments took place and by anxiety symptoms over time. The negative long-term trajectory of healthy behaviors suggests that tailored interventions are needed that sustain patients' capabilities to self-regulate their behaviors over time and consider patient preference in function of season.

Keywords: acute coronary syndrome; healthy behaviors; diet; legumes; fish; red/processed meat; physical activity; anxiety; depression; season

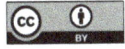

1. Introduction

Cardiovascular disease (CVD) is one of the most common causes of hospitalization in Western countries and is associated with high morbidity and mortality rates. CVD's burden is not only a health issue, but also a growing economic and societal challenge [1,2]. INTERHEART [3], a case-control study conducted in 52 countries, has identified nine risk factors and health behaviors (namely, hypertension, dyslipidemia, diabetes, obesity, smoking, alcohol, unhealthy diet, sedentary lifestyle, and psychosocial factors) that account for more than 90% of the population attributable risk of CVD. Based on scientific evidence that the virtuous management of these risk factors may reduce the incidence of CVD at the population level, eight of them (all except psychosocial factors) are the World Health

Organization targets for reduction by 2025 [4]. Nevertheless, according to a recent report from the European Society of Cardiology [2], based on current trends, only the reduction in smoking from 28% to 21% over the last 20 years appears to be able to meet the WHO target. This goal may be achieved for smoking, but other behaviors like unhealthy diet and sedentary lifestyle still need strong attention.

Regarding physical activity, international guidelines recommend that adults engage in at least 150 minutes per week of accumulated moderate-intensity or 75 minutes per week of vigorous-intensity aerobic physical activity to reduce CVD risk [1,2]. Encouraging leisure-time exercise has consistently been shown to promote cardiovascular health [5]. International guidelines recommend a diet emphasizing the intake of fruits and vegetables, whole grains, fish, and legumes, and minimizing the intake of processed meats and fats to decrease CVD risk factors [1]. The widespread popularity of high-protein diets has drawn controversy as well as scientific interest [6]. Many meta-analyses have shown a potential CVD benefit for mainly secondary prevention with increased fish intake [7] and decreased red/processed meat intake [8]. Data about the intake of legumes are less consistent but go in the same direction [9,10].

Despite the large amount of scientific evidence and recommendations described in the international guidelines, both in terms of primary and secondary prevention, there is poor compliance with regimens of a healthy diet and physical activity [5]. Studies focused on the longitudinal trajectories of healthy lifestyle highlighted that patients with established CVD after the initial adoption of healthier lifestyles tend to drop out within six months of hospital discharge [11–13].

The role of psychological factors is largely underestimated. Indeed, these risk factors are not currently recorded in the ESC Atlas [2], nor are they among the WHO's targets for management for 2025 [4], although they are well established as contributors to CVD risk [14–16]. In a previous study by the present research group, an association between lifestyle profiles and psychological factors of depression and anxiety was found [17], consistent with other empirical evidence showing a deleterious effect of depression and anxiety on changing unhealthy lifestyles [18]. In another study [19], we found that higher levels of depression six months after an acute coronary event were associated with subsequent unhealthy lifestyle six months later. However, higher levels of depression at baseline were not associated with subsequent unhealthy lifestyle six or twelve months later. These findings underscore the importance of investigating the long-term role of psychological factors in predicting healthy behavior trajectories that to date remain almost unknown.

Compliance with regimens of a healthy lifestyle may also be influenced, at least partially, by the seasons [20]. Indeed, bad weather can represent a barrier to carrying out physical activity, especially outdoors. Again, eating habits change considerably according to the season [21,22]. All these changes, by modifying physiological responses and metabolism, could affect cardiovascular function and disease [23]. These changes may be particularly pronounced in countries subject to four distinct seasons and with very different winter-to-summer weather conditions, like countries in the Mediterranean area. Nevertheless, seasonal variations have seldom been considered a factor that modulates compliance with healthy regimens in patients with established CVD [24,25].

The present study explores the longitudinal trajectories and underlying predictors associated with protein consumption and physical activity in a cohort of 275 consecutive patients with acute coronary syndrome (ACS) at their first coronary event. The aim was to assess whether these factors could play a significant role in predicting adherence to physicians' prescriptions to achieve and maintain a sufficient level of physical activity and a balanced protein intake. In addition to the most well-known demographic and clinical predictors, for the first time, this study has investigated the role played by both psychological factors, namely anxiety and depressive symptoms, and environmental factors, i.e., seasonal variation. Patients were assessed at six time points, i.e., at baseline, at six months, and at one, two, three, and five years after the first cardiovascular event. An advanced statistical technique, namely hierarchical linear models (HLMs) with a piecewise regression approach, was used to model the individual change rate from pre-event to five-year post-cardiovascular event. This technique allowed us to test the hypotheses that (1) patients experienced increases in healthy protein consumption and physical activity from pre- to six-months post-cardiovascular event; (2) patients decreased their healthy behaviors from six-months to five-years post-cardiovascular event. We trust that investigating the predictors of lifestyle changes in patients affected by CVD can be a useful tool for developing tailored cardiovascular rehabilitation programs to increase and stabilize healthy behaviors. This may have a great impact on the effectiveness of healthcare practices.

2. Materials and Methods

2.1. Study Design and Participants

A total of 275 consecutive patients affected by ACS at their first coronary event were recruited from February 2011 to October 2013, in three large public hospitals in Italy. Eligible patients were between 30 and 80 years of age, had sufficient Italian language skills, and had neither cognitive deficits nor comorbidity with other major pathologies such as cancer. Physicians recruited patients who met the eligibility criteria during their cardiovascular rehabilitation (CR) at the hospital, which took place between two and eight weeks after their first acute coronary event. Information on lifestyle before the onset of ACS was retrospectively collected during the first assessment (baseline). After the first data collection, patients were re-evaluated at five subsequent follow-ups (after six months, one, two, three, and five years). At each time-point, sociodemographic, clinical, psychological, and behavioral data were collected. The date of each of the six assessments was used to define the variable "season" at each time-point.

This study is part of a larger longitudinal study aimed at profiling patients with ACS and hypertension in terms of a series of behavioral, clinical, and psychological variables [13,17,19,26]. For the first time, this study has focused on a five-year period after the first cardiovascular event and has considered the role of both psychological (anxiety and depressive symptoms) and environmental (seasonal variations) factors as predictors of the longitudinal trajectories of healthy behaviors in terms of diet and physical activity.

The Bio-Ethics Committee of all the institutions involved in the research project approved the study. Each participant provided written informed consent before their enrollment.

2.2. Measures

2.2.1. Protein Consumption

Protein consumption was measured using three items (pertinent to fish, legumes, and red/processed meat intake) from the Italian version of the Mediterranean Diet Scale (MDS) [26,27]. The MDS is a nine-item self-report questionnaire that measures the weekly consumption of nine foods using a six-point Likert scale (from 1 = Never to 6 = More than three times per day). Each response was coded as a dichotomous variable following Trichopoulou and collaborators [27]; 1 indicates healthy (two or more servings of fish per week; two or more servings of legumes per week; two or fewer servings of red/processed meat per week) and 0 indicates unhealthy consumption.

2.2.2. Physical Activity

Physical activity was measured using the Italian version of the Rapid Assessment of Physical Activity Questionnaire (RAPA-Q) [28], a seven-item measure of the frequency and intensity of the participants' physical activity. The questionnaire uses a yes/no scale. The total score ranges from 1 (i.e., sedentary) to 7 (i.e., regular and vigorous activity), with higher scores indicating a healthier amount of physical activity. Scores of 6 or 7 (i.e., at least 30 min of moderate to vigorous aerobic exercise five times a week) indicate the target amount of physical activity for cardiovascular prevention.

2.2.3. Anxious and Depressive Symptoms

Anxious and depressive symptoms were measured using the Italian version of the Hospital Anxiety and Depression Scale (HADS) [29,30], a 14-item self-report questionnaire developed to screen for generalized symptoms of psychological distress in medical patients. Participants reported their feelings and mood on a four-point Likert scale (for example, "I've lost interest in my appearance", and the possible answers are 3 = "definitely", 2 = "I don't take as much care as I should", 1 = "I may not take quite as much care", and 0 = "I take just as much care as ever"). Two sum scores were calculated for anxiety and depressive symptoms; the total score ranges from 0 to 21, in which higher scores indicate a greater presence of symptoms. The scale showed adequate internal consistency (Cronbach's alphas: anxiety = 0.81, depression = 0.73).

2.3. Data Analysis

Levels of physical activity from pre-event to the five-year follow-up were evaluated using two-level Hierarchical Linear Models (HLMs), whilst changes in fish, legume, and red/processed meat consumption (three dichotomous variables) were analyzed using hierarchical generalized linear models (H(G)LMs). H(G)LMs are the best statistical methods to examine longitudinal changes in nested data [31]. Their main advantage is their flexibility in handling missing data [32], a common occurrence in longitudinal studies.

We tested the hypotheses on lifestyle behaviors using piecewise regression models in H(G)LM, in which two level-1 "time" parameters were included to model the slope discontinuity from pre- to six-months post-cardiovascular event (Time.D1), and from six-months to five-year post-cardiovascular event (Time.D2) [33].

H(G)LM analyses were adjusted for several confounding demographic and clinical variables, namely age, sex, working status (not working vs. working), educational level (less than high school vs. high school or higher), marital status (single/widowed/divorced vs. married), presence of hypertension, diabetes, dyslipidemia, obesity, and family history of CVD (not present vs. present). Additionally, both anxious and depressive symptoms and the season during which data were collected for each participant were added as time-varying covariates at level 1 of the H(G)LM models. We further assessed and reported pseudo-R^2, a measure of HLMs' effect sizes indicating the proportion of within-person variance accounted for by adding the linear parameters [31]. All multilevel models and further information on piecewise regressions are reported in the Appendix A.

Analyses were performed using the Statistical Package for Social Sciences (SPSS) version 26.0 and Hierarchical Linear Models (HLM) Professional version 8.0. All statistical tests were two-tailed, and a $p \leq 0.05$ was considered statistically significant.

3. Results

3.1. Study Population

The study population included 275 consecutive ACS patients at their first coronary event, aged 57.1 ± 7.87 years; 84% were men and 16% women. The proportion of men in the sample was a direct consequence of the incidence of ACS, which is more common among men than women [34]. The patients' mean BMI was 27.2 ± 4.1 kg/m², their mean waist circumference [WC] was 96.5 ± 11.1 cm. All of them were Caucasian. Almost all patients were prescribed pharmacological treatment for ACS, consisting of antiplatelet drugs (99% of patients), beta-blockers (89%), statins (97%), sartans, or ace-inhibitors (99%). Further demographic and clinical variables are reported in Tables 1 and 2.

Table 1. Sociodemographic characteristics of the sample (N = 275). Means and standard deviations (SD) are reported for age. Frequencies (n) and percentages are reported for gender, working status, educational level, and marital status.

Sociodemographic Variables	ACS Patients
Age, mean (SD)	57.1 (7.87)
Gender, n (%)	
Male	231 (84%)
Female	44 (16%)
Working status, n (%)	
working	111 (40.4%)
not working	163 (59.3%)
Educational level, n (%)	
less than high school	141 (51.3%)
high school or higher	134 (48.7%)
Marital status, n (%)	
single\widowed\divorced	78 (28.4%)
married	197 (71.6%)

Table 2. Clinical characteristics of the sample (N = 275). Frequencies (n) and percentages are reported for clinical presentation, percutaneous coronary intervention, patients with at least one stent, and risk factors. Means and standard deviations (SD) are reported for body mass index, systolic blood pressure, and diastolic blood pressure.

Clinical Variables	ACS Patients
Clinical Presentation, n (%)	
Non-ST elevation myocardial infarction (NSTEMI)	54 (19.8)
ST-elevation myocardial infarction (STEMI)	196 (71.8)
Unstable Angina	23 (8.5)
Percutaneous coronary intervention, n (%)	258 (94.5)
Patients with at least one stent, n (%)	263 (96)
Risk factors, n (%)	
Hypertension	127 (46.5)
Dyslipidemia	143 (52.4)
Smoking History	180 (66.4)
Diabetes	47 (17.2)
Obesity	43 (15.8)
Family History of CVD	108 (39.3)
Physical Inactivity	20 (7.3)
Body Mass Index, mean (SD)	27.2 (4.1)
Systolic Blood Pressure (SBP), mean (SD)	115.9 (13.9)
Diastolic Blood Pressure (DBP), mean (SD)	72.9 (8.5)

Regarding the psychological assessment, the results showed that, on average, patients were not affected by clinically significant anxiety (the mean score overtime was 5.78, with a cut-off of 7), or clinically significant depression (the mean score overtime was 3.16, with a cut-off of 7). Table 3 reports a detailed description of anxiety and depression scores across all time points.

Table 3. Sample size (N) and percentages of patients with a mean score above the cut-off of 7 for anxiety and depression during all time points (baseline, six-month, one-, two-, three- and five-year follow-up). The cut-off of 7 defines the presence of clinically significant symptoms of anxiety and depression. Means and standard deviations (SD) of the sample for each time point are also reported.

	Baseline		6 Months		1 Year		2 Years		3 Years		5 Years	
	N (%)	Mean (SD)	N (%)	Mean (SD)	N (%)	Mean (SD)	N (%)	Mean (SD)	N (%)	Mean (SD)	N (%)	Mean (SD)
Anxiety	274 39%	6.85 (3.88)	241 33%	6.23 (3.35)	233 26%	5.70 (3.45)	218 28%	5.99 (3.37)	183 26%	5.68 (3.34)	175 14%	4.21 (3.19)
Depression	274 21%	4.73 (3.42)	241 19%	4.45 (3.18)	233 11%	3.84 (2.98)	218 17%	4.45 (3.14)	183 15%	4.25 (3.29)	175 14%	2.90 (2.94)

Regarding drop-outs, 12.7% of patients were absent at the six-month follow-up, 14.9% at the one-year, 20.7% at the two-year, 33.1% at the three-year, and 35.3% at the five-year. In comparison, percentages of drop-outs at the one-year follow-up were similar to those reported in other European studies on ACS patients [35]. Causes of drop-out included: loss to follow-up, relocation, refusal, and, in a small minority of cases, inability to track down the patient. It is worth noting that this study's statistical techniques enabled us to use all the data available and not only those provided by completers. Therefore, the final number of participants remained 275.

3.2. Longitudinal Changes in Protein Intake

Preliminary analyses showed that both the time slopes (Time.D1 and Time.D2; see Appendix A for the multilevel model) for the variables Fish and Legume intake were non-significant and were therefore fixed in subsequent analyses. Similarly, the pre-to-post event time slope for the variable red/processed meat intake was non-significant, and its effect was treated as fixed. In both cases, this suggested that participants had similar changes over time in the aforementioned eating behaviors (i.e., the slopes were not significantly different between participants).

As regards fish intake, results showed that before the onset of cardiovascular disease (i.e., at the intercept), 66.4% of patients consumed two or more servings of fish per week. From pre-event to six months later (i.e., the "Time.D1" slope $\beta 1$), patients increased their fish intake. Those who had a family history of CVD had a greater increase in fish intake ($\beta = 1.31$; $p = 0.043$) than those without a family history of CVD. A significant longitudinal decrease in fish intake was found from the six-month to the five-year follow-up (i.e., the "Time.D2" slope $\beta 2$). Anxiety, depression, and seasonal variations were not significant predictors.

As regards legume intake, results showed that before the onset of CVD (i.e., at the intercept), a high percentage (79.1%) of patients consumed two or more servings of legumes per week. Older patients reported higher levels of legume intake ($\beta = 0.07$; $p = 0.007$). From pre-event to six months after (i.e., the "Time.D1" slope $\beta 1$), patients maintained stable levels of legume intake, except older patients, who decreased their consumption of legumes ($\beta = -0.13$; $p = 0.009$). A significant longitudinal decrease in legume intake was found from the six-month to the five-year follow-up (i.e., the "Time.D2" slope $\beta 2$). This decrease was smaller among patients affected by hypertension ($\beta = 0.15$; $p = 0.035$), and dyslipidemia ($\beta = 0.15$; $p = 0.041$). Anxiety, depression, and seasonal variations were not significant predictors.

Regarding the consumption of red/processed meat, results showed that before the onset of cardiovascular disease (i.e., at the intercept), only 8.4% of patients consumed two or fewer servings of red/processed meat per week. From pre-event to six months after (i.e., the "Time.D1" slope $\beta 1$), red meat consumption significantly declined; indeed, 33.5% of patients consumed two or fewer servings of red/processed meat per week. This decrease was greater among patients affected by hypertension ($\beta = 1.87$; $p = 0.031$).

From the six-month to the five-year follow-up (i.e., the "Time.D2" slope β2), a significant longitudinal decrease in red/processed meat consumption was found. Patients who were married decreased their consumption of red/processed meat more than patients who were single, widowed, or divorced (β = 0.20; p = 0.041). Patients affected by hypertension decreased their consumption of red/processed meat less than patients not affected by hypertension (β = −0.24; p = 0.004). Patients with higher levels of anxiety decreased their consumption of red/processed meat more than patients with lower anxiety levels (β = 0.09; p = 0.025). There was no statistically significant effect of depression on red/processed meat consumption. The decrease in red/processed meat consumption was significantly higher in spring (β = 0.47; p = 0.016) and in autumn (β = 0.43; p = 0.041) than in winter. Further, the consumption of red/processed meat was significantly lower in spring than in summer (β = 0.48; p = 0.027). The lowest consumption of red/processed meat was recorded in spring (frequency = 165, 39.3% of patients ate a healthy amount of meat); it increased in summer (frequency = 75, 28.8%), decreased in autumn (frequency = 120, 39.2%), and increased again in winter (frequency = 115, 34%).

3.3. Longitudinal Changes in Physical Activity

Regarding physical activity, results showed that before the onset of cardiovascular disease (i.e., at the intercept), patients affected by hypertension performed less physical activity (β = −0.63; p = 0.011) compared to patients not affected by hypertension. From pre-event to six months after (i.e., the "Time.D1" slope β1), patients increased their physical activity. Patients with higher educational levels had steeper increases (β = 0.99; p = 0.036) than those with less education. Patients affected by hypertension increased their levels of physical activity (β = 1.08; p = 0.025). A significant longitudinal decrease in levels of physical activity was found from the six-month to the five-year follow-up (i.e., the "Time.D2" slope β2). Patients who were married decreased their physical activity levels more than patients who were single, widowed, or divorced (β = −0.12; p = 0.048). Anxiety and depression were not significant predictors. Physical activity was significantly higher in autumn than in winter (β = 0.31; p = 0.015). The difference between the amount of physical activity in summer and winter approached significance (β = 0.28; p = 0.048). The highest amount of physical activity was recorded in autumn (mean = 5.11 ± 1.88); it decreased significantly in winter (mean = 4.65 ± 2.09), then rose in a variable manner in spring (mean = 4.92 ± 1.93) and summer (mean = 4.83 ± 2.06).

Frequencies, percentages, means, and standard deviations for all outcome variables across all time points are reported in Table 4. All regression coefficients, standard errors, t and p values for β1 and β2 slope parameters are reported in Table 5. All fixed effects are reported in the Supplementary Materials. Figure 1 illustrates the longitudinal trajectory of healthy protein consumption and the amount of physical activity.

Table 4. Descriptive statistics of the outcome measures at all time points (pre-event, six-month, one-, two-, three- and five-year follow-up). Frequencies (n) and percentages are reported for the protein consumption outcomes (fish, legumes, and healthy consumption of red/processed meat). Means and standard deviations (SD) are reported for physical activity.

	Pre		6 Months		1 Year		2 Years		3 Years		5 Years	
	N	n (%)	N	n (%)	N	n (%)	N	n (%)	N	n (%)	N	n (%)
Fish	274	182 (66.4)	239	185 (77.4)	233	186 (67.6)	216	124 (57.4)	183	105 (57.4)	176	109 (61.9)
Legumes	273	216 (79.1)	238	195 (81.9)	231	190 (82.3)	218	151 (69.3)	183	124 (67.8)	175	131 (74.9)
Red/processed meat	274	23 (8.4)	239	80 (33.5)	233	75 (32.2)	218	105 (48.2)	184	85 (46.2)	176	107 (60.8)
	N	Mean (SD)	N	Mean (SD)	N	Mean (SD)	N	Mean (SD)	N	Mean (SD)	N	Mean (SD)
Physical Activity	275	4.20 (2.02)	240	5.48 (1.79)	234	5.36 (1.80)	217	5.17 (1.89)	183	5.12 (1.94)	176	3.86 (1.96)

Data on lifestyle behaviors at pre-event were collected retrospectively once patients were hospitalized.

Table 5. Fixed effects for the longitudinal changes in behavioral outcomes (fish intake, legume intake, red/processed meat intake, physical activity).

Variables	Fixed Effects										
	β_1	SE	t Values	DF	p	β_2	SE	t Values	DF	p	R^2
Fish intake	0.902	0.324	2.783	1006	0.005	−0.213	0.040	−5.341	1006	<0.001	\
Legume intake	−0.035	0.339	−0.103	1003	0.918	−0.085	0.038	−2.240	1003	0.025	\
Red/processed meat intake	4.011	0.508	7.895	749	<0.001	0.276	0.044	6.351	260	<0.001	\
Physical Activity	2.334	0.229	10.217	260	<0.001	−0.240	0.025	−9.623	260	<0.001	34.4%

β_1 = unstandardized regression coefficient for the average growth rate from pre-event to six months after. β_2 = unstandardized regression coefficient for the average growth rate from the six-month follow-up to the five-year follow-up. SE = standard error of the regression coefficient; DF = degrees of freedom (df changes due to missing values or to the presence of fixed\random time slopes). R^2 refers to pseudo-R^2, indicating the proportion of within-person variance accounted for by adding the "Time.1" and "Time.2" parameter to the model; it cannot be analyzed for dichotomous variables.

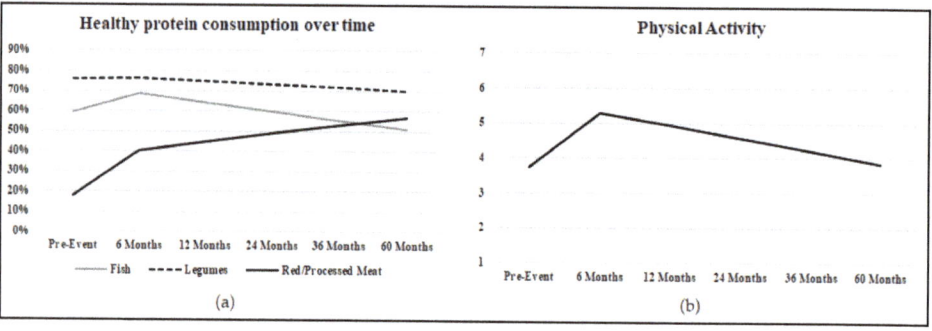

Figure 1. (a) The graph shows the longitudinal trajectory of healthy protein consumption (i.e., two or more portions of fish per week—grey line, two or more portions of legumes per week—dashed line, two or fewer portions of red meat per week/processed—black line). The time is represented on the horizontal axis, the percentage of patients showing healthy behavior is represented on the vertical axis; (b) the graph shows the longitudinal trajectory of the amount of physical activity. The time is represented on the horizontal axis; the average physical activity score is represented on the vertical axis. The total score ranges from 1 to 7, with higher scores indicating a healthier amount of physical activity. Scores higher than 6 indicate the target amount of physical activity for cardiovascular prevention.

4. Discussion

The present study explored the longitudinal trajectories of physical activity and protein consumption in a cohort of patients with ACS at their first event. The aim was to assess whether and which factors could play a significant role in predicting healthier behavior. For the first time, this study has investigated the role played by anxiety and depressive symptoms, and the change of seasons.

Our results are in agreement with previous studies showing that most patients affected by CVD fail to achieve healthy lifestyle targets [11,13,36,37]. They showed that, on average, patients experienced significant increases in the levels of healthy behaviors from pre- to post-cardiovascular event. However, from post-event to the five-year follow-up, patients showed a significant decline in their levels of healthy behaviors. This demonstrates the difficulty of patients not so much in assuming but maintaining the recommended healthy behaviors in the long term. In particular, as regards fish intake, results showed that a good percentage of patients consumed two or more servings of fish per week before the onset of the ACS, which has been related to positive health outcomes [27]. Immediately after the cardiovascular event, fish consumption increased, especially among patients with a family history of CVD. We could argue that patients with this risk factor received more health-related suggestions or were more sensitive to prescriptions received regarding fish intake, possibly due to a greater risk perception than patients with no family history of CVD. In support of this hypothesis, a cross-sectional study showed that a family history of CVD was associated with both higher risk perception and the adoption of a healthier lifestyle in people diagnosed with familial hypercholesterolemia [38]. Overall, the findings therefore suggest that healthcare professionals should be aware that some people may underestimate the risk of CVD and emphasize how behavior change can reduce risk [38]. This consideration is reinforced by the evidence that adherence declined over time in our sample, highlighting a great difficulty in maintaining positive behavior.

Similar results were obtained in the case of legume intake. Indeed, before the onset of the ACS, many patients consumed the recommended two or more servings of legumes per week [27], especially older adults. Immediately after the cardiovascular event, patients maintained stable levels of legume intake. Considering the high percentage of patients who consumed a quantity of legumes in line with recommendations before the cardiac event, it is not surprising that the behavior was maintained and did not increase further. This observation is reinforced by the fact that older patients decreased legume intake, regressing towards the mean. Over the five-year follow-up, legume consumption decreased, except for patients affected by hypertension and dyslipidemia. Again, the presence of multiple risk factors could be associated with higher risk perception. Previous studies have shown that reporting a high perceived CVD risk in the general population was strongly associated with treatment for hypertension, diabetes, or dyslipidemia [39]. This could make patients more alert and receptive to physicians' prescriptions during cardiovascular rehabilitation and have an effect, albeit weak, in the long term. Again, this finding underlines that healthcare professionals should be aware that some patients underestimate the risks associated with CVD and are therefore less likely to change their health-related behavior stably.

As regards the consumption of red and processed meat, results showed that a small percentage of patients consumed the recommended two or fewer servings of red and processed meat per week before the cardiovascular event [27]. Immediately after the cardiovascular event, patients significantly decreased red and processed meat intake. Consumption continued to decrease over time, especially among patients who were married. This result goes in the same direction as studies that showed this demographic variable's protective role in fostering a healthier diet [13,40], and it emphasizes the importance that the partner can have in motivating and supporting the patient to adopt a healthy diet. A second relevant observation is that immediately after the cardiovascular event, patients with hypertension adopted healthier behavior than patients without this risk factor. However, after the first follow-up, they decreased their red and processed meat intake less than patients without this risk factor, regressing towards the mean. This result underlines once again how the presence of multiple risk factors can make patients more alert and willing to follow medical indications to adopt a healthier lifestyle, although there is a difficulty in maintaining healthy behavior stably.

Interestingly, patients with higher anxiety levels decreased red and processed meat intake more than patients with lower levels of anxiety over the five-year follow-up. Among psychological disorders, anxiety, together with depression, is the most widely and frequently studied condition. Anxiety has been linked to health status and several risk factors predisposing CVD [41]. Previous studies have reported contrasting results of the impact of anxiety on manifold health-related outcomes [42,43]. In line with our findings, Grace and colleagues [14] found that patients with anxiety symptoms were more likely to participate in cardiovascular rehabilitation. Moreover, Parker and colleagues [44] found that patients who had been hospitalized for an ACS and suffered from generalized anxiety disorder had a superior five-year outcome than patients with different psychological symptoms. The group discussed the positive contribution of worry in medication adherence and a proactive approach to health practitioners. However, to the best of our knowledge, no studies have explored if a relatively high level of anxiety could play a role in promoting a positive long-term lifestyle change, specifically in adopting a healthier diet. Feeling "tense or wound up", getting "a sort of frightened feeling as if something awful were about to happen", experiencing "worrying thoughts" about one's health can somehow promote awareness of the risks to one's health and consequently motivate one to change one's behavior. Consistently, a study focused on sedentary young adults [45] found that the exposure to web-based images and information about cardiovascular risk could lead to higher levels of worry and risk perception, contributing to increase motivation in adopting a healthier behavior. Our findings suggest that cardiovascular rehabilitation programs would benefit from the introduction of psychological interventions aimed, on the one hand, at treating the emotional aspects related to anxiety, providing psychological support, and promoting coping [14,41], and on the other hand, at exploiting the concern patients express about their health to promote cognitive awareness of the risks associated to CVD recurrence. This awareness could sustain patients' abilities to self-regulate their behaviors and increase their beliefs about their self-efficacy [46–48]. Self-efficacy refers to the belief in one's capabilities to organize and execute the actions required to produce given attainments [49]. Such beliefs are particularly relevant with regard to health-related behaviors [50]. In the context of CVD, it has been shown that self-efficacy plays a crucial role in adopting and maintaining a healthy diet [26,51] and a physically active lifestyle [51,52]. Especially for maintenance, the confidence in one's abilities to preserve the newly developed behavior in spite of the possible barriers is pivotal. Indeed, as already suggested: "once an action has been taken, individuals with high maintenance self-efficacy invest more effort and persist longer than those who are less self-efficacious" [53]. Regarding depression, our results go in the same direction as a previous study in which we found that higher levels of depression at baseline were not associated with a subsequent unhealthy lifestyle six or twelve months later [19]. It should be noted that only a very small percentage of patients experienced anxiety and depressive symptoms, so it was probably not possible to capture any effects of this psychological variable.

The last observation regarding the longitudinal trajectory in red and processed meat consumption is that it was affected by seasonal variations. Red and processed meat intake was significantly lower in spring and autumn than in winter and summer. This result is not surprising if we consider the seasonal cultural habits of the Mediterranean area, where the patients of this study come from. Indeed, winter, especially Christmastime, and summer are the times when the longest holidays are taken in Italy. It is possible that it is more difficult to follow a healthy diet, particularly at these times. Similar trends have been described in a recent meta-analysis [21], suggesting a significant decrease of meat consumption from summer to autumn across different European countries. Interestingly, those food groups characterized by less healthy consumption (high consumption of unhealthy foods, or low consumption of healthy foods) were also characterized by consumption that varied with the season [22]. Consistent with this observation, in the present study, the role of seasonality emerged on the consumption of red and processed meat, whose intake was on average less healthy than the fish and legume intake. Maintaining a low consumption of red and processed meat was the eating behavior that saw the greatest effort, and in which the greatest change was observed. Perhaps for this reason, it is the behavior where a greater sensitivity to exceptions emerges. It is possible that patients were led to allow themselves exceptions, being more sensitive to contextual factors linked to the change in seasons in the case of red and processed meat consumption than in fish and legume consumption. This trend highlights, once again, the need for tailored cardiovascular rehabilitation programs. Patients' preference for red/processed meat intake may differ between seasons, and this variation may impact adherence to a healthy lifestyle. Patients should be aware that the incidence of CVDs has seasonal peaks [23], and the incidence of cardiovascular events could be, at least in part, associated with the difficulties they may encounter at different seasons of the year in adopting a healthy lifestyle. Patients should be supported in finding strategies that can compensate for variations in healthy behavior linked to contextual factors and seasonal variations (i.e., weather, holiday periods, or vice versa of greater workload). It is useful to underline once again that red/processed meat is the protein source for which the unhealthier behavior was recorded before the cardiovascular event and for which the most significant changes in consumption were observed over time; perhaps for this reason, among the protein sources examined in the present study, it is also the one in which the role of several predictors emerged.

Finally, as regards physical activity, the results of the present study showed that patients reported sub-optimal amounts of physical activity at each time-point. Accordingly, previous studies showed that adherence to good physical activity levels is one of the most difficult goals to reach and maintain among patients with CVDs [11,12,46]. Before the onset of cardiovascular disease, patients with hypertension were less physically active than those without hypertension. This observation is consistent with previous studies [54], and it is relevant considering that regular exercise is one of the most important activities for primary prevention of hypertension and improving long-term survival [54]. Immediately after the cardiovascular event, patients significantly increased their physical activity. This increase was higher among patients with hypertension, and those with higher educational levels. This last result goes in the same direction as studies that have shown that this demographic variable plays a protective role [55,56]. Low levels of education have been associated with low levels of health literacy [55]. Health literacy is defined as the set of skills to access, understand, and evaluate information to make health related decisions in everyday life. Poor health literacy has been linked to less healthy behaviors. Our results support, albeit indirectly, studies that emphasize the crucial role of health literacy in the success of cardiovascular rehabilitation programs [55]. After the first time-point, a significant longitudinal decrease in physical activity levels was found, decreeing a failure to adopt a healthier behavior stably. Patients who were married decreased their physical activity levels more than patients who were single, widowed, or divorced. This result may seem surprising when we generally consider being married as an indicator of social support. For red and processed meat consumption, we found the opposite pattern. This difference could lie in the fact that in the sample of the present study, made up mostly of men in their 60s, the wife represents the partner. In this generation and the Mediterranean area culture, it is common for women to cook, so we may infer that somehow their presence promotes a healthier diet [13,40]. In the case of physical activity, patients must actively engage themselves in doing more physical activity. It is also possible that partners hinder rather than encourage this behavior, which leads patients to choose between exercise time and family time. Indeed, our results may suggest that patient caregivers should also be included in the physical activity education programs. It is also important to underline that it is not so much being married (an indicator of structural social support), but rather the quality of the relationship (the so-called functional social support) that plays a protective role in the behavior of adherence to the prescriptions for one's health [57]. Therefore the "marital status" variable can only capture part of the phenomenon linked to social support.

The highest amount of physical activity was recorded in autumn; it decreased significantly in winter, and rose variably in spring and summer. These results show that patients tend to be more active after the summer; in winter, perhaps due to the cold, they have more difficulty maintaining a sufficient physical activity level. In spring, probably being able to resume physical activity outdoors, they become more active again, but with the heat of summer, the trend goes down once more. The seasonal variation of recreational physical activity has been reported in several studies [20]. In the CVD population, it has been argued that the decrease in physical activity from summer to winter was mainly due to an increase in symptom severity in winter, making exercise difficult to maintain over all the seasons [25]. Nevertheless, seasonal variations have seldom been considered a factor that modulates compliance with healthy regimens in this population [24,25]. Indeed, prior literature has also suggested taking seasonal differences in physical activity levels into consideration in future research, in order to better understand their influence on long-term adherence [58]. As discussed above, our findings suggest the need to pay attention to the role of environmental variations in CVD patients' adherence to healthy lifestyles, and they confirm the need for tailored cardiovascular rehabilitation programs that help patients overcome the difficulties they may face in adopting a healthy lifestyle in different seasons of the year. For example, at specific times of the year, it would be useful to suggest alternative activities, if those preferred by patients are outdoors (walking).

The present study has a series of limitations. First, despite using the piecewise regression approach, which allows for modeling the slope discontinuity from pre-event to six months after, information about diet and physical activity before the onset of the ACS was measured retrospectively by asking patients to report their habits before the acute event. This approach may limit the results' reliability, because patients may have over- or underestimated their real past healthy lifestyle. Second, both diet and physical activity were evaluated through self-report measures and not through an objective behavioral measure. Nevertheless, this methodology is widely adopted in the medical and psychological literature [26–28], and it has been proven to correlate with more objective measurement methods [59].

Despite these limitations, the present study reports several original findings and has important implications for behavioral intervention in cardiovascular disease patients. First, patients' protein consumption and physical activity were evaluated over a long period of time. Second, an advanced statistical technique (HLMs) with a piecewise regression approach was used to model the individual change rate from pre-event to five-year post-cardiovascular event. This technique allowed us to test the hypotheses that patients experienced both increases and decreases in healthy protein consumption and physical activity in subsequent periods of time. Overall, this approach allowed us to demonstrate that patients' main difficulty was not in assuming but in maintaining the recommended healthy behaviors in the long term. Third, the study focused on a homogeneous sample of patients at their first cardiovascular event. While the homogeneity of the sample may limit the generalizability of the results, it ensures that the inferences drawn from the study apply effectively to the population of ACS patients at their first cardiac event. Therefore, they assume an important significance for secondary cardiovascular prevention. Finally, by simultaneously considering several predictors of healthy behavior, our results confirmed the protective role of specific sociodemographic and clinical characteristics. For the first time, the roles of both environmental and psychological factors have been considered.

5. Conclusions

In summary, the present study shows that patients with ACS experience difficulties in achieving and mostly maintaining adequate levels of a healthy diet and physical activity over time. These difficulties are modulated by environmental conditions, and most importantly, by psychological characteristics. These findings suggest how to tailor diet and physical activity interventions. Tailoring should consider that patients' preference for diet and physical activity could differ between seasons, which could impact their adherence to a healthy lifestyle. Tailoring should also be aimed at promoting cognitive awareness of the risks associated with CVD recurrence. In fact, our study results showed that patients who were more anxious, therefore more concerned and somehow aware of their health, were more able to maintain healthy behavior over time. Cognitive awareness of the risks associated with CVD recurrence may be a useful tool to sustain patients' capabilities to self-regulate their behaviors and to ameliorate lifestyle behavior.

Supplementary Materials: The following are available online at https://www.mdpi.com/2072-6643/13/2/634/s1: Table S1: Fixed effects (with robust standard errors) for the dependent variable "Physical Activity" (MDS8); Table S2: Fixed effects (with robust standard errors) for the dependent variable "Legume intake"; Table S3: Fixed effects (with robust standard errors) for the dependent variable "Fish Intake"; Table S4: Fixed effects (with robust standard errors) for the dependent variable "Red/processed Meat Intake".

Author Contributions: Conceptualization: A.G., M.D., F.F., C.G. and P.S.; data curation: A.G. and A.M.; formal analysis: A.G. and A.B.; funding acquisition: P.S.; investigation: A.G. and A.B.; methodology: A.G., M.D., F.F., C.G. and P.S.; project administration: A.G., M.D. and P.S.; resources: A.G. and A.B.; supervision: P.S.; visualization: A.G., A.B., R.A., M.D., F.F., C.F., C.G., A.M., F.Z. and P.S.; writing—original draft: R.A.; writing—review and editing: A.G., A.B., R.A., M.D., F.F., C.F., C.G., A.M., F.Z. and P.S. All authors have read and agreed to the published version of the manuscript.

Funding: This research was funded by a FIRB ("Futuro in Ricerca") Grant from the Italian Ministry of Instruction, University, and Research (ref. RBFR08YVUL).

Institutional Review Board Statement: The study was conducted according to the guidelines of the Declaration of Helsinki, and approved by the Institutional Review Board (or Ethics Committee) of the University of Milano-Bicocca (protocol code 0021536, approved in 25 October 2010).

Informed Consent Statement: Informed consent was obtained from all subjects involved in the study.

Data Availability Statement: The data presented in this study are available on request from the corresponding author. The data are not publicly available due to privacy and ethical restrictions.

Conflicts of Interest: The authors declare no conflict of interest. The funders had no role in the study's design; in the collection, analyses, or interpretation of data; in the writing of the manuscript; or in the decision to publish the results.

Appendix A

HGLM 2-level models 1

Level-1 Model

$\text{Prob}(Y_{ti} = 1 \mid \pi_i) = \phi_{ti}$

$\log[\phi_{ti}/(1 - \phi_{ti})] = \eta_{ti}$

$\eta_{ti} = \pi_{0i} + \pi_{1i} * (\text{TIME.1}_{ti}) + \pi_{2i} * (\text{TIME.2}_{ti}) + \pi_{3i} * (\text{HADS.Anxiety}_{ti}) + \pi_{4i} * (\text{HADS.Depression}_{ti}) + \pi_{5i} * (\text{Season.Spring}_{ti}) + \pi_{6i} * (\text{Season.Summer}_{ti}) + \pi_{7i} * (\text{Season.Autumn}_{ti}) + e_{ti}$

Level-2 Model

$\pi_{0i} = \beta_{00} + \beta_{01} * (\text{AGE}_i) + \beta_{02} * (\text{SEX}_i) + \beta_{03} * (\text{WORKING\_STATUS}_i) + \beta_{04} * (\text{MARITAL\_STATUS}_i) + \beta_{05} * (\text{EDUCATION}_i) + \beta_{06} * (\text{LIVING\_STATUS}_i) + \beta_{07} * (\text{FAMILY\_HISTORY}_i) + \beta_{08} * (\text{HYPERTENSION}_i) + \beta_{09} * (\text{DIABETES}_i) + \beta_{010} * (\text{DYSLIPIDEMIA}_i) + \beta_{011} * (\text{OBESITY}_i) + r_{0i}$

$\pi_{1i} = \beta_{10} + \beta_{11} * (\text{AGE}_i) + \beta_{12} * (\text{SEX}_i) + \beta_{13} * (\text{WORKING\_STATUS}_i) + \beta_{14} * (\text{MARITAL\_STATUS}_i) + \beta_{15} * (\text{EDUCATION}_i) + \beta_{16} * (\text{LIVING\_STATUS}_i) + \beta_{17} * (\text{FAMILY\_HISTORY}_i) + \beta_{18} * (\text{HYPERTENSION}_i) + \beta_{19} * (\text{DIABETES}_i) + \beta_{110} * (\text{DYSLIPIDEMIA}_i) + \beta_{111} * (\text{OBESITY}_i) + r_{1i}$

$\pi_{2i} = \beta_{20} + \beta_{21} * (\text{AGE}_i) + \beta_{22} * (\text{SEX}_i) + \beta_{23} * (\text{WORKING\_STATUS}_i) + \beta_{24} * (\text{MARITAL\_STATUS}_i) + \beta_{25} * (\text{EDUCATION}_i) + \beta_{26} * (\text{LIVING\_STATUS}_i) + \beta_{27} * (\text{FAMILY\_HISTORY}_i) + \beta_{28} * (\text{HYPERTENSION}_i) + \beta_{29} * (\text{DIABETES}_i) + \beta_{210} * (\text{DYSLIPIDEMIA}_i) + \beta_{211} * (\text{OBESITY}_i) + r_{2i}$

$\pi_{3i} = \beta_{30}$

$\pi_{4i} = \beta_{40}$

$\pi_{5i} = \beta_{50}$

$\pi_{6i} = \beta_{60}$

$\pi_{7i} = \beta_{70}$

Note. Y = Dependent Variable (Fish intake, Legume intake, and Red/processed meat intake, dichotomized); The level-1 dummy-coded variable "Season" was uncentered, while HADS Anxiety and Depression were group-mean centered. All level-2 variables were centered around the grand mean.

HLM 2-level models 2

Level-1 Model

$Y_{ti} = \pi_{0i} + \pi_{1i} * (\text{TIME.1}_{ti}) + \pi_{2i} * (\text{TIME.2}_{ti}) + \pi_{3i} * (\text{HADS.Anxiety}_{ti}) + \pi_{4i} * (\text{HADS.Depression}_{ti}) + \pi_{5i} * (\text{Season.Spring}_{ti}) + \pi_{6i} * (\text{Season.Summer}_{ti}) + \pi_{7i} * (\text{Season.Autumn}_{ti}) + e_{ti}$

Level-2 Model

$\pi_{0i} = \beta_{00} + \beta_{01} * (AGE_i) + \beta_{02} * (SEX_i) + \beta_{03} * (WORKING\_STATUS_i) + \beta_{04} * (MARITAL\_STATUS_i) + \beta_{05} * (EDUCATION_i) + \beta_{06} * (LIVING\_STATUS_i) + \beta_{07} * (FAMILY\_HISTORY_i) + \beta_{08} * (HYPERTENSION_i) + \beta_{09} * (DIABETES_i) + \beta_{010} * (DYSLIPIDEMIA_i) + \beta_{011} * (OBESITY_i) + r_{0i}$

$\pi_{1i} = \beta_{10} + \beta_{11} * (AGE_i) + \beta_{12} * (SEX_i) + \beta_{13} * (WORKING\_STATUS_i) + \beta_{14} * (MARITAL\_STATUS_i) + \beta_{15} * (EDUCATION_i) + \beta_{16} * (LIVING\_STATUS_i) + \beta_{17} * (FAMILY\_HISTORY_i) + \beta_{18} * (HYPERTENSION_i) + \beta_{19} * (DIABETES_i) + \beta_{110} * (DYSLIPIDEMIA_i) + \beta_{111} * (OBESITY_i) + r_{1i}$

$\pi_{2i} = \beta_{20} + \beta_{21} * (AGE_i) + \beta_{22} * (SEX_i) + \beta_{23} * (WORKING\_STATUS_i) + \beta_{24} * (MARITAL\_STATUS_i) + \beta_{25} * (EDUCATION_i) + \beta_{26} * (LIVING\_STATUS_i) + \beta_{27} * (FAMILY\_HISTORY_i) + \beta_{28} * (HYPERTENSION_i) + \beta_{29} * (DIABETES_i) + \beta_{210} * (DYSLIPIDEMIA_i) + \beta_{211} * (OBESITY_i) + r_{2i}$

$\pi_{3i} = \beta_{30}$

$\pi_{4i} = \beta_{40}$

$\pi_{5i} = \beta_{50}$

$\pi_{6i} = \beta_{60}$

$\pi_{7i} = \beta_{70}$

Note. Y = Dependent Variable (Physical Activity, continuous); The level-1 dummy-coded variable "Season" was uncentered, while HADS Anxiety and Depression were group-mean centered. All level-2 variables were centered around the grand mean.

References

1. Arnett, D.K.; Blumenthal, R.S.; Albert, M.A.; Buroker, A.B.; Goldberger, Z.D.; Hahn, E.J.; Himmelfarb, C.D.; Khera, A.; Lloyd-Jones, D.; McEvoy, J.W.; et al. 2019 ACC/AHA Guideline on the Primary Prevention of Cardiovascular Disease: Executive Summary. *J. Am. Coll. Cardiol.* **2019**, *74*, 1376–1414. [CrossRef] [PubMed]
2. Timmis, A.; Townsend, N.; Gale, C.P.; Torbica, A.; Lettino, M.; Petersen, S.E.; Mossialos, E.A.; Maggioni, A.P.; Kazakiewicz, D.; May, H.T.; et al. European Society of Cardiology: Cardiovascular Disease Statistics 2019. *Eur. Heart J.* **2019**, *41*, 12–85. [CrossRef]
3. Yusuf, S.; Hawken, S.; Ounpuu, S.; Dans, T.; Avezum, A.; Lanas, F.; McQueen, M.; Budaj, A.; Pais, P.; Varigos, J.; et al. Effect of Potentially Modifiable Risk Factors Associated with Myocardial Infarction in 52 Countries (the INTERHEART Study): Case-Control Study. *Lancet* **2004**, *364*, 937–952. [CrossRef]
4. World Health Organization. *Global Action Plan for the Prevention and Control of Noncommunicable Diseases 2013–2020*; World Health Organization: Geneva, Switzerland, 2013.
5. Hamer, M.; O'Donovan, G.; Murphy, M. Physical Inactivity and the Economic and Health Burdens Due to Cardiovascular Disease: Exercise as Medicine. *Adv. Exp. Med. Biol.* **2017**, *999*, 3–18. [CrossRef]
6. Hu, F.B. Protein, Body Weight, and Cardiovascular Health. *Am. J. Clin. Nutr.* **2005**, *82*, 242S–247S. [CrossRef]
7. Zhang, B.; Xiong, K.; Cai, J.; Ma, A. Fish Consumption and Coronary Heart Disease: A Meta-Analysis. *Nutrients* **2020**, *12*, 2278. [CrossRef]
8. Cui, K.; Liu, Y.; Zhu, L.; Mei, X.; Jin, P.; Luo, Y. Association between Intake of Red and Processed Meat and the Risk of Heart Failure: A Meta-Analysis. *BMC Public Health* **2019**, *19*, 1–8. [CrossRef]
9. Widmer, R.J.; Flammer, A.J.; Lerman, L.O.; Lerman, A. The Mediterranean Diet, Its Components, and Cardiovascular Disease. *Am. J. Med.* **2015**, *128*, 229–238. [CrossRef]
10. Bechthold, A.; Boeing, H.; Schwedhelm, C.; Hoffmann, G.; Knüppel, S.; Iqbal, K.; De Henauw, S.; Michels, N.; Devleesschauwer, B.; Schlesinger, S.; et al. Food Groups and Risk of Coronary Heart Disease, Stroke and Heart Failure: A Systematic Review and Dose-Response Meta-Analysis of Prospective Studies. *Crit. Rev. Food Sci. Nutr.* **2019**, *59*, 1071–1090. [CrossRef] [PubMed]
11. Kotseva, K.; De Backer, G.; De Bacquer, D.; Rydén, L.; Hoes, A.; Grobbee, D.; Maggioni, A.; Marques-Vidal, P.; Jennings, C.; Abreu, A.; et al. Lifestyle and Impact on Cardiovascular Risk Factor Control in Coronary Patients across 27 Countries: Results from the European Society of Cardiology ESC-EORP EUROASPIRE V Registry. *Eur. J. Prev. Cardiol.* **2019**, *26*, 824–835. [CrossRef] [PubMed]
12. Tang, L.; Patao, C.; Chuang, J.; Wong, N.D. Cardiovascular Risk Factor Control and Adherence to Recommended Lifestyle and Medical Therapies in Persons with Coronary Heart Disease (from the National Health and Nutrition Examination Survey 2007–2010). *Am. J. Cardiol.* **2013**, *112*, 1126–1132. [CrossRef]
13. Greco, A.; Brugnera, A.; D'Addario, M.; Compare, A.; Franzelli, C.; Maloberti, A.; Giannattasio, C.; Fattirolli, F.; Steca, P. A Three-Year Longitudinal Study of Healthy Lifestyle Behaviors and Adherence to Pharmacological Treatments in Newly Diagnosed Patients with Acute Coronary Syndrome: Hierarchical Linear Modeling Analyses. *J. Public Health (Bangkok)* **2020**, 1–12. [CrossRef]
14. Grace, S.L.; Abbey, S.E.; Shnek, Z.M.; Irvine, J.; Franche, R.-L.; Stewart, D.E. Cardiac Rehabilitation II: Referral and Participation. *Gen. Hosp. Psychiatry* **2002**, *24*, 127–134. [CrossRef]

15. Jensen, M.T.; Marott, J.L.; Holtermann, A.; Gyntelberg, F. Living Alone Is Associated with All-Cause and Cardiovascular Mortality: 32 Years of Follow-up in the Copenhagen Male Study. *Eur. Heart J. Qual. Care Clin. Outcomes* **2019**, *5*, 208–217. [CrossRef]
16. May, H.T.; Horne, B.D.; Knight, S.; Knowlton, K.U.; Bair, T.L.; Lappé, D.L.; Le, V.T.; Muhlestein, J.B. The Association of Depression at Any Time to the Risk of Death Following Coronary Artery Disease Diagnosis. *Eur. Heart. J. Qual. Care Clin. Outcomes* **2017**, *3*, 296–302. [CrossRef]
17. Monzani, D.; D'Addario, M.; Fattirolli, F.; Giannattasio, C.; Greco, A.; Quarenghi, F.; Steca, P. Clustering of Lifestyle Risk Factors in Acute Coronary Syndrome: Prevalence and Change after the First Event. *Appl. Psychol. Health Well-Being* **2018**, *10*, 434–456. [CrossRef] [PubMed]
18. Kuhl, E.A.; Fauerbach, J.A.; Bush, D.E.; Ziegelstein, R.C. Relation of Anxiety and Adherence to Risk-Reducing Recommendations Following Myocardial Infarction. *Am. J. Cardiol.* **2009**, *103*, 1629–1634. [CrossRef]
19. Steca, P.; Monzani, D.; Greco, A.; Franzelli, C.; Magrin, M.E.; Miglioretti, M.; Sarini, M.; Scrignaro, M.; Vecchio, L.; Fattirolli, F.; et al. Stability and Change of Lifestyle Profiles in Cardiovascular Patients after Their First Acute Coronary Event. *PLoS ONE* **2017**, *12*, e0183905. [CrossRef]
20. Ma, Y.; Olendzki, B.C.; Li, W.; Hafner, A.R.; Chiriboga, D.; Hebert, J.R.; Campbell, M.; Sarnie, M.; Ockene, I.S. Seasonal Variation in Food Intake, Physical Activity, and Body Weight in a Predominantly Overweight Population. *Eur. J. Clin. Nutr.* **2006**, *60*, 519–528. [CrossRef]
21. Stelmach-Mardas, M.; Kleiser, C.; Uzhova, I.; Peñalvo, J.L.; La Torre, G.; Palys, W.; Lojko, D.; Nimptsch, K.; Suwalska, A.; Linseisen, J.; et al. Seasonality of Food Groups and Total Energy Intake: A Systematic Review and Meta-Analysis. *Eur. J. Clin. Nutr.* **2016**, *70*, 700–708. [CrossRef]
22. van der Toorn, J.E.; Cepeda, M. Seasonal Variation of Diet Quality in a Large Middle-Aged and Elderly Dutch Population-Based Cohort. *Eur. J. Nutr.* **2020**, *59*, 493–504. [CrossRef]
23. Bhatnagar, A. Environmental Determinants of Cardiovascular Disease. *Circ. Res.* **2017**, *121*, 162–180. [CrossRef] [PubMed]
24. Izawa, K.P.; Watanabe, S.; Oka, K.; Brubaker, P.H.; Hirano, Y.; Omori, Y.; Kida, K.; Suzuki, K.; Osada, N.; Omiya, K.; et al. Leisure-Time Physical Activity over Four Seasons in Chronic Heart Failure Patients. *Int. J. Cardiol.* **2014**, *177*, 651–653. [CrossRef] [PubMed]
25. Klompstra, L.; Jaarsma, T.; Strömberg, A.; van der Wal, M.H.L. Seasonal Variation in Physical Activity in Patients with Heart Failure. *Heart Lung* **2019**, *48*, 381–385. [CrossRef]
26. Steca, P.; Pancani, L.; Greco, A.; D'Addario, M.; Magrin, M.E.; Miglioretti, M.; Sarini, M.; Scrignaro, M.; Vecchio, L.; Cesana, F.; et al. Changes in Dietary Behavior among Coronary and Hypertensive Patients: A Longitudinal Investigation Using the Health Action Process Approach. *Appl. Psychol. Health Well Being* **2015**, *7*, 316–339. [CrossRef] [PubMed]
27. Trichopoulou, A.; Costacou, T.; Bamia, C.; Trichopoulos, D. Adherence to a Mediterranean Diet and Survival in a Greek Population. *N. Engl. J. Med.* **2003**, *348*, 2599–2608. [CrossRef]
28. Topolski, T.D.; LoGerfo, J.; Patrick, D.L.; Williams, B.; Walwick, J.; Patrick, M.B. The Rapid Assessment of Physical Activity (RAPA) among Older Adults. *Prev. Chronic Dis.* **2006**, *3*, A118.
29. Zigmond, A.S.; Snaith, R.P. The Hospital Anxiety and Depression Scale. *Acta Psychiatr. Scand.* **1983**, *67*, 361–370. [CrossRef] [PubMed]
30. Costantini, M.; Musso, M.; Viterbori, P.; Bonci, F.; Del Mastro, L.; Garrone, O.; Venturini, M.; Morasso, G. Detecting Psychological Distress in Cancer Patients: Validity of the Italian Version of the Hospital Anxiety and Depression Scale. *Support. Care Cancer* **1999**, *7*, 121–127. [CrossRef]
31. Raudenbush, S.W.; Bryk, A.S. *Hierarchical Linear Models: Applications and Data Analysis Methods*, 2nd ed.; Sage: Thousand Oaks, CA, USA, 2002; Volume 1.
32. Gallop, R.; Tasca, G.A. Multilevel Modeling of Longitudinal Data for Psychotherapy Researchers: II. The Complexities. *Psychother. Res.* **2009**, *19*, 438–452. [CrossRef]
33. Willet, J.; Singer, J. *Applied Longitudinal Data Analysis: Modeling Change and Event Occurrence*; Oxford University Press: New York, NY, USA, 2003.
34. Calabrò, P.; Gragnano, F.; Di Maio, M.; Patti, G.; Antonucci, E.; Cirillo, P.; Gresele, P.; Palareti, G.; Pengo, V.; Pignatelli, P.; et al. Epidemiology and Management of Patients With Acute Coronary Syndromes in Contemporary Real-World Practice: Evolving Trends from the EYESHOT Study to the START-ANTIPLATELET Registry. *Angiology* **2018**, *69*, 795–802. [CrossRef]
35. Munyombwe, T.; Hall, M.; Dondo, T.B.; Alabas, O.A.; Gerard, O.; West, R.M.; Pujades-Rodriguez, M.; Hall, A.; Gale, C.P. Quality of Life Trajectories in Survivors of Acute Myocardial Infarction: A National Longitudinal Study. *Heart* **2020**, *106*, 33–39. [CrossRef]
36. Peersen, K.; Munkhaugen, J.; Gullestad, L.; Liodden, T.; Moum, T.; Dammen, T.; Perk, J.; Otterstad, J.E. The Role of Cardiac Rehabilitation in Secondary Prevention after Coronary Events. *Eur. J. Prev. Cardiol.* **2017**, *24*, 1360–1368. [CrossRef]
37. Urbinati, S.; Olivari, Z.; Gonzini, L.; Savonitto, S.; Farina, R.; Del Pinto, M.; Valbusa, A.; Fantini, G.; Mazzoni, A.; Maggioni, A.P. Secondary Prevention after Acute Myocardial Infarction: Drug Adherence, Treatment Goals, and Predictors of Health Lifestyle Habits. The BLITZ-4 Registry. *Eur. J. Prev. Cardiol.* **2015**, *22*, 1548–1556. [CrossRef]
38. Claassen, L.; Henneman, L.; Kindt, I.; Marteau, T.M.; Timmermans, D.R. Perceived Risk and Representations of Cardiovascular Disease and Preventive Behaviour in People Diagnosed with Familial Hypercholesterolemia: A Cross-Sectional Questionnaire Study. *J. Health Psychol.* **2010**, *15*, 33–43. [CrossRef] [PubMed]

39. Alwan, H.; William, J.; Viswanathan, B.; Paccaud, F.; Bovet, P. Perception of Cardiovascular Risk and Comparison with Actual Cardiovascular Risk. *Eur. J. Cardiovasc. Prev. Rehabil.* **2009**, *16*, 556–561. [CrossRef]
40. Laursen, U.B.; Johansen, M.N.; Joensen, A.M.; Overvad, K.; Larsen, M.L. Is Cardiac Rehabilitation Equally Effective in Improving Dietary Intake in All Patients with Ischemic Heart Disease? *J. Am. Coll. Nutr.* **2020**, 1–8. [CrossRef] [PubMed]
41. Grace, S.L.; Abbey, S.E.; Shnek, Z.M.; Irvine, J.; Franche, R.-L.; Stewart, D.E. Cardiac Rehabilitation I: Review of Psychosocial Factors. *Gen. Hosp. Psychiatry* **2002**, *24*, 121–126. [CrossRef]
42. Tully, P.J.; Cosh, S.M.; Baune, B.T. A review of the affects of worry and generalized anxiety disorder upon cardiovascular health and coronary heart disease. *Psychol. Health Med.* **2013**, *18*, 627–644. [CrossRef]
43. Beckie, T.M.; Beckstead, J.W. Predicting Cardiac Rehabilitation Attendance in a Gender-Tailored Randomized Clinical Trial. *J. Cardiopulm. Rehabil. Prev.* **2010**, *30*, 147–156. [CrossRef]
44. Parker, G.; Hyett, M.; Hadzi-Pavlovic, D.; Brotchie, H.; Walsh, W. GAD is good? Generalized anxiety disorder predicts a superior five-year outcome following an acute coronary syndrome. *Psychiatry Res.* **2011**, *188*, 383–389. [CrossRef] [PubMed]
45. Lee, T.J.; Cameron, L.D.; Wünsche, B.; Stevens, C. A randomized trial of computer-based communications using imagery and text information to alter representations of heart disease risk and motivate protective behaviour. *Br. J. Health Psychol.* **2011**, *16*, 72–91. [CrossRef] [PubMed]
46. Conraads, V.M.; Deaton, C.; Piotrowicz, E.; Santaularia, N.; Tierney, S.; Piepoli, M.F.; Pieske, B.; Schmid, J.P.; Dickstein, K.; Ponikowski, P.P.; et al. Adherence of Heart Failure Patients to Exercise: Barriers and Possible Solutions: A Position Statement of the Study Group on Exercise Training in Heart Failure of the Heart Failure Association of the European Society of Cardiology. *Eur. J. Heart Fail.* **2012**, *14*, 451–458. [CrossRef] [PubMed]
47. Greco, A.; Steca, P.; Pozzi, R.; Monzani, D.; D'Addario, M.; Villani, A.; Rella, V.; Giglio, A.; Malfatto, G.; Parati, G. Predicting Depression from Illness Severity in Cardiovascular Disease Patients: Self-Efficacy Beliefs, Illness Perception, and Perceived Social Support as Mediators. *Int. J. Behav. Med.* **2014**, *21*, 221–229. [CrossRef]
48. Vellone, E.; Pancani, L.; Greco, A.; Steca, P.; Riegel, B. Self-Care Confidence May Be More Important than Cognition to Influence Self-Care Behaviors in Adults with Heart Failure: Testing a Mediation Model. *Int. J. Nurs. Stud.* **2016**, *60*, 191–199. [CrossRef]
49. Bandura, A. Self-Efficacy: Toward a Unifying Theory of Behavioral Change. *Psychol. Rev.* **1977**, *84*, 191. [CrossRef]
50. Schwarzer, R. Social-Cognitive Factors in Changing Health-Related Behaviors. *Curr. Dir. Psychol. Sci.* **2001**, *10*, 47–51. [CrossRef]
51. Sol, B.G.M.; van der Graaf, Y.; van Petersen, R.; Visseren, F.L.J. The Effect of Self-Efficacy on Cardiovascular Lifestyle. *Eur. J. Cardiovasc. Nurs.* **2011**, *10*, 180–186. [CrossRef]
52. Baretta, D.; Sartori, F.; Greco, A.; D'Addario, M.; Melen, R.; Steca, P. Improving Physical Activity MHealth Interventions: Development of a Computational Model of Self-Efficacy Theory to Define Adaptive Goals for Exercise Promotion. *Adv. Hum. Comput. Interact.* **2019**, *2019*, 3068748. [CrossRef]
53. Schwarzer, R. Modeling health behavior change: How to predict and modify the adoption and maintenance of health behaviors. *Appl. Psychol.* **2008**, *57*, 1–29. [CrossRef]
54. Sharman, J.E.; La Gerche, A.; Coombes, J.S. Exercise and Cardiovascular Risk in Patients with Hypertension. *Am. J. Hypertens.* **2015**, *28*, 147–158. [CrossRef] [PubMed]
55. Aaby, A.; Friis, K.; Christensen, B.; Rowlands, G.; Maindal, H.T. Health Literacy Is Associated with Health Behaviour and Self-Reported Health: A Large Population-Based Study in Individuals with Cardiovascular Disease. *Eur. J. Prev. Cardiol.* **2017**, *24*, 1880–1888. [CrossRef] [PubMed]
56. Veronesi, G.; Ferrario, M.M.; Kuulasmaa, K.; Bobak, M.; Chambless, L.E.; Salomaa, V.; Soderberg, S.; Pajak, A.; Jørgensen, T.; Amouyel, P.; et al. Educational Class Inequalities in the Incidence of Coronary Heart Disease in Europe. *Heart* **2016**, *102*, 958–965. [CrossRef] [PubMed]
57. Magrin, M.E.; D'addario, M.; Greco, A.; Miglioretti, M.; Sarini, M.; Scrignaro, M.; Steca, P.; Vecchio, L.; Crocetti, E. Social Support and Adherence to Treatment in Hypertensive Patients: A Meta-Analysis. *Ann. Behav. Med.* **2015**, *49*, 307–318. [CrossRef]
58. Wareheim, S.; Dinkel, D.; Alonso, W.; Pozehl, B. Long-term exercise adherence in patients with heart failure: A qualitative study. *Heart Lung* **2020**, *49*, 696–701. [CrossRef] [PubMed]
59. Prince, S.A.; Adamo, K.B.; Hamel, M.E.; Hardt, J.; Gorber, S.C.; Tremblay, M. A Comparison of Direct versus Self-Report Measures for Assessing Physical Activity in Adults: A Systematic Review. *Int. J. Behav. Nutr. Phys. Act.* **2008**, *5*, 1–24. [CrossRef] [PubMed]

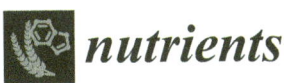

Article

Nutrition Status and Renal Function as Predictors in Acute Myocardial Infarction with and without Cancer: A Single Center Retrospective Study

Naoki Itaya [1], Ako Fukami [1], Tatsuyuki Kakuma [2] and Yoshihiro Fukumoto [1,*]

[1] Division of Cardiovascular Medicine, Department of Internal Medicine, Kurume University School of Medicine, Kurume 830-0011, Japan; itaya_naoki@kurume-u.ac.jp (N.I.); fukami_ako@kurume-u.ac.jp (A.F.)
[2] Biostatistics Center, Kurume University, Kurume 830-0011, Japan; tkakuma@med.kurume-u.ac.jp
* Correspondence: fukumoto_yoshihiro@med.kurume-u.ac.jp; Tel.: +81-94-231-7562

Abstract: *Background:* Clinical characteristics of nutrition status in acute myocardial infarction (AMI) patients with cancer remains unknown. Therefore, this study aimed to clarify the differences of clinical parameters, including nutrition status, between AMI patients with and without history of cancer. *Methods and Results:* This retrospective cohort study, using the database of AMI between 2014 and 2019 in Kurume University Hospital, enrolled 411 patients; AMI patients without cancer (*n* = 358, 87.1%) and with cancer (*n* = 53, 12.9%). AMI patients with cancer were significantly older with lower body weight, worse renal function, and worse nutrition status. Next, we divided the patients into 4 groups by cancer, age, and plaque area, detected by coronary image devices. The prediction model indicated that nutrition, lipid, and renal functions were significant predictors of AMI with cancer. The ordinal logistic regression model revealed that worse nutrition status, renal dysfunction, lower uric acid, and elevated blood pressure were significant predictors. Finally, we were able to calculate the probability of the presence of cancer, by combining each factor and scoring. *Conclusions:* Worse nutrition status and renal dysfunction were associated with AMI with cancer, in which nutrition status was a major different characteristic from those without cancer.

Keywords: onco-cardiology; nutrition status; cancer; acute myocardial infarction

Citation: Itaya, N.; Fukami, A.; Kakuma, T.; Fukumoto, Y. Nutrition Status and Renal Function as Predictors in Acute Myocardial Infarction with and without Cancer: A Single Center Retrospective Study. *Nutrients* 2021, *13*, 2663. https://doi.org/10.3390/nu13082663

Academic Editor: Pramod Khosla

Received: 22 June 2021
Accepted: 28 July 2021
Published: 30 July 2021

Publisher's Note: MDPI stays neutral with regard to jurisdictional claims in published maps and institutional affiliations.

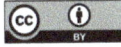

Copyright: © 2021 by the authors. Licensee MDPI, Basel, Switzerland. This article is an open access article distributed under the terms and conditions of the Creative Commons Attribution (CC BY) license (https://creativecommons.org/licenses/by/4.0/).

1. Introduction

Acute myocardial infarction (AMI) is mainly caused by coronary arteries thrombus due to atherosclerotic plaque rupture or endothelial erosion, and sometimes coronary artery spasm, microvascular thrombus, or others [1]. The formation of fibrofatty lesions in the atherosclerotic vulnerable plaques occurs during the atherosclerosis progression [2], which have been treated by lipid-lowering therapy to stabilize during these 2 decades [3,4]. Further, it has been reported that rapid plaque progression of moderately severe vulnerable plaques is the critical step prior to AMI in most patients [5–7]. Actually, accumulating evidence demonstrates that atherosclerotic risk factors, including hypertension, dyslipidemia, diabetes mellitus, and cigarette smoking, develop atherosclerotic lesions through immune system [2]. The atherosclerotic plaques often contain lipid core and fibrous cap, which consist of smooth muscle cells, macrophages, angiogenesis, and adventitial inflammation [8]. Taken together, when focused on vulnerable coronary atherosclerosis, not stable atheroma, it is considered that AMI most likely occurs due to rapidly progressed coronary atherosclerosis, caused by traditional atherosclerotic risk factors, including age; however, even small atherosclerotic plaques can cause AMI in some patients, which might be associated with some other risk factors.

In cancer patients, the mechanisms of atherosclerosis progression might be different. Especially, clonal hematopoiesis with indeterminate potential (CHIP) has been reported to increase the risk of AMI [9]. CHIP carriers had a 4.0-fold (95% confidence interval 2.4–6.7)

higher risk of myocardial infarction than non-carriers [9]. It has been also reported that each of DNA methyltransferase 3A (DNMT3A), ten-eleven translocation-2 (TET2), additional sex combs-like 1 (ASXL1), and Janus kinase 2 (JAK2) mutation was associated with coronary artery disease, and that CHIP carriers with these mutations also had high levels of coronary artery calcification [9]. Further, TET2-deficient bone marrow cells enlarge atherosclerotic plaques by infiltrating macrophages, and TET2-deficiency increases cytokines/chemokines such as C-X-C motif ligand (CXCL)-1, CXCL 2, CXCL 3, interleukin (IL)-6 and IL-1β [10]. Also, Heyde et al., have reported that CHIP causes hematopoietic stem cell proliferation, promotes arteriosclerosis, and leads to a vicious cycle of proliferation of hematopoietic stem cells [11]. Above all, CHIP is an independent coronary risk factor in patients with premature menopause, especially in patients with spontaneous premature menopause [12]. Thus, coronary risk factors in the clinical settings might be different between cancer and non-cancer patients.

During these 4 decades, cancer is the first cause of death in Japan, and cardiovascular diseases (CVDs) are the second [13]. Because of recent improvement of cancer prognosis due to the advancement of cancer early detection, surgery, and anticancer drug treatment, the number of cancer survivors has increased [6,7]. Cancer and CVDs have common risks of lifestyle factors, such as smoking, obesity, and unhealthy food intake, in which healthy lifestyle is oppositely associated with a longer life expectancy free from major chronic diseases, including cancer and CVDs [14]. However, the clinical characteristics, especially in the aspects of nutrition status, remains scant in AMI patients with cancer.

Therefore, the purpose of the present study was to clarify the differences of clinical parameters in AMI with and without history of cancer, focusing on traditional coronary risk factors and nutrition status, and to develop a statistical model to evaluate the presence of cancer in patients with AMI, using database of AMI in Kurume University Hospital.

2. Materials and Methods

2.1. Study Design

This study was retrospective cohort study using the database of AMI in Cardiovascular Medicine, Kurume University Hospital. We enrolled 437 patients, who were treated by primary percutaneous coronary intervention (PCI) due to AMI in Cardiovascular Medicine, Kurume University Hospital from January 2014 to December 2019. We excluded patients if the patients had following reasons; (1) AMI occurred due to PCI complication, (2) PCI due to acute stent thrombosis, (3) unsuccessful PCI, and (4) coronary bypass surgery due to multi-vessel coronary artery disease.

2.2. Data Collection

Baseline demographic data were collected based on the medical records, including age, sex, height, body weight, waist, medications, traditional risk factors (hypertension, glucose intolerance/diabetes mellitus and dyslipidemia), blood pressure (BP), pulse rate, heart rate, and comorbidities (coronary artery disease, hypertensive heart disease, cardiomyopathy, valvular heart diseases, and congenital heart diseases). All cardiovascular diseases were diagnosed by expert cardiologists. AMI was diagnosed according to fourth universal definition of myocardial infarction [15].

All patients were treated by PCI combined with the use of image devices, such as intravascular ultrasound (IVUS) or optical coherence tomography (OCT). We retrospectively measured the coronary atherosclerotic plaque area by image devices at the culprit lesions.

2.3. Blood Sampling

Peripheral blood was drawn from the antecubital vein for measurements of blood cell counts, lipid profiles including total cholesterol (T.chol), low-density lipoprotein cholesterol (LDL-c), high-density lipoprotein cholesterol (HDL-c), and triglyceride, liver and renal function markers including creatinine (Cr) and estimated glomerular filtration rate (eGFR), glycemic parameters of fasting plasma glucose (FPG) and hemoglobin A1c (HbA1c), uric acid, troponin, and N-terminal pro-brain natriuretic peptide (NT-pro-BNP). These chemistries were measured at a commercially available laboratory in Kurume University Hospital.

2.4. Definition of Comorbidities

Hypertension was defined as the use of antihypertensive drugs and/or systolic blood pressure ≥ 140 mmHg or diastolic blood pressure ≥ 90 mmHg. Dyslipidemia was defined as the use of lipid-lowering drugs and/or plasma LDL-c ≥ 140 mg/dL and/or triglycerides ≥ 150 mg/dL, and/or HDL-c < 40 mg/dL. Diabetes mellitus was diagnosed using antidiabetic drugs and/or fasting plasma glucose ≥ 110 mg/dL or HbA$_{1c}$ ≥ 6.5%.

2.5. Evaluation of Nutrition Status

The nutrition status was evaluated using the Glasgow Prognostic Score (GPS) [16], modified GPS (mGPS) [17,18] and Controlling Nutritional Status (CONUT) [19].

2.6. Statistical Analysis

All continuous variables were given as the mean ± standard deviations (SDs) or median with interquartile range. Categorical data were presented as number (*n*) or percentage (%). For intergroup univariate comparisons, an unpaired *t* test was applied in continuous variables and chi-square test in categorical variables.

The mean ± SDs and frequencies were presented by the two groups with and without cancer (Tables 1 and 2).

Table 1. Clinical characteristics of acute myocardial infarction patients with and without cancer.

	Non-Cancer (N = 358)	Cancer (N = 53)	*p* Value
Age, y	67.6 ± 12.3	74.0 ± 7.6	<0.0001
Male sex (*n*,%)	273.0 (80.0)	38.0 (70.0)	0.47
Height, cm	161.7 ± 9.4	157.9 ± 8.9	0.006
Body mass index	23.8 ± 3.6	22.8 ± 2.8	0.03
Weight, kg	62.8 ± 13.2	57.2 ± 9.4	0.0002
Systolic BP, mmHg	131.2 ± 26.6	131.5 ± 25.2	0.95
Diastolic BP, mmHg	78.2 ± 18.3	71.5 ± 15.5	0.01
Heart rate, bpm	80.5 ± 21.9	83.6 ± 20.0	0.34
Blood test			
Red blood cell count, ×10^4/mm^3	7.1 ± 35.8	3.9 ± 0.8	0.1
Hemoglobin, g/dL	13.6 ± 2.0	12.2 ± 2.2	<0.0001
Hematocrit, %	40.0 ± 5.5	36.0 ± 6.2	<0.0001
Platelet count, ×10^4/mm^3	218.7 ± 68.7	227.9 ± 110.3	0.56
White blood cell count, /mm^3	10.6 ± 4.3	9.2 ± 4.3	0.04
Lymphocytes, /mm^3	2126.7 ± 1470.1	1708.0 ± 1248.1	0.05
Total bilirubin, mg/dL	0.7 ± 0.3	0.8 ± 0.5	0.22
AST, U/L	133.0 (25–72.3)	62.8 (25.5–54)	0.21
ALT, U/L	56.3 (17–42)	31.4 (15–29.5)	0.05
LDH, U/L	355.9 (199.8–347.5)	297.7 (202–335.5)	0.17
ALP, U/L	234.3 ±79.9	316.8 ± 250.7	0.03
γ-GTP, U/L	41.7 (18.3–47.8)	45.8 (17–46)	0.66
C-reactive protein, mg/dL	0.8 ±2.0	1.9 ± 4.9	0.1
Creatinine kinase, U/L	492.6 (104.8–421.3)	319.6 (81.5–356)	0.03
Creatinine kinase -MB, U/L	45.1 (6–44)	31.9 (7–33.5)	0.1
NT-pro BNP, pg/mL	402.1 (75.3–2013.7)	5993.1 (212–3720)	0.54
Blood urea nitrogen, mg/dL	18.5 ± 9.5	21.7 ± 15.8	0.16
Creatinine, mg/dL	1.1 (0.64–1.01)	1.6 (0.69–1.11)	0.14
eGFR, mL/min/1.73 m^2	71.0 (54.3–88.5)	59.2 (46.8–74.7)	0.005
Sodium, mEq/L	139.3 ± 3.2	137.8 ± 4.0	0.01
Potassium, mEq/L	4.0 ± 0.6	4.2 ± 0.6	0.11
Chloride, mEq/L	104.0 ± 3.5	102.9 ± 3.8	0.03

Table 1. Cont.

	Non-Cancer (N = 358)	Cancer (N = 53)	p Value
Uric acid, mg/dL	5.9 ± 1.8	5.7 ± 1.8	0.37
Fasting plasma glucose, mg/dL	176.8 ± 79.1	164.6 ± 53.9	0.29
Hemoglobin A$_{1C}$, %	6.3 ± 1.2	6.4 ± 0.9	0.76
Total protein, g/dL	6.6 ± 0.6	6.4 ± 0.9	0.12
Albumin, g/dL	3.7 ± 0.5	3.5 ± 0.6	0.005
Total cholesterol, mg/dL	187.1 ± 44.5	169.5 ± 58.7	0.04
Triglyceride, mg/dL	131.8 (67.3–160.8)	123.0 (65.3–146.8)	0.62
HDL-cholesterol, mg/dL	48.2 ± 11.7	47.6 ± 13.6	0.72
LDL-cholesterol, mg/dL	121.2 ± 37.6	104.7 ± 45.8	0.02
PT-INR	1.1 ± 0.4	1.1 ± 0.3	0.92
APTT, sec	55.7 (26.2–50.2)	51.8 (27.7–39.2)	0.63
D-dimer, µg/mL	3.9 (0.6–1.8)	4.8 (0.9–2.1)	0.69
FDP, µg/mL	10.2 (2.5–5.6)	12.1 (2.9–7.6)	0.66
Cardiac ultrasonography			
AOD, mm	30.1 ± 4.2	29.1 ± 4.3	0.18
LAD, mm	33.7 ± 6.1	33.5 ± 6.0	0.87
IVST, mm	9.8 ± 2.1	9.5 ± 1.9	0.39
PWT, mm	10.3 ± 5.9	9.9 ± 1.7	0.32
LVDd, mm	45.1 ± 6.9	44.2 ± 5.8	0.39
LVDs, mm	32.9 ± 7.2	32.2 ± 7.5	0.54
EF, %	50.6 ± 14.2	52.6 ± 14.2	0.33
Nutrition status			
CONUT score	1.9 ± 2.0	3.2 ± 2.6	0.002
mGPS			
score 0, n (%)	233 (57.3)	21 (5.2)	
score 1, n (%)	83 (20.4)	18 (4.4)	0.0002
score 2, n (%)	38 (9.3)	13 (3.2)	
GPS			
score 0, n (%)	249 (61.3)	28 (6.8)	
score 1, n (%)	75 (18.5)	13 (3.2)	0.003
score 2, n (%)	30 (7.3)	11 (2.7)	
Intravascular ultrasound			
CSA, mm^2	14.7 ± 4.6	12.1 ± 2.9	<0.0001
MLA, mm^2	4.1 ± 1.3	3.5 ± 1.3	0.04
PA (CSA-MLA), mm^2	10.6 ± 4.2	8.6 ± 2.8	0.0001
Percentages of PA, % (%PA = (CSA-MLA)/CSA)	70.9 ± 9.7	69.7 ± 9.6	0.47

Data are mean ± SD or median (interquartile rage). Abbreviations: BP: blood pressure, AST: aspartate aminotransferase, ALT: alanine aminotransferase, LDH: Lactate dehydrogenase, γGTP:γ-Glutamyl transpeptidase, ALP: alkaline phosphatase, NT-pro BNP: N-terminal pro-brain natriuretic peptide, eGFR: estimated glomerular filtration rate, HDL: high-density lipoprotein, LDL: low-density lipoprotein, PT-INR: Prothrombin time-international normalized ratio, APTT: activated partial thromboplastin time, FDP: fibrin/fibrinogen degradation products, AOD: aortic dimension, LAD: left atrial dimension, IVST: interventricular septum thickness, PWT: posterior wall thickness, LVDd: left ventricular diameter at end diastole LVDs: left ventricular diameter at end systole, EF: ejection fraction, CONUT: Controlling Nutrition Status, mGPS: modified Glasgow Prognostic Score, GPS: Glasgow Prognostic Score, CSA: average reference lumen cross-sectional area, MLA: minimal lumen area, PA: plaque area.

Table 2. Comorbidities and medicine of acute myocardial infarction patients with and without cancer.

	Non-Cancer (N = 358)		Cancer (N = 53)		p Value
	Yes, n	%	Yes, n	%	
Acute myocardial infarction	319	89.1	45	84.9	0.37
Unstable angina pectoris	39	10.9	8	15.1	0.37
Responsible lesion					
Left anterior descending artery	190	53.1	30	56.6	0.63
Left circumflex artery	36	10.1	8	15.1	0.27
Multivessel disease	174	48.6	32	60.3	0.23
Right coronary artery	125	34.9	15	28.3	0.34
Smoking (Current and former)	229	64.0	35	66.0	0.76

Table 2. Cont.

	Non-Cancer (N = 358)		Cancer (N = 53)		p Value
	Yes, n	%	Yes, n	%	
Comorbidities					
Hypertension	265	74.0	41	77.4	0.60
Dyslipidemia	263	73.5	33	62.3	0.09
Diabetes mellitus	155	43.3	32	60.4	0.02
Hyperuricemia	91	25.4	13	24.5	0.89
Chronic kidney disease	117	32.7	25	47.2	0.04
Hemodialysis	13	3.6	4	7.5	0.18
Percutaneous coronary intervention	48	13.4	9	17.0	0.48
Coronary artery bypass graft	5	1.4	3	5.7	0.03
Aortic disease	10	2.8	3	5.7	0.26
Collagen disease	11	3.1	4	7.5	0.11
Peripheral artery disease	16	4.5	6	11.3	0.04
Cerebrovascular disease	45	12.6	10	18.9	0.21
Medication					
Angiotensin-converting enzyme inhibitor	25	7.0	5	9.4	0.52
Angiotensin II receptor blocker	102	28.5	15	28.3	0.97
Aspirin	65	18.2	15	28.3	0.08
Beta blocker	43	12.0	9	17.0	0.31
Antihyperuricemic	19	5.3	4	7.5	0.51
Calcium channel blocker	116	32.4	19	35.8	0.62
Diuretic	37	10.3	8	15.1	0.30
Clopidogrel	34	9.5	10	18.9	0.04
Prasugrel	3	0.8	0	0.0	0.50
Ticlopidine	1	0.3	2	3.8	0.01
Warfarin	9	2.5	3	5.7	0.20
Direct oral anticoagulants	5	1.4	0	0.0	0.39
Other antiplatelet agents	10	2.8	5	9.4	0.02
Dipeptidyl-peptidase IV inhibitor	54	15.1	13	24.5	0.08
Sodium glucose cotransporter II inhibitor	6	1.7	1	1.9	0.91
Insulin	20	5.6	4	7.5	0.57
Other oral hypoglycemic agent	59	16.5	12	22.6	0.26
Statin	83	23.2	16	30.2	0.27
Omega-3 fatty acid ethyl esters	4	1.1	1	1.9	0.63
Eicosapentaenoic acid	12	3.4	3	5.7	0.40
Ezetimibe	7	2.0	2	3.8	0.40
Anti-cancer agent	0	0.0	8	15.1	<0.0001
Immunosuppressant	6	1.7	2	3.8	0.30
Steroid	11	3.1	5	9.4	0.03
In-hospital mortality	17	4.7	4	7.5	0.38
Intravascular ultrasound	304	84.9	47	88.7	0.47

To evaluate the impact of various risk factors of myocardial infarction on cancer and non-cancer patients, following three analytical steps were taken. First, the classification and regression tree (CART) model was employed to define risk groups (Table 3). Cancer status (yes or no) was used as the response variable and plaque area, age and sex were used as predictors. The fitted probability for the levels of the response was calculated, and the split is chosen to minimize the residual log-likelihood chi-square. Second, principal component analyses were performed to derive synthetic variables based on five sets of risk factors. Specifically, three measurements of nutrition, two measurements for lipid, glucose, blood pressure and renal function were subjected in the principal component analyses which render a way to avoid collinearity problems among highly correlated measurements within each set of risk factor (Tables 4 and 5). Finally, ordinal logistic regression was employed to evaluate effect of each synthetic variables on the risk groups derived from the CART. Effect of each synthetic variable was interpreted based on the odds ratio (Tables 6 and 7), and the predicted probability of the risk groups were calculated (Figure 5). To compare the results with logistic regressing model with cancer/non-cancer as response variable, an additional table was added (Table 8).

Table 3. Divided groups by age and atherosclerotic plaque area.

Group	N	Cancer	Age	Plaque Area	Group Definition
G1	90	No	<60 years old	N/A	Non-cancer/Low risk
G2	122	No	≥60 years old	≥9.39 mm^2	Non-cancer/Middle risk
G3	146	No	≥60 years old	<9.39 mm^2	Non-cancer/High risk
G4	53	Yes	≥60 years old	N/A	Cancer

Table 4. Compartments of Synthetic variable with weights.

Synthetic Variable	Original Variables with Its Weight			
Nutrition	CONUT (0.243)	GPS (0.898)	mGPS (0.846)	cons * (−1.307)
Lipid	T.chol (0.015)	LDL-c (0.018)	-	cons * (−4.947)
Glucose	FPG (0.009)	HbA1c (0.594)	-	cons * (−4.45)
Blood pressure	sBP (0.027)	Pulse pressure (0.038)	-	cons * (−5.559)
Renal function	Cr (0.469)	eGFR (0.025)	-	cons * (1.151)

Abbreviations: CONUT; Controlling Nutrition Status, GPS; Glasgow Prognostic Score, mGPS; modified Glasgow Prognostic Score, T.chol; total cholesterol, LDL-c; low-density lipoprotein cholesterol, FPG; Fasting plasma glucose, HbA1c; hemoglobin A1c, sBP; systolic blood pressure, Cr; Creatinine, eGFR; estimated glomerular filtration rate, cons *; constant term used to calculate principal component score along with weight of each variable.

Table 5. Mean and SD of six risk variables by Four Groups.

	G1	G2	G3	G4	p Value *
Nutrition	−0.65 (1.13)	−0.15(1.43)	0.26(1.68)	0.76(1.85)	<0.0001
Lipid	0.44 (1.33)	0.001(1.19)	−0.09(1.39)	−0.50(1.69)	0.001
Glucose	−0.06 (1.15)	−0.09(0.95)	0.15(1.30)	−0.11(0.81)	0.27
Uric acid	6.33 (1.55)	5.86(1.76)	5.75(1.91)	5.70(1.82)	0.13
Blood pressure	−0.14 (1.23)	−0.01(1.38)	0.01(1.24)	0.22(1.49)	0.47
Renal function	−0.60 (0.83)	0.01(1.07)	0.19(1.36)	0.47(1.72)	<0.0001

p value * based on One-Way Analysis of Variance (ANOVA). Data are means (SD). The equation of nutrition was expressed as "Nutrition = (−1.307) + 0.243 * CONUT + 0.898 * GPS + 0.846 * mGPS". Similarly, other equations were expressed as "Lipid = (−4.947) + 0.018 * LDL-c + 0.015 * T.chol", "Glucose = (−5.448) + 0.594 * HbA1c + 0.0092 * FPG", "Blood pressure = (−5.559) + 0.038 * Pulse pressure + 0.027 * systolic BP", "Renal function = (1.151) + 0.469 * Cr + (−0.025) * eGFR". Nutrition, lipid, and renal functions were significant predictors of risk grouping.

Table 6. Estimate of the ordinal logistic regression model.

Parameter	Estimate	SE	Wald χ2	p Value
G4 (α1)	−0.985	0.362	7.39	0.01
G3 (α2)	1.157	0.359	10.39	0.00
G2 (α3)	2.658	0.376	50.00	<0.0001
Nutrition	0.232	0.071	10.64	0.00
Lipid	−0.134	0.080	2.80	0.09
Glucose	0.032	0.087	0.14	0.71
Blood pressure	0.157	0.074	4.53	0.03
Renal	0.363	0.091	16.00	<0.0001
Uric acid	−0.209	0.059	12.59	0.00
smoking (Yes)	−0.081	0.100	0.65	0.42

Table 7. Estimates of odds ratio from ordinal logistic regression model.

Variable	Odds Ratio *	95% CI	p Value
Nutrition	1.26	1.10–1.45	0.001
Lipid	0.88	0.75–1.02	0.09
Glucose	1.03	0.87–1.23	0.71
Uric acid	0.81	0.72–091	0.0004
Blood pressure	1.17	1.01–1.35	0.03
Renal function	1.44	1.20–1.72	<0.0001
Smoking (Yes vs. No)	0.85	0.58–1.26	0.42

Odds ratio *: G1 is used as reference group.

Table 8. Estimates of odds ratio from ordinal logistic regression model.

Variable	Odds Ratio *	95% CI	p Value
Nutrition	0.927	0.709–1.211	0.578
Lipid	0.700	0.477–1.026	0.068
Glucose	0.860	0.573–1.291	0.467
Blood pressure	1.002	0.753–1.334	0.987
Renal function	1.316	0.976–1.775	0.072
Uric acid	0.972	0.782–1.209	0.800
Smoking (Yes vs. No)	1.419	0.626–3.217	0.403
Age	1.036	0.996–1.079	0.079
Plaque area	0.855	0.759–0.964	0.011

Statistical significance was defined as p value < 0.05. All statistical analyses were performed using JMP Pro 13.0 and SAS software (Release 9.3; SAS Institute, Cary, NC, USA).

2.7. Description of Ordinal Logistic Regression Model

Each subject denoted by i ($i = 1, \ldots, N$) is classified into risk group denoted as "G1", "G2", "G3" or "G4", and group membership is represented by random variable Y. Y takes value = 1 if G1, $Y = 2$ if G2, $Y = 3$ if G3 and $Y = 3$ if G4. Ordinal logistic regression is used to model Y_i. Let X be a vector of covariate defined as $X = (X_1, \cdots, X_6, W)'$ where $X_1, \cdots, X_6$ are 6 risk variables. W is a dummy variable, which takes value 0 or 1 for non-smoker and smoker respectively. Given covariate vector X, cumulative probability of Y is written as $P(Y \leq k|X)$, and ordinal logistic regression model is defined as

$$\text{logit}(P(Y \leq k|X)) = \log\left\{\frac{P(Y \leq k|X)}{1 - P(Y \leq k|X)}\right\} = \alpha_k - X'\beta \quad (1)$$

where α_k is an intercept with $\alpha_4 = 0$, and β is 7×1 parameter vector. From definition of the model, the expected predicted probabilities for G1, G2, G3 and G4 are given by

$$\begin{aligned}
P_1 &= P(Y = 1|X) = \frac{exp(\alpha_1 - X'\beta)}{1 - exp(\alpha_1 - X'\beta)}, \\
P_2 &= P(Y = 2|X) = \frac{exp(\alpha_2 - X'\beta)}{1 - exp(\alpha_2 - X'\beta)} - \frac{exp(\alpha_1 - X'\beta)}{1 - exp(\alpha_1 - X'\beta)}, \\
P_3 &= P(Y = 3|X) = \frac{exp(\alpha_3 - X'\beta)}{1 - exp(\alpha_3 - X'\beta)} - \frac{exp(\alpha_2 - X'\beta)}{1 - exp(\alpha_2 - X'\beta)}, \\
P_4 &= P(Y = 4|X) = 1 - \frac{exp(\alpha_3 - X'\beta)}{1 - exp(\alpha_3 - X'\beta)}
\end{aligned} \quad (2)$$

Finally, the predicted probabilities $(\hat{P}_1, \hat{P}_2, \hat{P}_3, \hat{P}_4)$ were obtained by plugging in parameter estimates $(\hat{\alpha}_k, \hat{\beta})$ into the expected predicted probabilities, and $\hat{\alpha}_k - X'\hat{\beta}$ is referred to as the linear predicted score in the Figure 5.

Since our model is defined as $\text{logit}(P(Y \leq k|X)) = \alpha_k - X'\beta$, log odds ratio of belonging lower risk group when Nutrition score increase one unit is given by

$$\text{logit}(P(Y \leq k|X_1 = a+1)) - \text{logit}(P(Y \leq k|X_1 = a)) = -\beta_1 \quad (3)$$

where β_1 is the parameter estimate of "Nutrition", thus, odds ratio is given by exp $(-\beta_1)$. However, interpretation of odds ratio for a risk variable is easier for a subject being classified into higher risk group. To this end, we reversed the order of group membership (i.e., Y* = 5 − Y) and model Y* instead of Y where G1 was set as a reference group. Table 6 shown parameter estimates for modeling Y* where OR for nutrition is calculated as exp (0.232) = 1.26.

3. Results

3.1. Clinical Differences of Traditional Coronary Risk Factors and Nutrition Status with and without Cancer

Among 437 enrolled patients in the present study, 26 patients were excluded (Figure 1).

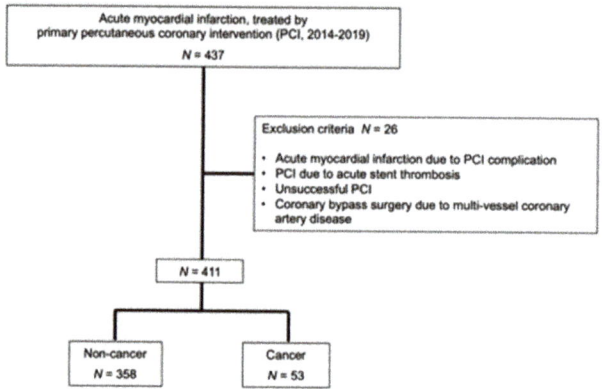

Figure 1. Enrollment of patients.

In the remaining 411 patients, there were 358 AMI patients without cancer (87.1%) and 53 with cancer (12.9%). To compare with AMI patients without cancer, those with cancer were significantly older with significantly lower body weight, lower diastolic blood pressure, anemia, worse renal function, lower albumin and cholesterol levels, and worse nutrition status, evaluated by CONUT score, GPS, and mGPS (Table 1).

Next in comorbidities, those with cancer had significantly higher prevalence of diabetes mellitus, chronic kidney disease, history of coronary artery bypass surgery treatment, and peripheral artery disease, who also had more frequent drug interventions by clopidogrel, ticlopidine, other antiplatelet agents, anti-cancer agents, and steroid (Table 2).

3.2. Risk Model of Cancer

To divide the patients into some groups to evaluate the presence of cancer, we first examined the association between age and coronary atherosclerotic plaque area (Figure 2).

Obviously, there was no cancer patient in Age < 60 years-old group. Then, the CART divided the patients by plaque area < 9.39 mm^2 and those ≥9.39 mm^2, which was the cut-off value of the presence and absence of cancer. According to this grouping process, we divided the whole patients into 4 groups to develop a new response variable to evaluate the presence of cancer (Figure 3 and Table 3). As we considered that if AMI occurred in patients with smaller coronary atherosclerotic plaques, the patients had higher risks, we defined the 4 groups as described in Figure 3 and Table 3.

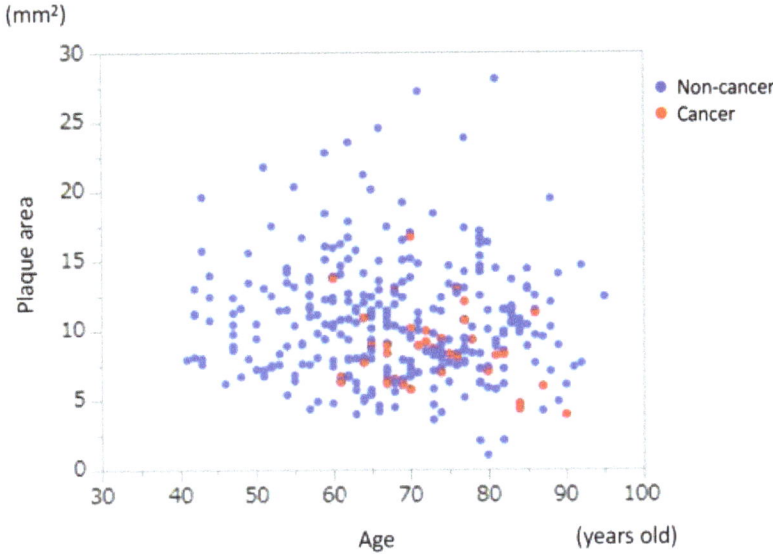

Figure 2. Association between age and coronary atherosclerotic plaque area. There was no significant association between age and coronary plaque area.

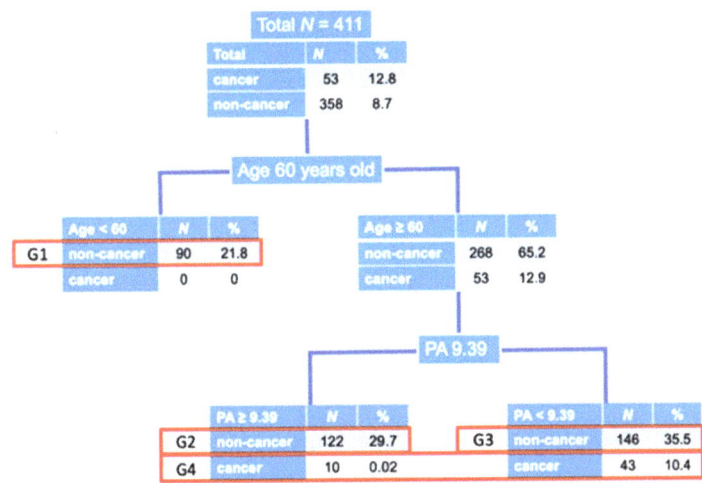

Figure 3. Disposition of patients. As there was no cancer patient in age < 60 years old, we first divided the patients into 2 groups according to age of 60 years old. Next, the CART defined that the cut-off value of coronary atherosclerotic plaque area (PA) to divide the patients into with and without cancer was 9.39 mm². Then, we divided the patients ≥ 60 years old into 2 groups according to plaque area of 9.39 mm², with and without cancer. Due to the small number of cancer patients, we made 4 groups as shown above. Group 1; non-cancer, age < 60 years old, Group 2; non-cancer, age ≥ 60 years old, plaque area ≥ 9.39 mm², Group 3; non-cancer, age ≥ 60 years old, plaque area < 9.39 mm², Group 4; cancer, age ≥ 60 years old.

Next, we have developed the prediction model, which consisted of nutrition, lipid, glucose, blood pressure, and renal function (Table 4).

The equation of nutrition was expressed as "Nutrition = (−1.307) + 0.243 * CONUT + 0.898 * GPS + 0.846 * mGPS". Similarly, other equations were expressed as "Lipid = (−4.947) + 0.018 * LDL-c + 0.015 * T.chol", "Glucose = (−5.448) + 0.594 * HbA1c + 0.0092 * FPG", "Blood pressure = (−5.559) + 0.038 * Pulse pressure + 0.027 * systolic BP", "Renal function = (1.151) + 0.469 * Cr + (−0.025) * eGFR". Using these equations, we performed analysis of variance, which indicated that nutrition, lipid, and renal functions were significant predictors of risk grouping (Table 5, Figure 4).

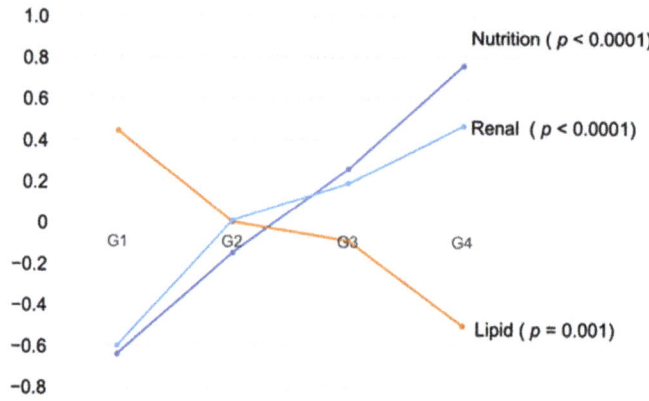

Figure 4. Mean of synthetic variable by Four Groups.

The odds of a subject being classified into higher risk group (i.e., group membership j (=1,2,3,4) increase) were 1.26 times when value of the synthetic variable "Nutrition" increased 1 point (Table 7).

Variables with odds ratio greater than 1 had similar interpretation. On the other hand, variables with odds ratio less than 1 had reverse effects. For example, when value of the synthetic variable "Lipid" increased 1 point, the odds of a subject being classified into higher risk group were 0.88 times compared with odds of being classified into lower risk group (Table 7). The additional logistic regression model, where cancer/non-cancer was used a response factor with age and plaque area as adjusting variables, showed the insignificant increase in nutrition (Table 8). Direction of effect of each synthetic variable could be also seen in the Table 5. Finally, we were able to calculate the probability of the presence of cancer, by combining each factor and scoring (Figure 5).

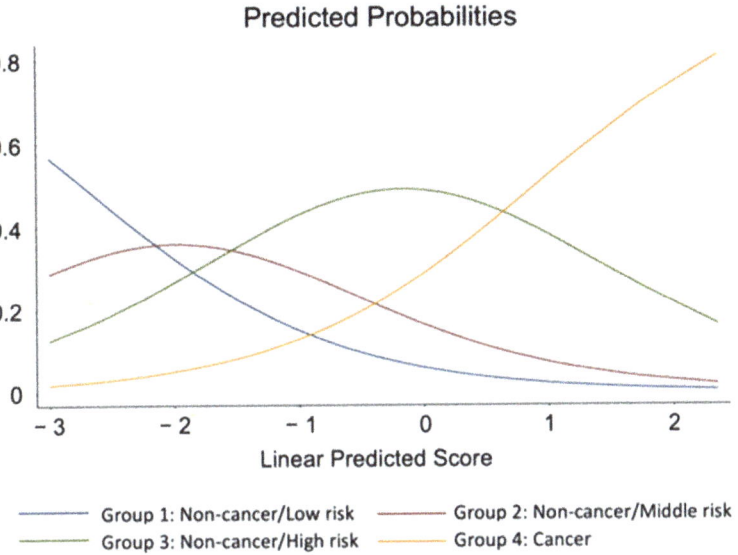

Figure 5. Predicted probabilities of classification to 4 risk groups. Linear predicted Score is referred to as linear combination of parameter estimates with its corresponding variable scores in the ordinal logistic regression model.

4. Discussion

The major findings of the present study were that (a) the prevalence of cancer in AMI patients was 13%, (b) AMI patients with cancer were older with worse nutrition status and renal dysfunction, (c) nutrition status and renal function were consistent predictors for obtaining cancer in AMI, and (d) we were able to calculate the probability of the presence of cancer, by combining each factor and scoring. To the best of our knowledge, this is the first study that provides the evidence of differential risk factors including nutrition status in AMI patients between with and without cancer in details.

4.1. Prevalence of Cancer in AMI

In the US National Inpatient Sample database between 2004 and 2014 report, among 6,563,255 AMI patients, there were 5,966,955 with no cancer, 186,604 with current cancer (2.8%), and 409,697 with a historical diagnosis of cancer (6.2%) [20]. Among 175,146 patients in Swedish registries of first AMI between 2001 and 2014, there were 16,237 patients (9.3%), who had received care for cancer in the 5 years before AMI [21]. The prevalence of cancer in AMI patients was 13% in the present study, which was relatively higher that these nationwide data, probably because the enrolled patients in the study might have complicated conditions such as being hospitalized in our University Hospital.

4.2. Differences of Traditional Risk Factors and Nutrition Status in AMI between with and without Cancer

Hypertension, diabetes, current smoking, family history, and dyslipidemia are well known as traditional risk factors in AMI [22], and it has been recently reported that aging, higher prevalence of dyslipidemia and hypertension, and lower prevalence of obesity, diabetes mellitus, and smoking were risk factors in breast cancer survivors compared with general female population [23]. However, the differential risk factors for AMI with cancer compared with non-cancer remains scant. The present study indicated for the first time that renal dysfunction and worse nutrition status were the strongest risk factors in AMI patients with cancer. Besides these factors, univariate analyses (Table 1) showed that AMI with cancer patients had significantly lower levels of albumin, T.chol, and LDL-c than those without cancer, which seemed to be caused by deterioration of nutrition status, which were different from traditional coronary risk factors.

4.3. Prediction and Scoring of Cancer in AMI

In the present study, we have developed formulas regarding nutrition status, lipid, glucose blood pressure, and renal function (Table 4). Using these formulas, we are able to avoid to evaluate several data separately, such as T.chol and LDL-c, or Cr and eGFR, and to consider these factors as whole. Further, we have established the predicted scoring system for AMI with cancer (Figure 5), which means that we are able to predict if the patients with AMI have cancer, by calculating this score. This might be useful in clinical settings to recognize the presence of cancer.

4.4. Limitations

Several limitations should be acknowledged in the present study. First, the present study was an observational retrospective cohort study from a single center. Thus, there might be some bias. Second, we were not able to divide cancer patients into active cancer and history of cancer, due to the limited number of patients with cancer. Also, we were not able to evaluate cancer stage in this study. Third, we were not able to distinguish coronary plaque rupture from coronary artery erosion as causes of AMI. Fourth, the enrolled patients in the present study were hospitalized in University Hospital, which may also cause some bias. Fifth, due to the limited number of enrolled patients, we were not able to examine sex-difference in the present study. Taken together, further investigations should be necessary in larger multi-center cohort studies.

5. Conclusions

The present study demonstrates that the prevalence of cancer in AMI was 13%, and that worse nutrition status and renal dysfunction were associated with AMI with cancer, in which nutrition status was a major different characteristic from non-cancer. Further, we have developed formulas to predict the presence of cancer in AMI.

Author Contributions: Conceptualization, N.I. and Y.F.; methodology, A.F. and T.K.; software, A.F. and T.K.; validation, T.K.; formal analysis, A.F.; investigation, N.I.; resources, Y.F.; data curation, N.I.; writing—original draft preparation, N.I.; writing—review and editing, Y.F.; visualization, A.F.; supervision, Y.F.; project administration, Y.F.; funding acquisition, Y.F. All authors have read and agreed to the published version of the manuscript.

Funding: This research received no external funding.

Institutional Review Board Statement: The study was conducted according to the guidelines of the Declaration of Helsinki, and approved by the institutional review board at Kurume University (No. 20181, 18 November 2020 approved).

Informed Consent Statement: Informed consent was waved due to the retrospective nature and opt-out was used in the study.

Data Availability Statement: The data presented in this paper are available on request from the corresponding author.

Conflicts of Interest: The authors declare no conflict of interest.

References

1. Crea, F.; Libby, P. Acute Coronary Syndromes: The Way Forward From Mechanisms to Precision Treatment. *Circulation* **2017**, *136*, 1155–1166. [CrossRef] [PubMed]
2. Libby, P.; Buring, J.E.; Badimon, L.; Hansson, G.K.; Deanfield, J.; Bittencourt, M.S.; Tokgozoglu, L.; Lewis, E.F. Atherosclerosis. *Nat. Rev. Dis. Primers* **2019**, *5*, 56. [CrossRef]
3. Fukumoto, Y.; Libby, P.; Rabkin, E.; Hill, C.C.; Enomoto, M.; Hirouchi, Y.; Shiomi, M.; Aikawa, M. Statins alter smooth muscle cell accumulation and collagen content in established atheroma of watanabe heritable hyperlipidemic rabbits. *Circulation* **2001**, *103*, 993–999. [CrossRef] [PubMed]

4. Libby, P.; Aikawa, M. Mechanisms of plaque stabilization with statins. *Am. J. Cardiol.* **2003**, *91*, 4B–8B. [CrossRef]
5. Ahmadi, A.; Leipsic, J.; Blankstein, R.; Taylor, C.; Hecht, H.; Stone, G.W.; Narula, J. Do plaques rapidly progress prior to myocardial infarction? The interplay between plaque vulnerability and progression. *Circ. Res.* **2015**, *117*, 99–104. [CrossRef]
6. Mayer, D.K.; Nasso, S.F.; Earp, J.A. Defining cancer survivors, their needs, and perspectives on survivorship health care in the USA. *Lancet Oncol.* **2017**, *18*, e11–e18. [CrossRef]
7. Takahashi, M. Cancer survivorship: Current status of research, care, and policy in Japan. *Jpn. J. Clin. Oncol.* **2016**, *46*, 599–604. [CrossRef]
8. Falk, E. Pathogenesis of atherosclerosis. *J. Am. Coll. Cardiol.* **2006**, *47*, C7–C12. [CrossRef]
9. Jaiswal, S.; Natarajan, P.; Silver, A.J.; Gibson, C.J.; Bick, A.G.; Shvartz, E.; McConkey, M.; Gupta, N.; Gabriel, S.; Ardissino, D.; et al. Clonal Hematopoiesis and Risk of Atherosclerotic Cardiovascular Disease. *N. Engl. J. Med.* **2017**, *377*, 111–121. [CrossRef] [PubMed]
10. Pardali, E.; Dimmeler, S.; Zeiher, A.M.; Rieger, M.A. Clonal hematopoiesis, aging, and cardiovascular diseases. *Exp. Hematol.* **2020**, *83*, 95–104. [CrossRef]
11. Heyde, A.; Rohde, D.; McAlpine, C.S.; Zhang, S.; Hoyer, F.F.; Gerold, J.M.; Cheek, D.; Iwamoto, Y.; Schloss, M.J.; Vandoorne, K.; et al. Increased stem cell proliferation in atherosclerosis accelerates clonal hematopoiesis. *Cell* **2021**, *184*, 1348–1361.e1322. [CrossRef] [PubMed]
12. Honigberg, M.C.; Zekavat, S.M.; Niroula, A.; Griffin, G.K.; Bick, A.G.; Pirruccello, J.P.; Nakao, T.; Whitsel, E.A.; Farland, L.V.; Laurie, C.; et al. Premature Menopause, Clonal Hematopoiesis, and Coronary Artery Disease in Postmenopausal Women. *Circulation* **2021**, *143*, 410–423. [CrossRef] [PubMed]
13. Ministry of Health, Labour and Welfare. Available online: https://www.mhlw.go.jp/toukei/saikin/hw/jinkou/geppo/nengai18/dl/gaikyou30.pdf (accessed on 22 June 2021).
14. Li, Y.; Schoufour, J.; Wang, D.D.; Dhana, K.; Pan, A.; Liu, X.; Song, M.; Liu, G.; Shin, H.J.; Sun, Q.; et al. Healthy lifestyle and life expectancy free of cancer, cardiovascular disease, and type 2 diabetes: Prospective cohort study. *BMJ* **2020**, *368*, l6669. [CrossRef] [PubMed]
15. Thygesen, K.; Alpert, J.S.; Jaffe, A.S.; Chaitman, B.R.; Bax, J.J.; Morrow, D.A.; White, H.D. Executive Group on behalf of the Joint European Society of Cardiology/American College of Cardiology/American Heart Association/World Heart Federation Task Force for the Universal Definition of Myocardial, I. Fourth Universal Definition of Myocardial Infarction (2018). *Circulation* **2018**, *138*, e618–e651. [CrossRef]
16. Forrest, L.M.; McMillan, D.C.; McArdle, C.S.; Angerson, W.J.; Dunlop, D.J. Evaluation of cumulative prognostic scores based on the systemic inflammatory response in patients with inoperable non-small-cell lung cancer. *Br. J. Cancer* **2003**, *89*, 1028–1030. [CrossRef]
17. Toiyama, Y.; Miki, C.; Inoue, Y.; Tanaka, K.; Mohri, Y.; Kusunoki, M. Evaluation of an inflammation-based prognostic score for the identification of patients requiring postoperative adjuvant chemotherapy for stage II colorectal cancer. *Exp. Ther. Med.* **2011**, *2*, 95–101. [CrossRef]
18. Inoue, Y.; Iwata, T.; Okugawa, Y.; Kawamoto, A.; Hiro, J.; Toiyama, Y.; Tanaka, K.; Uchida, K.; Mohri, Y.; Miki, C.; et al. Prognostic significance of a systemic inflammatory response in patients undergoing multimodality therapy for advanced colorectal cancer. *Oncology* **2013**, *84*, 100–107. [CrossRef]
19. de Ulibarri, J.I.; Gonzalez-Madrono, A.; de Villar, N.G.; Gonzalez, P.; Gonzalez, B.; Mancha, A.; Rodriguez, F.; Fernandez, G. CONUT: A tool for controlling nutritional status. First validation in a hospital population. *Nutr. Hosp.* **2005**, *20*, 38–45.
20. Bharadwaj, A.; Potts, J.; Mohamed, M.O.; Parwani, P.; Swamy, P.; Lopez-Mattei, J.C.; Rashid, M.; Kwok, C.S.; Fischman, D.L.; Vassiliou, V.S.; et al. Acute myocardial infarction treatments and outcomes in 6.5 million patients with a current or historical diagnosis of cancer in the USA. *Eur. Heart J.* **2020**, *41*, 2183–2193. [CrossRef]
21. Velders, M.A.; Hagstrom, E.; James, S.K. Temporal Trends in the Prevalence of Cancer and Its Impact on Outcome in Patients With First Myocardial Infarction: A Nationwide Study. *J. Am. Heart Assoc.* **2020**, *9*, e014383. [CrossRef]
22. Kawano, H.; Soejima, H.; Kojima, S.; Kitagawa, A.; Ogawa, H.; Japanese Acute Coronary Syndrome Study (JACSS) Investigators. Sex differences of risk factors for acute myocardial infarction in Japanese patients. *Circ. J.* **2006**, *70*, 513–517. [CrossRef] [PubMed]
23. Yandrapalli, S.; Malik, A.H.; Pemmasani, G.; Gupta, K.; Harikrishnan, P.; Nabors, C.; Aronow, W.S.; Cooper, H.A.; Panza, J.A.; Frishman, W.H.; et al. Risk Factors and Outcomes During a First Acute Myocardial Infarction in Breast Cancer Survivors Compared with Females Without Breast Cancer. *Am. J. Med.* **2020**, *133*, 444–451. [CrossRef] [PubMed]

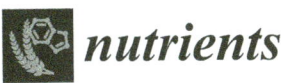

Article

High Plasma Docosahexaenoic Acid Associated to Better Prognoses of Patients with Acute Decompensated Heart Failure with Preserved Ejection Fraction

Naoaki Matsuo [1], Toru Miyoshi [1,*], Atsushi Takaishi [2], Takao Kishinoue [2], Kentaro Yasuhara [2], Masafumi Tanimoto [2], Yukari Nakano [3], Nobuhiko Onishi [2], Masayuki Ueeda [4] and Hiroshi Ito [1]

1. Department of Cardiovascular Medicine, Okayama University Graduate School of Medicine, Dentistry and Pharmaceutical Sciences, Okayama 700-8558, Japan; naoaki.matsuo.1985@gmail.com (N.M.); itomd@md.okayama-u.ac.jp (H.I.)
2. Department of Cardiovascular Medicine, Mitoyo General Hospital, Kagawa 769-1601, Japan; takaishi1013@ybb.ne.jp (A.T.); takao.nakayama.0922@gmail.com (T.K.); ilovesukuramu@yahoo.co.jp (K.Y.); kpggp925@gmail.com (M.T.); nobuohnishi@mitoyo-hosp.jp (N.O.)
3. Nakano Cardiovascular Clinic, Kagawa 762-0012, Japan; nakanocc.20200129@gmail.com
4. Ueeda Cardiovascular Clinic, Kagawa 769-1504, Japan; ueedacvc@gmail.com
* Correspondence: miyoshit@cc.okayama-u.ac.jp; Tel.: +81-86-235-7351

Abstract: The clinical relevance of polyunsaturated fatty acids (PUFAs) in heart failure remains unclear. The aim of this study was to investigate the association between PUFA levels and the prognosis of patients with heart failure with preserved ejection fraction (HFpEF). This retrospective study included 140 hospitalized patients with acute decompensated HFpEF (median age 84.0 years, 42.9% men). The patients' nutritional status was assessed, using the geriatric nutritional risk index (GNRI), and their plasma levels of eicosapentaenoic acid (EPA), docosahexaenoic acid (DHA), arachidonic acid (AA), and dihomo-gamma-linolenic acid (DGLA) were measured before discharge. The primary outcome was all-cause mortality. During a median follow-up of 23.3 months, the primary outcome occurred in 37 patients (26.4%). A Kaplan–Meier analysis showed that lower DHA and DGLA levels, but not EPA or AA levels, were significantly associated with an increase in all-cause death (log-rank; $p < 0.001$ and $p = 0.040$, respectively). A multivariate Cox regression analysis also revealed that DHA levels were significantly associated with the incidence of all-cause death (HR: 0.16, 95% CI: 0.06–0.44, $p = 0.001$), independent of the GNRI. Our results suggest that low plasma DHA levels may be a useful predictor of all-cause mortality and potential therapeutic target in patients with acute decompensated HFpEF.

Keywords: heart failure with preserved ejection fraction; docosahexaenoic acid; geriatric nutritional risk index

1. Introduction

Heart failure (HF) is a common and growing public health problem with an estimated prevalence of over 37.7 million cases worldwide [1]. Despite recent developments of HF treatments, including pharmacological and device therapy, HF still results in high mortality and re-hospitalization rates [2]. HF clinically manifests in two modes, which are defined by ventricular function: HF with reduced ejection fraction (HFrEF) and HF with preserved ejection fraction (HFpEF) [3]. Unfortunately, standard pharmacological therapies for HFrEF such as angiotensin-converting enzyme inhibitors and β-blockers show a lack of efficacy in the treatment of HFpEF [4]. Patients with HFpEF are more likely to be older, female, and have hypertension, renal disease, atrial fibrillation, and malnutrition [5]. Malnutrition, in particular, is a common problem in elderly patients with HFpEF and is a known risk factor for a poor prognosis [6].

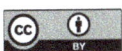

Polyunsaturated fatty acids (PUFAs) play structural and functional roles as membrane components and precursors of physiologically active substances involved in inflammation [7]. Fish oils, sunflower, safflower, and corn oils are rich in omega-3 PUFAs, while meat from farm animals are rich in omega-6 PUFAs [8]. Omega-3 PUFAs, such as eicosapentaenoic acid (EPA) and docosahexaenoic acid (DHA), and oemga-6 PUFAs, such as arachidonic acid (AA) and dihomo-gamma-linolenic acid (DGLA), have been shown to have opposite effect [9]. It has been reported that AA-derived metabolites are pro-inflammatory, while EPA- and DHA-derived metabolites are pro-resolution/anti-inflammatory [10–12]. Some metabolites have been reported to play a critical role in the development of cardiac hypertrophy and heart failure by regulating inflammatory reactions [12–14]. However, omega-7 and omega-9 monounsaturated fatty acids, such as palmitoleic acid and oleic acid, are components of complex lipids, such as sphingosines and phospholipids, and could interfere with cellular injury [15–17].

Several clinical trials and meta-analysis have demonstrated that omega-3 PUFAs are beneficial for patients with cardiovascular events [18–20]. Regarding the association between omega-3 PUFAs and heart failure, a meta-analysis of seven prospective studies with 176,441 subjects and 5480 cases of HF found a lower risk of HF in patients that took high amounts of marine omega-3 PUFAs [21]. Another study including 6562 patients, in over 13 years, found that plasma EPA levels were significantly lower in HF patients, compared to HF-free patients [22]. Small-scale clinical trials have indicated that omega-3 PUFAs may improve the outcomes of patients with HF [23–26]. However, recent large-scale randomized controlled studies investigating cardiovascular benefit of omega-3 supplementation showed conflicting findings [27,28].

The aim of this study was to investigate the role of PUFAs in the prognosis of patients with acute decompensated HFpEF. In addition, the impact of the patients' nutritional status on the association between PUFAs and their prognosis was evaluated.

2. Materials and Methods

2.1. Study Design and Participants

This study was a retrospective single-center cohort study. The study protocol was approved by the Institutional Review Board of Mitoyo General Hospital (19CR01-122) and conducted in accordance with the principles of the Declaration of Helsinki. The requirement for informed consent was waived because of the low-risk nature of the study and inability to obtain consent directly from all the study subjects. Instead, we announced this study protocol extensively at Mitoyo General Hospital and on the hospital website (http://mitoyo-hosp.jp) and provided patients with the opportunity to withdraw from the study. We initially enrolled 301 consecutive patients with acute decompensated HFpEF that were not receiving hemodialysis and who were admitted to Mitoyo General Hospital between August 2015 and January 2019. Acute decompensated HF was diagnosed based on the Framingham's criteria. [29]. A diagnosis of HF was made if a patient had at least two major criteria or one major criterion and two minor criteria. The major criteria are acute pulmonary edema, cardiomegaly, hepatojugular reflex, distended neck veins, paroxysmal nocturnal dyspnea, pulmonary rales, and third heart sound. The minor criteria are ankle edema, dyspnea on exertion, hepatomegaly, nocturnal cough, pleural effusion, and tachycardia [29]. HFpEF was defined as HF with a left ventricular ejection fraction $\geq$50%. Patients with HFrEF and those receiving omega-3 PUFA therapy were excluded. Figure 1 shows the flow diagram of this study. Follow-ups were performed by referring to patient electronic medical records, direct contact with the patients' physicians in the outpatient clinic, and telephone interviews with patients or family members. A total of 140 patients were ultimately included in the final analysis.

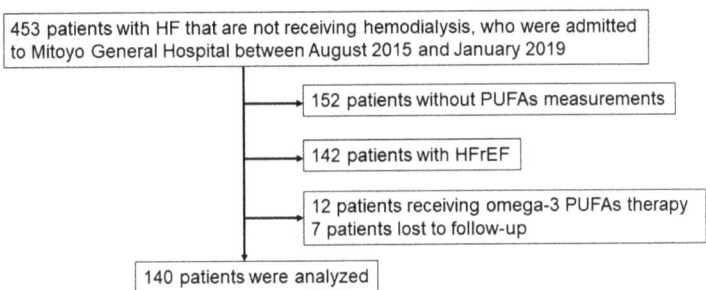

Figure 1. Flowchart of study population. Heart failure (HF) was defined based on the Framingham criteria. Heart failure with reduced ejection fraction (HFrEF); Heart failure with preserved ejection fraction (HFpEF) was defined as HF with a left ventricular ejection fraction ≥50%. PUFAs, polyunsaturated fatty acids.

2.2. Blood Sampling and Equations

Whole blood samples were collected within 24 h of admission. Approximately 20 mL of blood was collected by venipuncture and separated into tubes containing clot activator, gel serum separator, ethylenediaminetetraacetic acid dipotassium, and heparin sodium. Plasma levels of EPA, DHA, AA, and DGLA were measured by using gas chromatography (SRL Inc., Tokyo, Japan) [30]. Routine laboratory tests were performed, using an automated analyzer, at Mitoyo General Hospital. The estimated glomerular filtration rate (eGFR) was calculated based on the Japanese equation that uses serum creatinine level, age, and sex as follows: eGFR (mL/min/1.73 m^2) = 194 × serum creatinine$^{-1.094}$ × age$^{-0.287}$ (for females = ×0.739) [31]. The geriatric nutritional risk index (GNRI) was calculated as follows, using the serum albumin level, body weight, and height obtained on admission: GNRI = 14.89 × serum albumin (g/dL) + 41.7 × (actual body weight/ideal body weight). GNRI is a nutrition-related risk index that makes it possible to classify patients according to a risk of morbidity and mortality, and the GNRI ≥98 means no nutritional-related risk [32]. The ideal body weight in the present study was calculated by using a body mass index of 22 kg/m^2.

2.3. Assessment of Additional Risk Factors

Hypertension was defined as having a seated blood pressure >140/90 mmHg or undergoing current treatment with antihypertensive medications. Diabetes mellitus was defined as having a previous diagnosis of diabetes mellitus in the medical records, a hemoglobin A1C (national glycohemoglobin standardization program calculation) level ≥6.5%, or receiving treatment with oral antidiabetic agents or insulin. Dyslipidemia was defined as one or more of the following characteristics: ≥150 mg/dL serum triglyceride, <40 mg/dL high-density lipoprotein cholesterol (HDL-cholesterol), ≥140 mg/dL low-density lipoprotein cholesterol (LDL-cholesterol), or current treatment with a lipid-lowering drug. Smoking status was defined as "currently smoking".

2.4. Study Outcomes

The primary endpoint was all-cause mortality. Furthermore, as an ad hoc analysis, patients were divided into four groups, based on the median DHA level and median GNRI, so that the association between the primary endpoint and each group could be evaluated. The secondary endpoints were cardiac death and re-hospitalization for HF.

2.5. Statistical Analyses

The results are presented as the mean ± standard deviation when they are normally distributed, and as the median and interquartile range (IQR) when they are non-normally distributed. The normality of distribution was determined by the Kolmogorov–Smirnov test. Differences between the groups were analyzed by using the unpaired Student's t-test or Mann–Whitney U test for continuous variables, and the chi-squared test or Fisher's exact test for dichotomous variables, as appropriate. For the survival analyses, Kaplan–Meier survival plots were constructed by dividing the patients' PUFA levels on admission into two groups, according to the median values, and log-rank testing was performed to study the influence of PUFA levels on primary and secondary endpoints. To evaluate the influence of PUFA levels on the primary endpoint, Cox proportional-hazards regression models were used to estimate the hazard ratio (HR) and 95% confidence interval (CI). To avoid overfitting, variables that were included in the principal multivariate models were adjusted for age, sex, hypertension, dyslipidemia, diabetes mellitus, and GNRI. All the tests were two-tailed, and a value of $p < 0.05$ was considered statistically significant. All the analyses were performed by using IBM SPSS statistics version 24.0 (IBM Corp., Armonk, NY, USA).

3. Results

3.1. Baseline Characteristics

Table 1 shows the baseline characteristics of the patients in this study and a comparison of those characteristics between the patients with and without primary endpoints. The median age of all the patients was 84.0 years, 42.9% were male, and 56.4% had atrial fibrillation. The prevalence of hypertension and diabetes mellitus within the group of patients was 90.0% and 22.9%, respectively.

During the median follow-up of 23.3 months, 37 (26.4%) of the patients exhibited the primary endpoint. Patients experiencing the primary endpoint were older; had lower BMI and GNRI values; had a lower prevalence of hypertension and dyslipidemia; had lower statin use; and had lower hemoglobin, albumin, HDL-cholesterol, and LDL-cholesterol levels than those who did not experience the primary endpoint. No significant differences in the prevalence of atrial fibrillation, prior hospitalization for HF, or medication use, except for statins, were observed between the two groups. The median levels of EPA, DHA, DGLA, and AA, as well as the ratio of EPA to AA (EPA/AA), DHA to AA (DHA/AA), and AA + DGLA to EPA + DHA (AA + DGLA/EPA + DHA), on admission were 46.6 μg/mL, 116.1 μg/mL, 23.6 μg/mL, 159.8 μg/mL, 0.26, 0.74, and 1.15, respectively. The levels of DHA, DGLA, and AA for the patients with adverse events were significantly lower than for those patients without adverse events. The levels of EPA, EPA/AA, DHA/AA, and AA+DGLA/EPA+DHA did not differ between the two groups.

3.2. Cumulative Event Rates Based on PUFA Levels

The Kaplan–Meier analyses showed that lower levels of DHA and DGLA on admission were significantly associated with the incidence of adverse events (log-rank; $p < 0.001$ and $p = 0.040$, respectively) (Figure 2B,D). However, the EPA and AA levels and the EPA/AA, DHA/AA, and AA + DGLA/ EPA + DHA were not associated (log-rank; $p = 0.051$, $p = 0.154$, $p = 0.649$, $p = 0.887$, $p = 0.712$, respectively) (Figure 2A,C,E–G).

3.3. Univariate and Multivariate Analyses of Parameters Contributing to the Primary and Secondary Endpoints

The univariate Cox regression analyses showed that age, body mass index, statin use, hemoglobin, albumin, LDL-cholesterol, GNRI, DGLA level, and DHA level were associated with the incidence of the primary endpoint (Table 2). The multivariate Cox regression analyses revealed that patients with high DHA levels was significantly associated with a low incidence of the primary endpoint after an adjustment for age, sex, hypertension, dyslipidemia, diabetes mellitus, and GNRI (HR: 0.16, 95% CI: 0.06–0.44, $p = 0.001$). However, the DGLA level was not significantly associated with the primary endpoint after an adjustment for confounding variables.

Table 1. Baseline characteristics according to the presence or absence of the primary endpoint.

Variables	All (n = 140)	Primary Endpoint Absent (n = 103)	Primary Endpoint Present (n = 37)	p
Men	60 (42.9)	40 (38.8)	20 (54.1)	0.110
Age, years	84.0 (77.0, 88.0)	82.0 (76.0, 88.0)	86.0 (83.0, 89.0)	0.018
Body mass index, kg/m^2	23.3 (20.4, 26.6)	22.4 (20.8, 27.5)	22.1 (19.9, 24.1)	0.008
Hypertension	126 (90.0)	96 (93.2)	30 (81.1)	0.035
Diabetes Mellitus	32 (22.9)	22 (21.4)	10 (27.0)	0.485
Dyslipidemia	45 (32.1)	38 (36.9)	7 (18.9)	0.045
Current smoker	49 (35.0)	33 (32.0)	16 (43.2)	0.223
Prior hospitalization for heart failure	19 (13.6)	13 (12.6)	6 (16.2)	0.587
Ischemic heart disease	18 (12.9)	15 (14.6)	3 (8.1)	0.318
Atrial fibrillation	79 (56.4)	59 (57.3)	20 (54.1)	0.736
Prior PCI	14 (10.0)	12 (11.7)	2 (5.4)	0.281
Prior CABG	5 (3.6)	5 (4.9)	0 (0)	0.175
Valve repair/placement	14 (10.0)	12 (11.7)	2 (5.4)	0.281
Pacemaker implantation	14 (10.0)	7 (6.8)	7 (18.9)	0.035
Medications				
ACEIs/ARBs	55 (39.3)	43 (41.7)	12 (32.4)	0.323
β-blockers	48 (34.3)	39 (37.9)	9 (24.3)	0.139
CCBs	72 (51.4)	55 (53.4)	17 (45.9)	0.440
Loop diuretics	79 (56.4)	54 (52.4)	25 (67.6)	0.113
MRAs	26 (18.6)	16 (15.5)	10 (27.0)	0.125
Antiplatelets	31 (22.1)	27 (26.2)	4 (10.8)	0.053
Oral antidiabetic agents	22 (15.7)	17 (16.5)	5 (13.5)	0.671
Statins	35 (25.0)	31 (30.1)	4 (10.8)	0.020
Anticoagulants	22 (15.7)	46 (44.7)	17 (45.9)	0.894
Laboratory findings				
Hemoglobin (g/dL)	11.0 ± 2.09	11.2 ± 2.10	10.3 ± 1.94	0.017
Creatinine (mg/dL)	1.08 (0.82, 1.62)	1.03 (0.83, 1.56)	1.27 (0.79, 1.75)	0.364
eGFR (ml/min/1.73 m^2)	42.2 (29.0, 56.0)	43.0 (29.0, 55.0)	41.0 (26.2, 59.6)	0.530
Albumin (g/dL)	3.6 (3.2, 3.9)	3.6 (3.4, 3.9)	3.4 (2.9, 3.7)	0.001
hsCRP (mg/dL)	0.43 (0.17, 1.45)	0.36 (0.15, 1.08)	0.86 (0.24, 1.59)	0.581
BNP (pg/mL)	453.0 (260.4, 699.0)	464.0 (246.8, 739.4)	411.0 (269.9, 659.5)	0.107
Troponin I (pg/mL)	32.7 (15.2, 84.7)	33.0 (14.3, 84.7)	28.9 (16.3, 70.8)	0.520
Hemoglobin A1C (%)	5.9 (5.6, 6.5)	5.9 (5.6, 6.5)	5.9 (5.6, 6.6)	0.871
Triglycerides (mg/dL)	76 (57, 98)	78 (62, 98)	67 (50, 94)	0.110
HDL-C (mg/dL)	46 ± 14.4	48 ± 13.8	41 ± 15.5	0.047
LDL-C (mg/dL)	97 ± 36.7	102 ± 37.1	81 ± 30.8	0.014
EPA (μg/mL)	46.6 (30.7, 64.2)	48.0 (31.9, 67.8)	39.6 (28.0, 55.0)	0.076
DHA (μg/mL)	116.1 (96.7, 144.9)	126.7 (99.1, 149.8)	102.8 (94.3, 119.5)	0.009
AA (μg/mL)	159.8 (133.8, 194.5)	167.1 (144.2, 195.0)	139.1 (110.5, 180.7)	0.001
DGLA (μg/mL)	23.6 (19.6, 30.5)	24.2 (20.1, 32.5)	22.2 (18.4, 27.1)	0.019
EPA/AA	0.26 (0.20, 0.40)	0.27 (0.20, 0.40)	0.26 (0.21, 0.39)	0.812
DHA/AA	0.74 (0.62, 0.89)	0.74 (0.60, 0.90)	0.78 (0.63, 0.88)	0.287
AA + DGLA/EPA + DHA	1.15 (0.90, 1.38)	1.15 (0.90, 1.42)	1.14 (0.95, 1.32)	0.481
GNRI	97.7 ± 12.03	99.9 ± 11.59	90.8 ± 10.84	< 0.001

Categorical variables are presented as number of patients (%). Continuous variables are presented as the mean ± standard deviation or median (interquartile range). PCI, percutaneous coronary intervention; CABG, coronary artery bypass grafting; ACEs, angiotensin-converting enzyme inhibitors; ARBs, angiotensin II receptor blockers; CCBs, calcium channel blockers; MRAs, mineralocorticoid receptor antagonists; eGFR, estimated glomerular filtration rate; hsCRP, high-sensitivity C-reactive protein; BNP, brain natriuretic peptide; HDL-C, high-density lipoprotein cholesterol; LDL-C, low-density lipoprotein cholesterol; EPA, eicosapentaenoic acid; DHA, docosahexaenoic acid; DGLA, dihomo-gamma-linolenic acid; AA, arachidonic acid; DHA/AA, ratio of DHA to AA; AA+DGLA/EPA+DHA, ratio of AA+DGLA to EPA+DHA; GNRI, geriatric nutritional risk index.

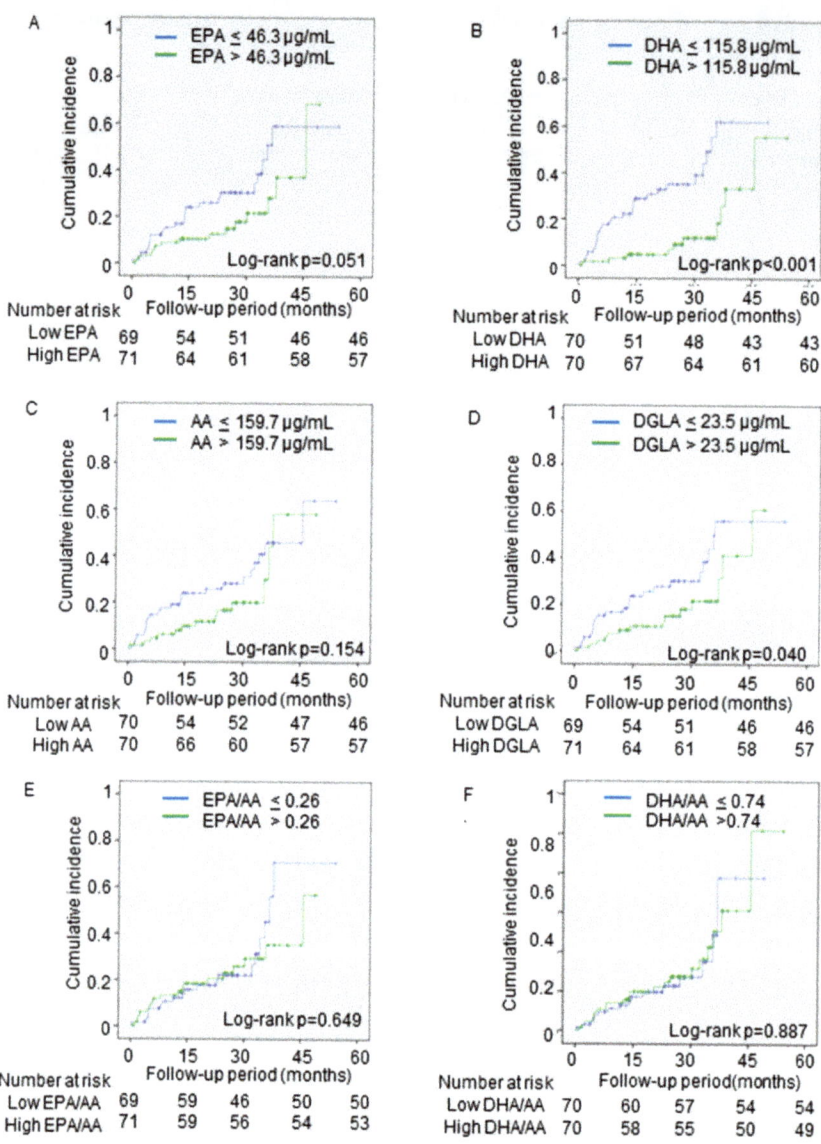

Figure 2. Cont.

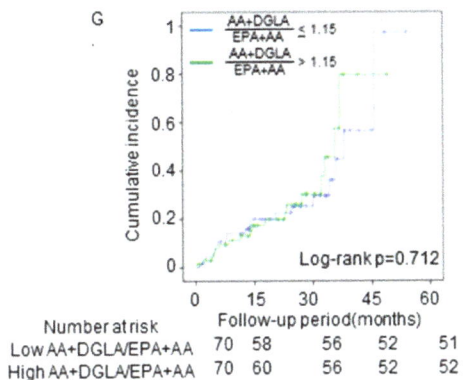

Figure 2. The associations between the primary outcomes and PUFA levels. The cumulative incidences of the primary endpoint (all-cause death) were estimated by using the Kaplan–Meier method. The patients were divided into two groups, based on the median levels of (**A**) EPA, (**B**) DHA, (**C**) AA, (**D**) DGLA, (**E**) EPA/AA, (**F**) DHA/AA, and (**G**) AA + DGLA/ EPA + DHA. Log-rank testing was performed to study the influence of PUFA levels on primary endpoint. EPA, eicosapentaenoic acid; DHA, docosahexaenoic acid; DGLA, dihomo-gamma-linolenic acid; AA, arachidonic acid; EPA/AA, ratio of EPA to AA; DHA/AA, ratio of DHA to AA; AA + DGLA/EPA + DHA; ratio of AA + DGLA to EPA + DHA.

Table 2. The association between PUFAs and the primary endpoint analyzed with Cox proportional hazards models.

	Univariate			Multivariate-1			Multivariate-2		
	HR	95% CI	p	HR	95% CI	p	HR	95% CI	p
Age, per 1 year	1.06	1.01–1.11	0.009	1.05	0.99–1.10	1.102	1.06	1.00–1.13	0.042
Male	1.76	0.92–3.37	0.087	1.76	0.81–3.83	0.155	1.98	0.91–4.29	0.083
Body mass index, per 1.0 kg/m^2	0.90	0.82–0.98	0.017	-	-	-	-	-	-
Hypertension	0.52	0.26–1.06	0.071	0.65	0.26–1.59	0.342	1.13	0.45–2.82	0.793
Dyslipidemia	0.45	0.20–1.03	0.060	0.72	0.25–2.12	0.549	0.66	0.23–1.91	0.441
Diabetes mellitus	1.54	0.74–3.21	0.249	1.99	0.87–4.58	0.104	1.86	0.78–4.46	0.164
Statin use	0.34	0.12–0.95	0.040	-	-	-	-	-	-
Hemoglobin, per 1.0 mg/dL	0.82	0.70–0.96	0.013	-	-	-	-	-	-
Albumin, per 1.0 g/dL	0.34	0.18–0.63	0.001	-	-	-	-	-	-
HDL-C, per 1 mg/dL	0.96	0.93–1.00	0.054	-	-	-	-	-	-
LDL-C, per 1 mg/dL	0.98	0.96–0.99	0.004	-	-	-	-	-	-
GNRI, per 1 index	0.94	0.91–0.97	<0.001	0.95	0.91–0.99	0.010	0.95	0.91–0.98	0.002
High DGLA	0.50	0.26–0.98	0.044	1.02	0.47–2.19	0.969	-	-	-
High AA	0.61	0.31–1.21	0.158	-	-	-	-	-	-
High EPA	0.52	0.27–1.01	0.055	-	-	-	-	-	-
High DHA	0.25	0.12–0.53	<0.001	-	-	-	0.16	0.06–0.44	<0.001
High EPA/AA	0.86	0.45–1.65	0.650	-	-	-	-	-	-
High DHA/AA	1.05	0.54–2.02	0.887	-	-	-	-	-	-
High AA + DGLA/ EPA + DHA	1.13	0.59–2.17	0.712	-	-	-	-	-	-

The multivariate model-1 and model-2 were adjusted for age, sex, hypertension, dyslipidemia, diabetes mellitus, and GNRI. HR, hazard ratio; CI, confidence interval; GNRI, geriatric nutritional risk index; EPA, eicosapentaenoic acid; DHA, docosahexaenoic acid; DGLA, dihomo-gamma-linolenic acid; AA, arachidonic acid. EPA/AA, ratio of EPA to AA; DHA/AA, ratio of DHA to AA; AA + DGLA/EPA + DHA; ratio of AA + DGLA to EPA + DHA.

As an ad hoc analysis, the patients were divided into four groups, based on the median DHA and GNRI values. As shown in Figure 3, the low-GNRI and low-DHA groups showed the greatest incidence of the primary endpoint, compared to the other groups (log-rank; $p < 0.001$). In the multivariate Cox regression analyses, the low-GNRI and low-DHA groups had a significantly higher risk of the primary endpoint, compared with the high-GNRI and high-DHA groups, after an adjustment of age and sex (HR: 8.48, 95% CI: 2.47–29.07, $p = 0.001$) (Table 3).

The secondary endpoints occurred in 63 patients (cardiac death ($n = 15$) and rehospitalization for HF ($n = 480$)). As shown in Figure 4, none of the PUFA levels was associated with the secondary endpoints.

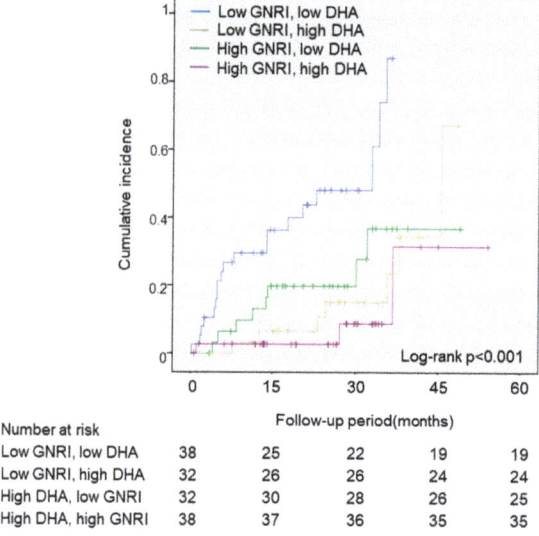

Figure 3. The associations between the primary outcomes and the DHA and GNRI values. The cumulative incidences of the primary endpoint (all-cause death) were estimated by using the Kaplan–Meier method. Log-rank testing was performed to study the influence of PUFA levels on primary endpoint. The patients were divided into four groups, based on the median DHA and GNRI values. DHA, docosahexaenoic acid; GNRI, geriatric nutritional risk index.

Table 3. The association between the DHA and GNRI values and primary endpoints analyzed with Cox proportional hazards models.

Variables	Multivariate Analysis		
	HR	95% CI	p
Age, per 1-year	1.07	1.02–1.13	0.006
Male	1.67	0.87–3.22	0.123
High DHA and high GNRI		Reference	
High DHA and low GNRI	1.14	0.28–4.64	0.858
Low DHA and high GNRI	3.03	0.80–11.48	0.104
Low DHA and low GNRI	8.48	2.47–29.07	0.001

Multivariate analysis was adjusted by age, sex, hemoglobin, and GNRI. HR, hazard ratio; CI, confidence interval; DHA, docosahexaenoic acid; GNRI, geriatric nutritional risk index.

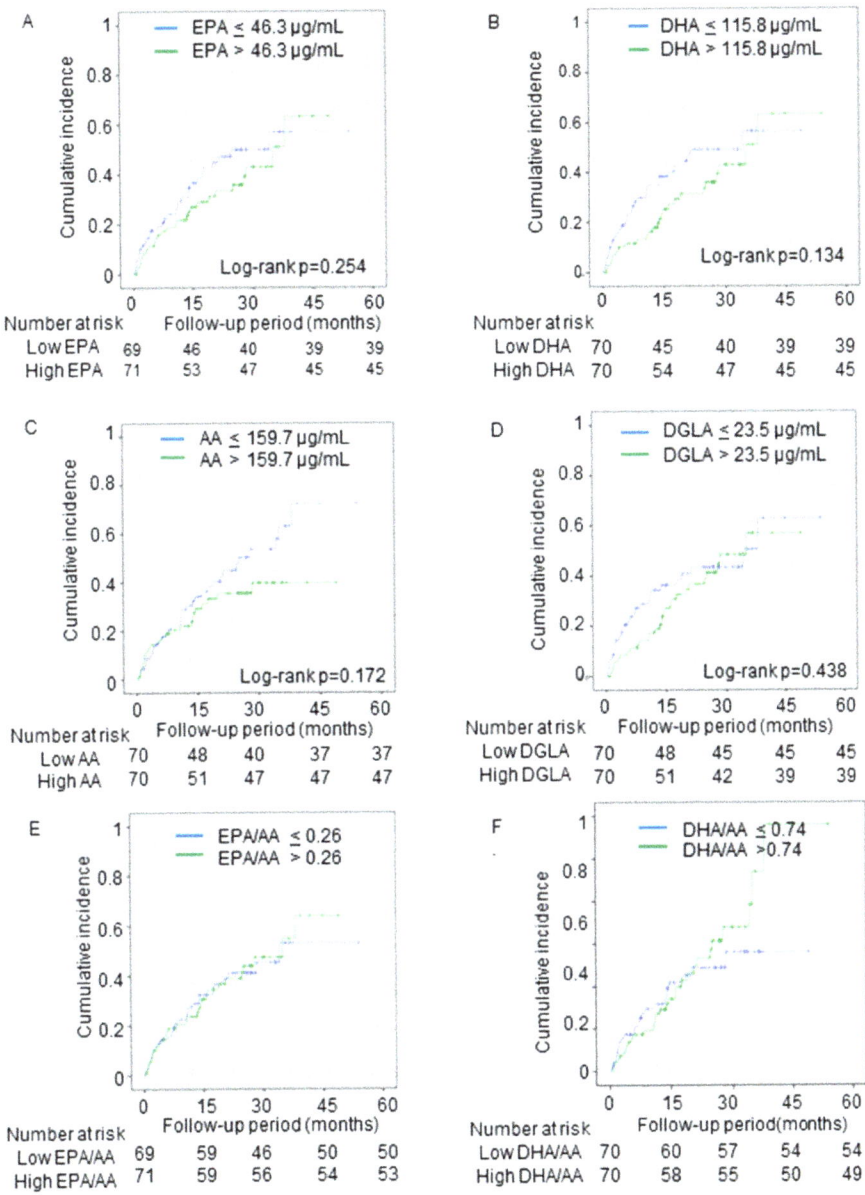

Figure 4. *Cont.*

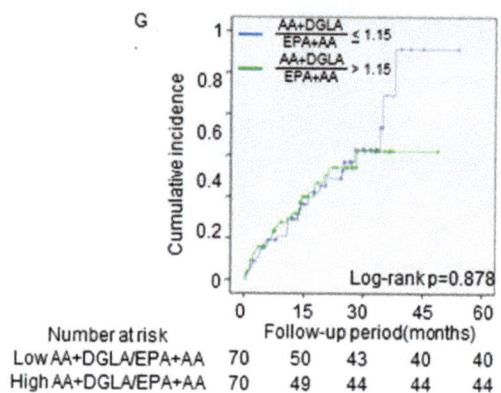

Figure 4. The associations between the secondary outcomes and PUFA levels. The cumulative incidences of the secondary endpoints (cardiac death and re-hospitalization for heart failure) were estimated by using the Kaplan–Meier method. Log-rank testing was performed to study the influence of PUFA levels on primary endpoint. The patients were divided into two groups, based on the median levels of (**A**) EPA, (**B**) DHA, (**C**) AA, (**D**) DGLA, and (**E**) EPA/AA, (**F**) DHA/AA, and (**G**) AA + DGLA/EPA + DHA. PUFA, polyunsaturated fatty acid; EPA, eicosapentaenoic acid; DHA, docosahexaenoic acid; AA, arachidonic acid; DGLA, dihomo-gamma-linolenic acid; EPA/AA, ratio of EPA to AA; DHA/AA, ratio of DHA to AA; AA + DGLA/EPA + DHA; ratio of AA + DGLA to EPA + DHA.

4. Discussion

The data from the present study showed that the acute decompensated HFpEF patients with lower plasma DHA levels had a significantly higher incidence of all-cause death, independent of GNRI. These findings suggest that plasma DHA levels are an important factor associated with prognosis, regardless of the nutritional status of patients with acute decompensated HFpEF. This suggests that measuring plasma DHA levels may be useful for the detection of high-risk patients hospitalized with HFpEF.

Several studies have shown the association between circulating concentrations of PUFAs and the incidence of HF. A previous cohort study, which included 2735 adults in the Cardiovascular Health Study from 1992 to 2006, reported that the total concentrations of omega-3 fatty acid were associated with the incidence of primary congestive HF [19]. A recent report from the Multi-Ethnic Study of Atherosclerosis (MESA) trial indicated that higher plasma EPA levels were significantly associated with a reduced risk of HF (for both reduced and preserved EF) [22]. In addition, regarding the association between PUFAs and the prognosis of patients with acute decompensated HF, a study showed that decreased plasma levels of DHA, DGLA, and AA were independently associated with long-term mortality in patients with acute decompensated HF [33]. Other studies have shown that lower omega-6 PUFAs levels were related to worse clinical outcomes in patients with acute decompensated HF [34,35]. However, most of the patients included in these studies had HFrEF. Thus, to the best of our knowledge, this is the first study to evaluate the correlation between PUFA levels and the prognosis of patients with HFpEF.

This study showed that lower DHA levels, but not EPA levels, were independently associated with all-cause mortality in patients with acute decompensated HFpEF. PUFAs play an important role in cellular membrane function [36]. While DHA is abundant in the cell membranes of cardiomyocytes [25], EPA is scarce. This difference may contribute to the distinct effects that DHA and EPA have on cardiac health. It should be noted, however, that while DHA can be obtained from the diet, it can also be synthesized from EPA [37]. In fact, the data from MESA suggested that EPA was more important than DHA for HF [19]. Therefore, any interpretation of the differences between the effects of DHA and EPA on the prognosis of HFpEF patients should be made with caution.

Although the present study showed a relationship between lower plasma DHA levels and a higher incidence of all-cause death, there was no significant association between DHA levels and composite events of cardiac death and re-hospitalization for HF. According to a Japanese cohort study called the Chronic Heart Failure Analysis and Registry in the Tohoku (CHART), the temporal trend in the mode of death in symptomatic HF has changed. As the prevalence of HFpEF in symptomatic HF increased from CHART-1 (2000–2005) to CHART-2 (2006–2010), the proportion of non-cardiac deaths increased from 23% in CHART-1 to 40% in CHART-2 [5]. In this study [5], those factors that were significantly associated with all-cause death were reported to be advanced age, low BMI, high systolic blood pressure, and absence of dyslipidemia. This is in line with our data shown in Table 1. Patients with HFpEF had more comorbidities than HFrEF patients, and noncardiac deaths occurred more frequently in HFpEF patients than in HFrEF patients [38].

Thus, the characteristics inherent to HFpEF patients specifically may be involved in the significant impact that DHA levels have on all-cause death, as opposed to cardiac death or re-hospitalization for HF.

Malnutrition is frequently observed and an important risk factor for poor outcomes in patients with HF. The GNRI is a simple and objective nutritional index, and a GNRI < 92 is generally used to evaluate the increased risk of morbidity and mortality in hospitalized elderly patients [21]. In our study, patients with the primary endpoint had an average GNRI of 90.8, suggesting a poor nutritional status. Although the patients with the primary endpoint also showed lower omega-3 PUFA levels, which were affected by oral intake, the Cox regression analyses revealed that the impact of the DHA levels on the patients' prognoses was independent of the GNRI. Even in the patients with a poor nutritional status, lower DHA levels were shown to be an independent predictor of all-cause mortality in HFpEF patients.

Inflammation is a normal process that is part of the body's defense and tissue-healing mechanism. However, excessive or unresolved inflammation can lead to uncontrolled tissue injury, and disease. Omega-6-derived metabolites, such as prostaglandins and leukotrienes, have pro-inflammatory effects, while omega-3-derived metabolites, such as resolvins and protectins, have anti-inflammatory and pro-resolving effects [10,11]. In this context, several clinical studies showed that the ratio of omega-3 to omega-6 PUFAs is a powerful predictor of heart disease [39–41]. Therefore, active screening of PUFAs would be beneficial in identifying patients at high risk of cardiovascular disease.

The GISSI-HF (Gruppo Italiano per lo Studio della Sopravvivenza nell'Infarto Miocardico Heart Failure) trial was a large-scale, placebo-controlled, randomized study that showed that 1 g daily of omega-3 fatty acid administration reduced the risk of all-cause death by 9% and the risk of hospitalization due to cardiovascular reasons by 8% in patients with chronic heart failure [42]. Other clinical trials have indicated that omega-3 fatty acids might improve outcomes in patients with HF [23–26]. In addition, animal studies have shown that omega-3 fatty acids, including EPA and DHA, at supraphysiological levels, preserve left ventricular function and prevent interstitial fibrosis in a mouse model of pressure overload-induced HF [39,43,44]. Despite these potential benefits, the use of omega-3 fatty acids in patients with HF remains controversial. Future large-scale randomized clinical trials to investigate the benefit of high dosages of omega-3 fatty acids, on top of the guideline-directed medical therapy for patients with documented overt HF, will be needed.

This study had several limitations. First, the study was conducted in a single center, the sample size was small, and the follow-up period was short. Therefore, it may be difficult to generalize these results. Second, the PUFAs were not measured in the cell membrane. PUFAs in the cell membrane have been reported to be direct precursors of pro- and anti-inflammatory eicosanoids. However, it has also been reported that cell-membrane PUFAs are significantly correlated with serum PUFAs in the Japanese population [30]. Third, food intake is associated with blood levels of PUFAs; however, measurement of dietary intake by using a frequency food questionnaire was not performed in this study. Moreover, the multivariate cox regression model included a limited number of variates to avoid statistical overfitting, because of the small number of the primary outcome. Therefore, large-scale studies will be needed to confirm our findings. Finally, the study was an observational study, so the causal relationship between DHA levels and prognosis is uncertain.

5. Conclusions

Lower levels of DHA are significantly associated with an increase in all-cause death in patients with acute decompensated HFpEF, independent of nutritional status. Measurement of plasma DHA levels may be useful in identifying high-risk patients with HFpEF, and supplementation with DHA may be a potential therapeutic target in these patients.

Author Contributions: Conceptualization, A.T.; formal analysis, N.M. and T.M.; data curation, N.M.; T.K., K.Y., M.T., Y.N., N.O., and M.U.; investigation, N.M.; A.T.; T.K., K.Y., M.T., Y.N., N.O., and M.U.; writing—original draft preparation, N.M.; writing—Review and Editing, T.M.; A.T.; T.K., K.Y., M.T., Y.N., N.O., and M.U.; project administration, H.I. All authors have read and agreed to the published version of the manuscript.

Funding: This research received no external funding.

Institutional Review Board Statement: The study protocol was approved by the Institutional Review Board of Mitoyo General Hospital (19CR01-122).

Informed Consent Statement: Patient consent was waived because of the low-risk nature of the study and inability to obtain consent directly from all the study subjects.

Data Availability Statement: The data presented in this study are available on request from the corresponding author.

Conflicts of Interest: The authors declare no conflict of interest.

References

1. Ziaeian, B.; Fonarow, G.C. Epidemiology and aetiology of heart failure. *Nat. Rev. Cardiol.* **2016**, *13*, 368–378. [CrossRef] [PubMed]
2. Virani, S.S.; Alonso, A.; Benjamin, E.J.; Bittencourt, M.S.; Callaway, C.W.; Carson, A.P.; Chamberlain, A.M.; Chang, A.R.; Cheng, S.; Delling, F.N.; et al. Heart Disease and Stroke Statistics-2020 Update: A Report From the American Heart Association. *Circulation* **2020**, *141*, e139–e596. [CrossRef] [PubMed]
3. Butler, J.; Fonarow, G.C.; Zile, M.R.; Lam, C.S.; Roessig, L.; Schelbert, E.B.; Shah, S.J.; Ahmed, A.; Bonow, R.O.; Cleland, J.G.; et al. Developing therapies for heart failure with preserved ejection fraction: Current state and future directions. *JACC Heart Fail.* **2014**, *2*, 97–112. [CrossRef] [PubMed]
4. Yancy, C.W.; Jessup, M.; Bozkurt, B.; Butler, J.; Casey, D.E., Jr.; Colvin, M.M.; Drazner, M.H.; Filippatos, G.S.; Fonarow, G.C.; Givertz, M.M.; et al. 2017 ACC/AHA/HFSA Focused Update of the 2013 ACCF/AHA Guideline for the Management of Heart Failure: A Report of the American College of Cardiology/American Heart Association Task Force on Clinical Practice Guidelines and the Heart Failure Society of America. *Circulation* **2017**, *136*, e137–e161. [CrossRef]
5. Ushigome, R.; Sakata, Y.; Nochioka, K.; Miyata, S.; Miura, M.; Tadaki, S.; Yamauchi, T.; Sato, S.; Onose, T.; Tsuji, K.; et al. Temporal trends in clinical characteristics, management and prognosis of patients with symptomatic heart failure in Japan—Report from the CHART Studies. *Circ. J.* **2015**, *79*, 2396–2407. [CrossRef]
6. Narumi, T.; Arimoto, T.; Funayama, A.; Kadowaki, S.; Otaki, Y.; Nishiyama, S.; Takahashi, H.; Shishido, T.; Miyashita, T.; Miyamoto, T.; et al. Prognostic importance of objective nutritional indexes in patients with chronic heart failure. *J. Cardiol.* **2013**, *62*, 307–313. [CrossRef]
7. Sokoła-Wysoczańska, E.; Wysoczański, T.; Wagner, J.; Czyż, K.; Bodkowski, R.; Lochyński, S.; Patkowska-Sokoła, B. Polyunsaturated Fatty Acids and Their Potential Therapeutic Role in Cardiovascular System Disorders—A Review. *Nutrients* **2018**, *10*, 1561. [CrossRef]
8. Russo, G.L. Dietary n-6 and n-3 polyunsaturated fatty acids: From biochemistry to clinical implications in cardiovascular prevention. *Biochem. Pharmacol.* **2009**, *77*, 937–946. [CrossRef]
9. Sakamoto, A.; Saotome, M.; Iguchi, K.; Maekawa, Y. Marine-Derived Omega-3 Polyunsaturated Fatty Acids and Heart Failure: Current Understanding for Basic to Clinical Relevance. *Int. J. Mol.* **2019**, *20*, 4025. [CrossRef]
10. Innes, J.K.; Calder, P.C. Omega-6 fatty acids and inflammation. *Prostaglandins Leukot. Essent. Fatty Acids* **2018**, *132*, 41–48. [CrossRef]
11. Serhan, C.N. Pro-resolving lipid mediators are leads for resolution physiology. *Nature* **2014**, *510*, 92–101. [CrossRef] [PubMed]
12. Frigolet, M.E.; Gutierrez-Aguilar, R. The Role of the Novel Lipokine Palmitoleic Acid in Health and Disease. *Adv. Nut.* **2017**, *8*, 173S–181S. [CrossRef] [PubMed]
13. Carrillo, C.; Cavia, M.D.M.; Alonso-Torre, S. Role of oleic acid in immune system; mechanism of action; a review. *Nutr. Hosp.* **2012**, *27*, 978–990. [CrossRef] [PubMed]

14. Sales-Campos, H.; Souza, P.R.; Peghini, B.C.; da Silva, J.S.; Cardoso, C.R. An overview of the modulatory effects of oleic acid in health and disease. *Mini Rev. Med. Chem.* **2013**, *13*, 201–210. [CrossRef]
15. Kayama, Y.; Minamino, T.; Toko, H.; Sakamoto, M.; Shimizu, I.; Takahashi, H.; Okada, S.; Tateno, K.; Moriya, J.; Yokoyama, M.; et al. Cardiac 12/15 lipoxygenase-induced inflammation is involved in heart failure. *J. Exp. Med.* **2009**, *206*, 1565–1574. [CrossRef]
16. Endo, J.; Sano, M.; Isobe, Y.; Fukuda, K.; Kang, J.X.; Arai, H.; Arita, M. 18-HEPE, an n-3 fatty acid metabolite released by macrophages, prevents pressure overload-induced maladaptive cardiac remodeling. *J. Exp. Med.* **2014**, *211*, 1673–1687. [CrossRef]
17. Kunapuli, P.; Lawson, J.A.; Rokach, J.A.; Meinkoth, J.L.; FitzGerald, G.A. Prostaglandin F2alpha (PGF2alpha) and the isoprostane, 8,12-iso-isoprostane F2alpha-III, induce cardiomyocyte hypertrophy. Differential activation of downstream signaling pathways. *J. Biol. Chem.* **1998**, *273*, 22442–22452. [CrossRef]
18. GISSI-Prevenzione Investigators (Gruppo Italiano per lo Studio della Sopravvivenza nell'Infarto miocardico). Dietary supplementation with n-3 polyunsaturated fatty acids and vitamin E after myocardial infarction: Results of the GISSI-Prevenzione trial. *Lancet* **1999**, *354*, 447–455. [CrossRef]
19. Mozaffarian, D.; Lemaitre, R.N.; King, I.B.; Song, X.; Spiegelman, D.; Sacks, F.M.; Rimm, E.B.; Siscovick, D.S. Circulating long-chain ω-3 fatty acids and incidence of congestive heart failure in older adults: The cardiovascular health study: A cohort study. *Ann. Intern. Med.* **2011**, *155*, 160–170. [CrossRef]
20. Bernasconi, A.A.; Wiest, M.M.; Lavie, C.J.; Milani, R.V.; Laukkanen, J.A. Effect of Omega-3 Dosage on Cardiovascular Outcomes: An Updated Meta-Analysis and Meta-Regression of Interventional Trials. *Mayo Clin. Proc.* **2020**. [CrossRef]
21. Djousse, L.; Akinkuolie, A.O.; Wu, J.H.; Ding, E.L.; Gaziano, J.M. Fish consumption, omega-3 fatty acids and risk of heart failure: A meta-analysis. *Clin. Nutr.* **2012**, *31*, 846–853. [CrossRef] [PubMed]
22. Block, R.C.; Liu, L.; Herrington, D.M.; Huang, S.; Tsai, M.Y.; O'Connell, T.D.; Shearer, G.C. Predicting Risk for Incident Heart Failure With Omega-3 Fatty Acids: From MESA. *JACC Heart Fail.* **2019**, *7*, 651–661. [CrossRef] [PubMed]
23. Nodari, S.; Triggiani, M.; Campia, U.; Manerba, A.; Milesi, G.; Cesana, B.M.; Gheorghiade, M.; Dei Cas, L. Effects of n-3 polyunsaturated fatty acids on left ventricular function and functional capacity in patients with dilated cardiomyopathy. *J. Am. Coll. Cardiol.* **2011**, *57*, 870–879. [CrossRef]
24. Chrysohoou, C.; Metallinos, G.; Georgiopoulos, G.; Mendrinos, D.; Papanikolaou, A.; Magkas, N.; Pitsavos, C.; Vyssoulis, G.; Stefanadis, C.; Tousoulis, D. Short term omega-3 polyunsaturated fatty acid supplementation induces favorable changes in right ventricle function and diastolic filling pressure in patients with chronic heart failure; A randomized clinical trial. *Vasc. Pharmacol.* **2016**, *79*, 43–50. [CrossRef] [PubMed]
25. Kohashi, K.; Nakagomi, A.; Saiki, Y.; Morisawa, T.; Kosugi, M.; Kusama, Y.; Atarashi, H.; Shimizu, W. Effects of eicosapentaenoic acid on the levels of inflammatory markers, cardiac function and long-term prognosis in chronic heart failure patients with dyslipidemia. *J. Atheroscler. Thromb.* **2014**, *21*, 712–729. [CrossRef]
26. Moertl, D.; Hammer, A.; Steiner, S.; Hutuleac, R.; Vonbank, K.; Berger, R. Dose-dependent effects of omega-3-polyunsaturated fatty acids on systolic left ventricular function, endothelial function, and markers of inflammation in chronic heart failure of nonischemic origin: A double-blind, placebo-controlled, 3-arm study. *Am. Heart. J.* **2011**, *161*, 915.e1–915.e9. [CrossRef]
27. O'Keefe, E.L.; Harris, W.S.; DiNicolantonio, J.J.; Elagizi, A.; Milani, R.V.; Lavie, C.J.; O'Keefe, J.H. Sea Change for Marine Omega-3s: Randomized Trials Show Fish Oil Reduces Cardiovascular Events. *Mayo Clin. Proc.* **2019**, *94*, 2524–2533. [CrossRef]
28. Elagizi, A.; Lavie, C.J.; O'Keefe, E.; Marshall, K.; O'Keefe, J.H.; Milani, R.V. An Update on Omega-3 Polyunsaturated Fatty Acids and Cardiovascular Health. *Nutrients* **2021**, *13*, 204. [CrossRef]
29. McKee, P.A.; Castelli, W.P.; McNamara, P.M.; Kannel, W.B. The natural history of congestive heart failure: The Framingham study. *N. Engl. J. Med.* **1971**, *285*, 1441–1446. [CrossRef]
30. Yanagisawa, N.; Shimada, K.; Miyazaki, T.; Kume, A.; Kitamura, Y.; Ichikawa, R.; Ohmura, H.; Kiyanagi, T.; Hiki, M.; Fukao, K.; et al. Polyunsaturated fatty acid levels of serum and red blood cells in apparently healthy Japanese subjects living in an urban area. *J. Atheroscler. Thromb.* **2010**, *17*, 285–294. [CrossRef]
31. Matsuo, S.; Imai, E.; Horio, M.; Yasuda, Y.; Tomita, K.; Nitta, K.; Yamagata, K.; Tomino, Y.; Yokoyama, H.; Hishida, A.; et al. Revised equations for estimated GFR from serum creatinine in Japan. *Am. J. Kidney Dis.* **2009**, *53*, 982–992. [CrossRef] [PubMed]
32. Bouillanne, O.; Morineau, G.; Dupont, C.; Coulombel, I.; Vincent, J.P.; Nicolis, I.; Benazeth, S.; Cynober, L.; Aussel, C. Geriatric Nutritional Risk Index: A new index for evaluating at-risk elderly medical patients. *Am. J. Clin. Nutr.* **2005**, *82*, 777–783. [CrossRef] [PubMed]
33. Ouchi, S.; Miyazaki, T.; Shimada, K.; Sugita, Y.; Shimizu, M.; Murata, A.; Kato, T.; Aikawa, T.; Suda, S.; Shiozawa, T.; et al. Low Docosahexaenoic Acid, Dihomo-Gamma-Linolenic Acid, and Arachidonic Acid Levels Associated with Long-Term Mortality in Patients with Acute Decompensated Heart Failure in Different Nutritional Statuses. *Nutrients* **2017**, *9*, 956. [CrossRef] [PubMed]
34. Nagai, T.; Honda, Y.; Sugano, Y.; Nishimura, K.; Nakai, M.; Honda, S.; Iwakami, N.; Okada, A.; Asaumi, Y.; Aiba, T.; et al. Circulating Omega-6, But Not Omega-3 Polyunsaturated Fatty Acids, Are Associated with Clinical Outcomes in Patients with Acute Decompensated Heart Failure. *PLoS ONE* **2016**, *11*, e0165841. [CrossRef]
35. Ouchi, S.; Miyazaki, T.; Shimada, K.; Sugita, Y.; Shimizu, M.; Murata, A.; Kato, T.; Aikawa, T.; Suda, S.; Shiozawa, T.; et al. Decreased circulating dihomo-gamma-linolenic acid levels are associated with total mortality in patients with acute cardiovascular disease and acute decompensated heart failure. *Lipids Health Dis.* **2017**, *16*, 150. [CrossRef]
36. Nieman, D.C.; Mitmesser, S.H. Potential Impact of Nutrition on Immune System Recovery from Heavy Exertion: A Metabolomics Perspective. *Nutrients* **2017**, *9*, 513. [CrossRef]

37. Saito, M.; Ueno, M.; Kubo, K.; Yamaguchi, M. Dose-Response Effect of Dietary Docosahexaenoic Acid on Fatty Acid Profiles of Serum and Tissue Lipids in Rats. *J. Agric. Food Chem.* **1998**, *46*, 184–193. [CrossRef]
38. Hamaguchi, S.; Kinugawa, S.; Sobirin, M.A.; Goto, D.; Tsuchihashi-Makaya, M.; Yamada, S.; Yokoshiki, H.; Tsutsui, H.; JCARE-CARD Investigators. Mode of death in patients with heart failure and reduced vs. preserved ejection fraction: Report from the registry of hospitalized heart failure patients. *Circ. J.* **2012**, *76*, 1662–1669. [CrossRef]
39. Fukuhara, M.; Kitazono, T.; Kiyohara, Y. Association between ratio of serum eicosapentaenoic acid to arachidonic acid and risk of cardiovascular disease: The Hisayama Study. *Atherosclerosis* **2013**, *231*, 261–267.
40. Domei, T.; Yokoi, H.; Kuramitsu, S.; Soga, Y.; Arita, T.; Ando, K.; Shirai, S.; Kondo, K.; Sakai, K.; Goya, M.; et al. Ratio of serum n-3 to n-6 polyunsaturated fatty acids and the incidence of major adverse cardiac events in patients undergoing percutaneous coronary intervention. *Circ. J.* **2012**, *76*, 423–429. [CrossRef]
41. Ueeda, M.; Doumei, T.; Takaya, Y.; Ohnishi, N.; Takaishi, A.; Hirohata, S.; Miyoshi, T.; Shinohata, R.; Usui, S.; Kusachi, S. Association of serum levels of arachidonic acid and eicosapentaenoic acid with prevalence of major adverse cardiac events after acute myocardial infarction. *Heart Vessel.* **2011**, *26*, 145–152. [CrossRef] [PubMed]
42. Tavazzi, L.; Maggioni, A.P.; Marchioli, R.; Barlera, S.; Franzosi, M.G.; Latini, R.; Lucci, D.; Nicolosi, G.L.; Porcu, M.; Tognoni, G.; et al. Effect of n-3 polyunsaturated fatty acids in patients with chronic heart failure (the GISSI-HF trial): A randomised, double-blind, placebo-controlled trial. *Lancet* **2008**, *372*, 1223–1230. [PubMed]
43. Madingou, N.; Gilbert, K.; Tomaro, L.; Prud'homme Touchette, C.; Trudeau, F.; Fortin, S.; Rousseau, G. Comparison of the effects of EPA and DHA alone or in combination in a murine model of myocardial infarction. *Prostaglandins Leukot. Essent. Fat. Acids* **2016**, *111*, 11–16. [CrossRef] [PubMed]
44. Chen, J.; Shearer, G.C.; Chen, Q.; Healy, C.L.; Beyer, A.J.; Nareddy, V.B.; Gerdes, A.M.; Harris, W.S.; O'Connell, T.D.; Wang, D. Omega-3 fatty acids prevent pressure overload-induced cardiac fibrosis through activation of cyclic GMP/protein kinase G signaling in cardiac fibroblasts. *Circulation* **2011**, *123*, 584–593. [CrossRef] [PubMed]

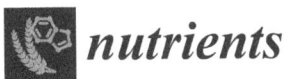

Article

Impact of Inadequate Calorie Intake on Mortality and Hospitalization in Stable Patients with Chronic Heart Failure

Yoshikuni Obata [1], Naoya Kakutani [1], Shintaro Kinugawa [1,2,*], Arata Fukushima [1], Takashi Yokota [1,3], Shingo Takada [1], Taisuke Ono [4], Takeshi Sota [5], Yoshiharu Kinugasa [6], Masashige Takahashi [7], Hisashi Matsuo [8], Ryuichi Matsukawa [9], Ichiro Yoshida [10], Isao Yokota [11], Kazuhiro Yamamoto [6] and Miyuki Tsuchihashi-Makaya [12]

1. Department of Cardiovascular Medicine, Faculty of Medicine, Graduate School of Medicine, Hokkaido University, Sapporo 060-8638, Japan; obata4492@yahoo.co.jp (Y.O.); kakutaninaoya@gmail.com (N.K.); arata.fukushima@gmail.com (A.F.); t-yokota@med.hokudai.ac.jp (T.Y.); s-takada@hokusho-u.ac.jp (S.T.)
2. Department of Cardiovascular Medicine, Faculty of Medical Sciences, Kyusyu University, Fukuoka 812-8582, Japan
3. Clinical Research and Medical Innovation Center, Hokkaido University Hospital, Sapporo 060-8648, Japan
4. Department of Cardiology, Kitami Red Cross Hospital, Kitami 090-8666, Japan; ono_taisuke@kitami.jrc.or.jp
5. Division of Rehabilitation, Tottori University Hospital, Tottori 683-8504, Japan; tsota@med.tottori-u.ac.jp
6. Department of Cardiovascular Medicine and Endocrinology and Metabolism, Faculty of Medicine, Tottori University, Tottori 683-8503, Japan; ykinugasa-circ@umin.ac.jp (Y.K.); ykazuhiro@med.tottori-u.ac.jp (K.Y.)
7. Department of Cardiology, Kushiro City General Hospital, Kushiro 085-0822, Japan; circ.masashiget@gmail.com
8. Department of Cardiology, Keiwakai Ebetsu Hospital, Ebetsu 069-0817, Japan; matsuo@keiwakai-ebetsu.or.jp
9. Division of Cardiology, Cardiovascular and Aortic Center, Saiseikai Fukuoka General Hospital, Fukuoka 810-0001, Japan; matukawa@cardiol.med.kyushu-u.ac.jp
10. Department of Cardiology, Obihiro Kyokai Hospital, Obihiro 080-0805, Japan; i-yoshida@obihiro-kyokai-hsp.jp
11. Department of Biostatistics, Faculty of Medicine, Graduate School of Medicine, Hokkaido University, Sapporo 060-8638, Japan; yokotai@pop.med.hokudai.ac.jp
12. School of Nursing, Kitasato University, Sagamihara 252-0373, Japan; miyuki-m@nrs.kitasato-u.ac.jp
* Correspondence: kinugawa@cardiol.med.kyushu-u.ac.jp; Tel.: +81-92-642-5360

Citation: Obata, Y.; Kakutani, N.; Kinugawa, S.; Fukushima, A.; Yokota, T.; Takada, S.; Ono, T.; Sota, T.; Kinugasa, Y.; Takahashi, M.; et al. Impact of Inadequate Calorie Intake on Mortality and Hospitalization in Stable Patients with Chronic Heart Failure. *Nutrients* 2021, 13, 874. https://doi.org/10.3390/nu13030874

Academic Editor: Yoshihiro Fukumoto

Received: 26 January 2021
Accepted: 4 March 2021
Published: 8 March 2021

Publisher's Note: MDPI stays neutral with regard to jurisdictional claims in published maps and institutional affiliations.

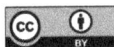

Copyright: © 2021 by the authors. Licensee MDPI, Basel, Switzerland. This article is an open access article distributed under the terms and conditions of the Creative Commons Attribution (CC BY) license (https://creativecommons.org/licenses/by/4.0/).

Abstract: Malnutrition is highly prevalent in patients with heart failure (HF), but the precise impact of dietary energy deficiency on HF patients' clinical outcomes is not known. We investigated the associations between inadequate calorie intake and adverse clinical events in 145 stable outpatients with chronic HF who had a history of hospitalization due to worsening HF. To assess the patients' dietary pattern, we used a brief self-administered diet-history questionnaire (BDHQ). Inadequate calorie intake was defined as <60% of the estimated energy requirement. In the total chronic HF cohort, the median calorie intake was 1628 kcal/day. Forty-four patients (30%) were identified as having an inadequate calorie intake. A Kaplan–Meier analysis revealed that the patients with inadequate calorie intake had significantly worse clinical outcomes including all-cause death and HF-related hospitalization during the 1-year follow-up period versus those with adequate calorie intake (20% vs. 5%, $p < 0.01$). A multivariate logistic regression analysis showed that inadequate calorie intake was an independent predictor of adverse clinical events after adjustment for various factors that may influence patients' calorie intake. Among patients with chronic HF, inadequate calorie intake was associated with an increased risk of all-cause mortality and rehospitalization due to worsening HF. However, our results are preliminary and larger studies with direct measurements of dietary calorie intake and total energy expenditure are needed to clarify the intrinsic nature of this relationship.

Keywords: calorie intake; heart failure; hospitalization; malnutrition; mortality

1. Introduction

Heart failure (HF) is common in adults and is associated with increased morbidity and mortality. Its prevalence is increasing due to the aging of the population in many countries [1]. Despite recent advances in pharmacological and non-pharmacological treatments for HF, the prognosis of individuals with chronic HF remains poor, and diet and exercise interventions are thus recognized as essential treatments for the prevention of HF progression.

Although obesity is a risk of incident HF, a low body mass index (BMI) is more closely associated with poor clinical outcomes in chronic HF patients, in a phenomenon known as the obesity paradox [2,3]. As one of the possible mechanisms of this paradox, malnutrition is a recent focus of attention among healthcare providers who are engaged in HF management. Malnutrition is highly prevalent in patients with chronic HF, and it increases their risk of death and hospitalization [4]. Patients with chronic HF have been demonstrated to have an increased energy expenditure compared to healthy sedentary subjects, but HF patients' dietary energy intake is often insufficient to meet their energy requirements for daily activities, even in a stable condition [5]. The negative energy balance leads to a catabolic state and causes protein–energy malnutrition, which results in muscle wasting and sarcopenia [6,7]. In addition, dietary guidance for HF patients has traditionally focused on reducing their salt and fluid intake; the patients' intake of dietary nutrients has tended to be less of a concern [8]. Restrictive diets for HF patients may cause a reduced intake of macronutrients and micronutrients, leading to increased morbidity and mortality [8].

We conducted the present study to determine whether calorie intake that is inadequate for the energy needed for daily activities is associated with adverse clinical events including all-cause death and HF-related hospitalization in stable patients with chronic HF. The patients' daily calorie intake was calculated by a brief self-administered diet-history questionnaire (BDHQ), which is a well-validated questionnaire for determining a patient's dietary pattern.

2. Materials and Methods

2.1. Study Design

This study was part of a multicenter, prospective observational investigation of the effects of dietary patterns on clinical outcomes in patients with chronic HF, and thus some of the data used herein were obtained from the same patients whose data were published previously but in a different context [9]. The study was approved by the ethics committees of Hokkaido University Hospital (approval no. 012-0224) and the other nine participating research institutes—Hakodate National Hospital, Hikone Municipal Hospital, Kitami Red Cross Hospital, Keiwakai Ebetsu Hospital, Kushiro City General Hospital, Obihiro Kyokai Hospital, Otaru Kyokai Hospital, Saiseikai Fukuoka General Hospital, and Tottori University Hospital. The study was conducted in accordance with the ethical principles described in the Declaration of Helsinki. Written informed consent was obtained from each patient before his or her participation in the study.

2.2. Patients

A total of 145 stable patients with chronic HF who were regularly visiting an outpatient ward for >1 month were enrolled between December 2012 and September 2014. These patients had a history of hospitalization due to worsening HF at least once within the 5 years before enrollment. The exclusion criteria included nephrotic syndrome, liver cirrhosis, cancer, a history of gastrointestinal surgery within the prior 3 months, or poorly controlled diabetes, i.e., glycosylated hemoglobin (HbA1c) >7.0%. We also excluded patients who were taking steroids or antidepressants, which could influence their appetite.

2.3. Study Protocol

At baseline, the patients underwent clinical and anthropometric measurements, blood testing, echocardiography, a 6-min walk test to assess exercise capacity, and the evaluation of their dietary pattern and calorie intake. The patients were then followed up for 1 year to evaluate adverse clinical events including all-cause death and hospitalization due to worsening HF.

2.4. Anthropometric Measurements

To assess the patients' muscle mass, we measured the circumferences of the upper arm and the thigh at the level of the muscle belly.

2.5. Laboratory Measurements

After blood collection, the patients' hemoglobin, serum albumin, HbA1c, and plasma levels of B-type natriuretic peptide (BNP) were determined by routine in-house analyses. The estimated glomerular filtration rate (eGFR) was calculated from the serum creatinine values and the patient's age with the use of the Japanese equation [10]: eGFR = $194 \times$ (serum creatinine, mg/dL)$^{-1.094} \times$ (age, years)$^{-0.287} \times$ (0.739 if female).

2.6. Assessment of Dietary Calorie Intake

Each patient's dietary pattern was evaluated using a BDHQ adjusted to typical Japanese diets. The BDHQ is a four-page fixed-portion questionnaire that calculates the frequency of the consumption of selected foods to estimate the intake of 58 food and beverage items during the preceding month, as described [11,12]. The BDHQ consists of five sections—(1) the intake frequency of food and nonalcoholic beverage items, (2) the daily intake of rice and miso soup, (3) the frequency of alcoholic beverage consumption and the amount per drink, (4) usual cooking methods, and (5) general dietary behavior. The dietary calorie intake was calculated as the sum of each energy conversion factor from the fats, proteins, and carbohydrates whose amount is estimated using the BDHQ, as described previously [13,14]. Dietary salt intake was estimated according to the diet history method using the quantitative information. In this estimation, intakes of table salt and salt-containing seasoning at the table, calculated using the qualitative information of general dietary behavior, were also considered, as described [12].

2.7. Estimation of the Dietary Calorie Requirement

The dietary calorie requirement was estimated using the Japanese Dietary Reference Intakes published by the Ministry of Health, Labour and Welfare (Japan) in 2015, as described previously [15,16]. Briefly, each patient's estimated dietary calorie requirement was determined in consideration of his or her age, gender, and physical activity level (low, moderate, or high). Since most of the patients were in a stable condition with New York Heart Association (NYHA) functional class I or II (normal or mild HF) and all the patients were ambulant and regularly visited an outpatient ward, the daily calorie requirement was estimated with the assumption that all of the patients were engaged in moderate physical activity (categorized as level II). This level requires the ability to do self-care activities (e.g., washing and dressing) and walk outside without any support. We then calculated the dietary energy adequacy (%) as the ratio of the individual patient's daily calorie intake to the estimated daily calorie requirement.

2.8. Assessment of Nutritional Status

Each patient's nutritional status was assessed by determining his or her controlling nutritional status (CONUT) score [17] and score on a geriatric nutritional risk index (GNRI) [18]. Briefly, the CONUT score was calculated based on the serum albumin level, total peripheral lymphocyte count, and total cholesterol level, and the scores are classified into normal (0–1 points), mild risk (2–4), moderate risk (5–8), and severe risk (9–12) of malnutrition. The GNRI was calculated from the patient's BMI and albumin concentration according to the modified version—GNRI = 14.89 × serum albumin (g/dL) + 41.7 × BMI/22. The GNRI values are classified into four grades of malnutrition-related risk—major risk (GNRI < 82), moderate risk (GNRI 82–91), low risk (GNRI 92–98), and no risk (GNRI > 98).

2.9. Statistical Analyses

Continuous variables are expressed as medians (interquartile range), and categorical variables are expressed as numbers (percentages). We divided the 145 patients into two groups based on their dietary calorie intake adequacy—the adequate calorie intake group (dietary calorie intake adequacy ≥60%; N = 101) and the inadequate calorie intake group (dietary calorie intake adequacy <60%; N = 44). The cut-off value of dietary calorie intake adequacy rate (60%) was predetermined by the results of the multivariate analysis. Continuous variables were compared between these groups with a Mann–Whitney U-test, and the χ^2-test was used for group comparisons of categorical variables. We performed a multivariate analysis to identify the decrease in dietary calorie intake adequacy that independently predicts adverse clinical events in chronic HF patients with other confounding factors that may influence dietary calorie intake, including age, BMI, NYHA functional class III, diabetes, left ventricular ejection fraction (LVEF), serum albumin, eGFR, and log BNP. The odds ratios (ORs) and 95% confidence intervals (CIs) were calculated for each variable from the logistic regression model. A Kaplan–Meier analysis with log-rank test was performed to assess the rates of all-cause death and rehospitalization due to worsening HF for 1 year. All analyses were performed using JMP Pro 13.1.0 software (SAS Institute, Cary, NC, USA). Probability (p)-values < 0.05 were considered significant.

3. Results

3.1. Characteristics of the Total Chronic HF Cohort

The characteristics of the total chronic HF cohort (N = 145) are summarized in Table 1. The median age of the patients with chronic HF was 67 years, and the median BMI was 22.9 kg/m². We recruited stable outpatients with chronic HF, and 90% of the patients had an NYHA functional class I or II. The median LVEF was 45%, and both HF patients with a reduced LVEF and those with a preserved LVEF were included in this cohort. The majority of the chronic HF patients were being treated with an angiotensin-converting enzyme (ACE) inhibitor or an angiotensin II receptor blocker (ARB) and a β-blocker. For the total chronic HF cohort, the median value of dietary calorie intake was 1628 kcal/day and the dietary calorie intake adequacy rate was 75%. The distribution of the dietary calorie intake adequacy rates of the patients is shown in Figure 1.

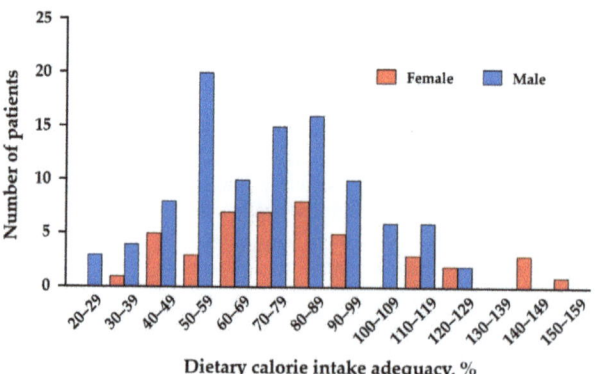

Figure 1. Distribution of dietary calorie intake adequacy rate of the female and male patients with chronic HF.

Table 1. Characteristics of total chronic heart failure (HF) cohort ($N = 145$).

Demographic Findings:	
Age, year	67 (60–77)
Female	45 (31%)
BMI, kg/m^2	22.9 (20.5–25.7)
Upper arm circumference, cm	27.5 (24.9–29.7)
Thigh circumference, cm	44.4 (40.8–47.0)
NYHA functional class:	
I–II	130 (90%)
III	15 (10%)
Primary cause of HF:	
Ischemic cause	46 (32%)
Dilated cardiomyopathy	45 (31%)
Others	54 (37%)
Hypertension	80 (55%)
Diabetes	38 (26%)
Dyslipidemia	100 (69%)
Echocardiographic findings:	
LVEF, %	45 (30–56)
Laboratory measurements:	
Hemoglobin, g/dL	13.3 (11.9–14.3)
Serum albumin, g/dL	4.2 (3.9–4.4)
eGFR, mL/min/1.73 m^2	54.2 (40.3–67.7)
HbA1c, %	5.8 (5.6–6.2)
Plasma BNP, pg/mL	154 (76–368)
Medications:	
ACE inhibitor or ARB	110 (76%)
β-blocker	128 (88%)
MRA	83 (57%)
Statin	69 (48%)
6-min walk test, m	433 (349–499)
Nutritional assessments:	
CONUT score	2 (1–2)
GNRI	106 (100–113)
Dietary calorie intake, kcal/day	1628 (1274–1996)
Estimated calorie requirement, kcal/day	2300 (1956–2425)
Dietary calorie intake adequacy, %	75 (58–91)

Data are median (1st–3rd quartile) or n (%). ACE: angiotensin-converting enzyme; ARB: angiotensin II receptor blocker; BMI: body mass index; BNP: B-type natriuretic peptide; CONUT: controlling nutritional status; eGFR: estimated glomerular filtration rate; GNRI: geriatric nutritional risk index; LVEF: left ventricular ejection fraction; MRA: mineralocorticoid receptor antagonist; NYHA: New York Heart Association.

3.2. Characteristics of the Chronic HF Patients with and without Adequate Calorie Intake

We divided the total chronic HF cohort into two groups—the adequate calorie intake group ($N = 101$) and the inadequate calorie intake group ($N = 44$). Inadequate calorie intake was defined as <60% of the estimated calorie requirement according to the results of the multivariate analysis. The baseline data of each group are summarized in Table 2. The median age of the chronic HF patients with inadequate calorie intake was younger than that of the patients with adequate calorie intake, but there was no significant difference in BMI or muscle mass (i.e., upper arm and thigh circumferences) between the groups. The percentage of diabetes was greater in the inadequate calorie intake group compared to the adequate calorie intake group. The LVEF, a parameter of LV systolic function, was significantly lower in the chronic HF patients with inadequate calorie intake. Renal function (i.e., eGFR) was more often impaired in the patients with inadequate calorie intake.

Table 2. Characteristics of chronic HF patients with adequate calorie intake and those with inadequate calorie intake.

	Adequate Calorie Intake (N = 101)	Inadequate Calorie Intake (N = 44)	p-Value
Demographic findings:			
Age, yrs	68 (61–78)	65 (55–73)	0.04
Female	35 (35%)	9 (20%)	0.07
BMI, kg/m^2	22.8 (20.3–26.1)	23.4 (20.7–25.4)	0.74
Upper arm circumference, cm	27.8 (24.7–30.0)	26.8 (24.9–29.4)	0.61
Thigh circumference, cm	44.4 (40.4–47.2)	43.9 (41.5–46.9)	0.99
NYHA functional class:			0.07
I–II	94 (93%)	36 (82%)	
III	7 (7%)	8 (18%)	
Primary cause of HF:			
Ischemic cause	33 (33%)	13 (30%)	0.71
Dilated cardiomyopathy	28 (28%)	17 (39%)	0.19
Others	40 (40%)	14 (32%)	0.37
Hypertension	55 (54%)	25 (57%)	0.79
Diabetes	21 (21%)	17 (39%)	0.02
Dyslipidemia	68 (67%)	32 (73%)	0.52
Echocardiographic findings:			
LVEF, %	49 (37–59)	34 (25–48)	<0.01
Laboratory measurements:			
Hemoglobin, g/dL	12.9 (11.7–14.2)	13.6 (12.4–14.4)	0.09
Serum albumin, g/dL	4.1 (4.0–4.3)	4.3 (3.9–4.5)	0.39
eGFR, mL/min/1.73 m^2	57.5 (42.9–71.1)	45.7 (34.5–56.5)	<0.01
HbA1c, %	5.8 (5.5–6.2)	5.9 (5.7–6.5)	0.17
Plasma BNP, pg/mL	153 (78–346)	156 (57–431)	0.88
Medications:			
ACE inhibitor or ARB	75 (74%)	35 (80%)	0.49
β-blocker	87 (86%)	41 (93%)	0.23
MRA	53 (52%)	30 (68%)	0.08
Statin	47 (47%)	22 (50%)	0.7
6-min walk test, m	435 (364–502)	424 (335–456)	0.15
Nutritional assessments:			
CONUT score	2 (1–2)	2 (1–3)	0.86
GNRI	106 (99–113)	107 (102–111)	0.54
Dietary calorie intake, kcal/day	1824 (1566–2276)	1145 (950–1308)	<0.01
Estimated calorie requirement, kcal/day	2238 (1913–2419)	2350 (2200–2469)	0.02
Dietary calorie intake adequacy, %	83 (73–99)	51 (42–57)	<0.01

Data are median (1st–3rd quartile) or n (%). Inadequate calorie intake was defined as <60% of estimated calorie requirement. ACE: angiotensin-converting enzyme; ARB: angiotensin II receptor blocker; BMI: body mass index; BNP: B-type natriuretic peptide; CONUT: controlling nutritional status; eGFR: estimated glomerular filtration rate; GNRI: geriatric nutritional risk index; LVEF: left ventricular ejection fraction; MRA: mineralocorticoid receptor antagonist; NYHA: New York Heart Association.

The nutritional parameters including the CONUT score and GNRI value were similar between the two groups. As expected, the chronic HF patients with inadequate calorie intake had a reduced daily calorie intake compared to those with an adequate calorie intake. In addition, most of foods and nutrients were less frequently consumed by the patient with inadequate calorie intake (Supplementary Tables S1 and S2). The daily salt intake was significantly reduced in the inadequate calorie intake group compared to the adequate calorie intake group (median (1st–3rd quartile range) 6.6 (5.4–8.3) vs. 10.2 (8.8–13.3) g/day, $p<0.01$) (Supplementary Table S2).

3.3. Adverse Clinical Events

During the 1-year follow-up period, the combined clinical events of all-cause death and HF-related hospitalization occurred in 14 patients (10%) (four deaths and 10 hospitalizations). The Kaplan–Meier analysis revealed that the patients with an inadequate calorie intake had a significantly higher risk of adverse clinical events than those with an adequate calorie intake (20% vs. 5%, respectively; $p < 0.01$) (Figure 2).

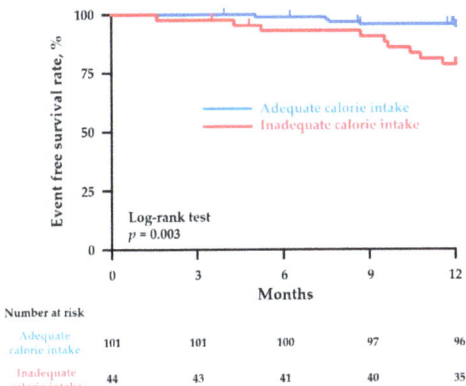

Figure 2. Kaplan–Meier curves for the cumulative event (all-cause death and HF-related hospitalization)-free ratio in the chronic HF patients with an adequate calorie intake (dietary calorie intake adequacy ≥60%) and those with an inadequate calorie intake (dietary calorie intake adequacy <60%).

3.4. Predictors of Adverse Clinical Events in Patients with Chronic HF

The results of the multivariate analysis revealed that after the adjustment for age, BMI, NYHA functional class III, LVEF, serum albumin, eGFR, and log BNP, inadequate calorie intake defined as <60% of the estimated calorie requirement was a significantly independent predictor of adverse clinical events including all-cause death and HF-related hospitalization over 1 year in the patients with chronic HF (Table 3).

Table 3. Multivariate analysis of predictors of adverse clinical events including all-cause death and HF-related hospitalization in patients with chronic HF.

	Dietary Calorie Intake Adequacy	OR	95% CI	*p*-Value
Inadequate calorie intake	<80%	2.16	0.33–14.2	0.42
	<70%	4.89	0.68–35.1	0.11
	<60%	7.39	1.02–53.5	0.04

As confounding factors that may influence patient's dietary calorie intake, age, BMI, NYHA functional class III, diabetes, LVEF, serum albumin, eGFR, and log BNP were included in each analysis. OR: odds ratio; CI: confidence interval.

4. Discussion

In the present cohort of 145 patients with chronic HF, the inadequate calorie intake group had a significantly higher risk of adverse clinical events including all-cause death and hospitalization due to worsening HF for the 1-year follow-up period compared to the adequate calorie intake group, when we defined inadequate calorie intake as <60% of estimated calorie requirement. The multivariate logistic regression analysis showed that dietary calorie intake adequacy <60% was an independent predictor of worse clinical outcomes after adjustment for age, BMI, NYHA functional class III, diabetes, LVEF, serum albumin, eGFR, and log BNP in chronic HF patients. To the best of our knowledge, this is the first study that revealed the impact of dietary energy deficiency on mortality and hospitalization in stable outpatients with chronic HF.

Although several nutritional assessment tools such as the CONUT score and the GNRI are used in clinical practice, we here focused on a questionnaire-based assessment of the daily calorie intake in patients with chronic HF. All of the patients were in stable condition at baseline, and most of them were categorized as having no risk or only a mild risk of malnutrition when they were evaluated using the CONUT score or the GNRI. The malnutrition risk scores calculated by these nutritional assessment tools did not differ between the patients with inadequate calorie intake and those with adequate calorie intake. Accordingly, our present finding that the lowered dietary calorie intake adequacy was associated with increased risks of death and hospitalization in chronic HF patients indicates that the dietary calorie intake can be a useful nutritional assessment tool to detect the early stage of malnutrition in stable patients with chronic HF.

Cardiac cachexia, characterized by weight loss, is a major contributor to a poor prognosis in chronic HF patients [19]. The negative energy balance caused by an inadequate dietary calorie intake that does not support energy needs may lead to protein breakdown, which results in muscle wasting and sarcopenia [6,7]. Although in the present investigation, the BMI and muscle mass measured at baseline were not reduced in the patients with inadequate calorie intake, a sustained dietary energy deficiency may contribute to the future onset of cardiac cachexia and sarcopenia.

Our analyses revealed that the daily intakes of macronutrients and micronutrients were significantly decreased in the chronic HF patients with inadequate calorie intake, and this pattern might lead to worse clinical outcomes. Deficiencies of micronutrients such as minerals and vitamins have been reported to potentially impair cardiac and systemic functional capacity, which results in reduced quality of life and poor prognosis [20,21]. Oxidative stress also plays a crucial role in the progression of HF [22–25], and in the present cohort, the patients with inadequate calorie intakes had lowered consumptions of antioxidative nutrients such as vitamin C, vitamin E, and carotenoids, which might also affect the increased rate of adverse clinical events.

Although we could not quantify the patient's appetite, intestinal congestion may cause appetite loss, which results in inadequate calorie intake in chronic HF patients. It is reported that cachectic patients with chronic HF had a larger bowel wall thickness (i.e., intestinal congestion) in the entire colon [26]. In addition, decreased hunger sensation and HF-related symptoms (such as fatigue, nausea, and anxiety) may be related to reduced calorie intake in chronic HF patients [27]. Taken together, digestive disturbance and HF-related symptoms may affect inadequate calorie intake in these patients.

Dietary salt restriction is widely recommended to HF patients as a dietary intervention. Unexpectedly, we observed that the daily salt intake was significantly lower in the patients with an inadequate calorie intake, who had a higher risk of adverse clinical events. It has been reported that strict adherence to salt restriction may lead to appetite loss and reduced calorie intake, which results in a dietary nutritional deficiency in chronic HF patients [28]. Accordingly, more comprehensive dietary interventions in consideration of dietary calorie intake adequacy and nutritional balance as well as salt restriction are necessary for the prevention of HF progression.

There are some study limitations to consider. First, the number of patients with inadequate calorie intake was small ($N = 44$). Second, the dietary calorie and nutritional intake were evaluated on the basis of the patient's self-reported information about dietary patterns, and we thus could not directly measure their dietary calorie intake. In addition, each patient's calorie requirement was estimated using the Japanese Dietary Reference Intakes for the general population. Because HF patients' energy expenditure is likely to be higher than that of healthy subjects, we cannot completely exclude the possibility that our patients' calorie requirement might be underestimated. Direct measurements of calorie intake and energy expenditure considering the patients' daily physical activity level might increase the accuracy of the estimations of dietary calorie intake adequacy. Finally, we did not evaluate the social, economic, or environmental conditions of patients, although these factors may also affect dietary calorie intake.

5. Conclusions

In stable patients with chronic HF, inadequate dietary calorie intake was independently associated with an increased risk of adverse clinical events including all-cause death and hospitalization due to worsening HF.

Supplementary Materials: The following are available online at https://www.mdpi.com/2072-6643/13/3/874/s1. Table S1: Daily intakes of foods and beverages estimated using a BDHQ, Table S2: Daily intakes of nutrients estimated using a BDHQ.

Author Contributions: S.K. and M.T.-M. designed the study. S.K., A.F., T.Y., T.O., T.S., Y.K., M.T., H.M., R.M., I.Y. (Ichiro Yoshida), and K.Y. collected the data and contributed to the discussion. Y.O., N.K., S.K., A.F., T.Y., S.T., and I.Y. (Isao Yokota) contributed to the data analysis. Y.O., N.K., and T.Y. wrote the manuscript. S.K., A.F., S.T., I.Y. (Isao Yokota), and M.T.-M. reviewed and edited the manuscript. All authors have read and agreed to the published version of the manuscript.

Funding: This study was partly supported by a Grant-in-Aid for Scientific Research from KAKENHI (no. JP24614001 to M.T.-M. and no. 18K08022 to T.Y.) and the Center of Innovation Program from the Japan Science and Technology Agency (no. JPMJCE1301 to T.Y.).

Institutional Review Board Statement: The study was approved by the ethics committees of Hokkaido University Hospital (approval no. 012-0224) and the other nine participating research institutes—Hakodate National Hospital, Hikone Municipal Hospital, Kitami Red Cross Hospital, Keiwakai Ebetsu Hospital, Kushiro City General Hospital, Obihiro Kyokai Hospital, Otaru Kyokai Hospital, Saiseikai Fukuoka General Hospital, and Tottori University Hospital.

Informed Consent Statement: The study was conducted in accordance with the ethical principles described in the Declaration of Helsinki. Written informed consent was obtained from each patient before his or her participation in the study.

Data Availability Statement: Data supporting the findings of this work are available from the corresponding author upon reasonable request. All the data are obtained from subjects and are not publicly available due to ethical reasons.

Acknowledgments: We thank Yoshihiro Himura (Hikone Municipal Hospital), Shigeo Kakinoki (Otaru Kyokai Hospital), Kazuya Yonezawa (National Hospital Organization Hakodate National Hospital), and Yoko Ikeda and Ayako Muramoto (Hokkaido University Hospital) for their kind support of this study. We also thank all of the participating patients, cardiologists, nurses, and dieticians who contributed to this study.

Conflicts of Interest: I.Y. received a speaking fee from Japan Tobacco, Inc. (Pharmaceutical Division). The other authors declare no conflict of interest relevant to this article.

References

1. Metra, M.; Teerlink, J.R. Heart failure. *Lancet* **2017**, *390*, 1981–1995. [CrossRef]
2. Sharma, A.; Lavie, C.J.; Borer, J.S.; Vallakati, A.; Goel, S.; Lopez-Jimenez, F.; Arbab-Zadeh, A.; Mukherjee, D.; Lazar, J.M. Meta-analysis of the relation of body mass index to all-cause and cardiovascular mortality and hospitalization in patients with chronic heart failure. *Am. J. Cardiol.* **2015**, *115*, 1428–1434. [CrossRef]
3. Hamaguchi, S.; Tsuchihashi-Makaya, M.; Kinugawa, S.; Goto, D.; Yokota, T.; Goto, K.; Yamada, S.; Yokoshiki, H.; Takeshita, A.; Tsutsui, H. Body mass index is an independent predictor of long-term outcomes in patients hospitalized with heart failure in Japan. *Circ. J.* **2010**, *74*, 2605–2611. [CrossRef] [PubMed]
4. Wawrzenczyk, A.; Anaszewicz, M.; Budzynski, J. Clinical significance of nutritional status in patients with chronic heart failure-a systematic review. *Heart Fail. Rev.* **2019**, *24*, 671–700. [CrossRef]
5. Pasini, E.; Opasich, C.; Pastoris, O.; Aquilani, R. Inadequate nutritional intake for daily life activity of clinically stable patients with chronic heart failure. *Am. J. Cardiol.* **2004**, *93*, 41A–43A. [CrossRef]
6. Doehner, W.; Frenneaux, M.; Anker, S.D. Metabolic impairment in heart failure: The myocardial and systemic perspective. *J. Am. Coll. Cardiol.* **2014**, *64*, 1388–1400. [CrossRef]
7. Springer, J.; Springer, J.I.; Anker, S.D. Muscle wasting and sarcopenia in heart failure and beyond: Update 2017. *ESC Heart Fail.* **2017**, *4*, 492–498. [CrossRef]
8. Vest, A.R.; Chan, M.; Deswal, A.; Givertz, M.M.; Lekavich, C.; Lennie, T.; Litwin, S.E.; Parsly, L.; Rodgers, J.E.; Rich, M.W.; et al. Nutrition, obesity, and cachexia in patients with heart failure: A consensus statement from the Heart Failure Society of America Scientific Statements Committee. *J. Card. Fail.* **2019**, *25*, 380–400. [CrossRef] [PubMed]
9. Nakano, I.; Tsuda, M.; Kinugawa, S.; Fukushima, A.; Kakutani, N.; Takada, S.; Yokota, T. Loop diuretic use is associated with skeletal muscle wasting in patients with heart failure. *J. Cardiol.* **2020**, *76*, 109–114. [CrossRef]
10. Matsuo, S.; Imai, E.; Horio, M.; Yasuda, Y.; Tomita, K.; Nitta, K.; Yamagata, K.; Tomino, Y.; Yokoyama, H.; Hishida, A.; et al. Revised equations for estimated GFR from serum creatinine in Japan. *Am. J. Kidney Dis.* **2009**, *53*, 982–992. [CrossRef]

11. Kobayashi, S.; Honda, S.; Murakami, K.; Sasaki, S.; Okubo, H.; Hirota, N.; Notsu, A.; Fukui, M.; Date, C. Both comprehensive and brief self-administered diet history questionnaires satisfactorily rank nutrient intakes in Japanese adults. *J. Epidemiol.* **2012**, *22*, 151–159. [CrossRef]
12. Kobayashi, S.; Murakami, K.; Sasaki, S.; Okubo, H.; Hirota, N.; Notsu, A.; Fukui, M.; Date, C. Comparison of relative validity of food group intakes estimated by comprehensive and brief-type self-administered diet history questionnaires against 16 d dietary records in Japanese adults. *Public Health Nutr.* **2011**, *14*, 1200–1211. [CrossRef] [PubMed]
13. Kagawa, M.; Hills, A.P. Preoccupation with body weight and under-reporting of energy intake in female Japanese nutrition students. *Nutrients* **2020**, *12*, 830. [CrossRef] [PubMed]
14. Komada, Y.; Narisawa, H.; Ueda, F.; Saito, H.; Sakaguchi, H.; Mitarai, M.; Suzuki, R.; Tamura, N.; Inoue, S.; Inoue, Y. Relationship between self-reported dietary nutrient intake and self-reported sleep duration among Japanese adults. *Nutrients* **2017**, *9*, 134. [CrossRef]
15. Kobayashi, S.; Asakura, K.; Suga, H.; Sasaki, S. Living status and frequency of eating out-of-home foods in relation to nutritional adequacy in 4,017 Japanese female dietetic students aged 18-20 years: A multicenter cross-sectional study. *J. Epidemiol.* **2017**, *27*, 287–293. [CrossRef] [PubMed]
16. Matsumoto, M.; Hatamoto, Y.; Masumoto, A.; Sakamoto, A.; Ikemoto, S. Mothers' nutrition knowledge is unlikely to be related to adolescents' habitual nutrient intake inadequacy in Japan: A cross-sectional study of Japanese junior high school students. *Nutrients* **2020**, *12*, 2801. [CrossRef]
17. Ignacio de Ulibarri, J.; Gonzalez-Madrono, A.; de Villar, N.G.; Gonzalez, P.; Gonzalez, B.; Mancha, A.; Rodriguez, F.; Fernandez, G. CONUT: A tool for controlling nutritional status. First validation in a hospital population. *Nutr. Hosp.* **2005**, *20*, 38–45.
18. Kinugasa, Y.; Kato, M.; Sugihara, S.; Hirai, M.; Yamada, K.; Yanagihara, K.; Yamamoto, K. Geriatric nutritional risk index predicts functional dependency and mortality in patients with heart failure with preserved ejection fraction. *Circ. J.* **2013**, *77*, 705–711. [CrossRef]
19. Argiles, J.M.; Fontes-Oliveira, C.C.; Toledo, M.; Lopez-Soriano, F.J.; Busquets, S. Cachexia: A problem of energetic inefficiency. *J. Cachexia Sarcopenia Muscle* **2014**, *5*, 279–286. [CrossRef]
20. Witte, K.K.; Clark, A.L.; Cleland, J.G. Chronic heart failure and micronutrients. *J. Am. Coll. Cardiol.* **2001**, *37*, 1765–1774. [CrossRef]
21. Sciatti, E.; Lombardi, C.; Ravera, A.; Vizzardi, E.; Bonadei, I.; Carubelli, V.; Gorga, E.; Metra, M. Nutritional deficiency in patients with heart failure. *Nutrients* **2016**, *8*, 442. [CrossRef]
22. Shirakawa, R.; Yokota, T.; Nakajima, T.; Takada, S.; Yamane, M.; Furihata, T.; Maekawa, S.; Nambu, H.; Katayama, T.; Fukushima, A.; et al. Mitochondrial reactive oxygen species generation in blood cells is associated with disease severity and exercise intolerance in heart failure patients. *Sci. Rep.* **2019**, *9*, 14709. [CrossRef]
23. Tang, W.H.; Tong, W.; Troughton, R.W.; Martin, M.G.; Shrestha, K.; Borowski, A.; Jasper, S.; Hazen, S.L.; Klein, A.L. Prognostic value and echocardiographic determinants of plasma myeloperoxidase levels in chronic heart failure. *J. Am. Coll. Cardiol.* **2007**, *49*, 2364–2370. [CrossRef]
24. Tang, W.H.; Wu, Y.; Mann, S.; Pepoy, M.; Shrestha, K.; Borowski, A.G.; Hazen, S.L. Diminished antioxidant activity of high-density lipoprotein-associated proteins in systolic heart failure. *Circ. Heart Fail.* **2011**, *4*, 59–64. [CrossRef]
25. Yokota, T.; Kinugawa, S.; Hirabayashi, K.; Yamato, M.; Takada, S.; Suga, T.; Nakano, I.; Fukushima, A.; Matsushima, S.; Okita, K.; et al. Systemic oxidative stress is associated with lower aerobic capacity and impaired skeletal muscle energy metabolism in heart failure patients. *Sci. Rep.* **2021**, *11*, 2272. [CrossRef]
26. Valentova, M.; von Haehling, S.; Bauditz, J.; Doehner, W.; Ebner, N.; Bekfani, T.; Elsner, S.; Sliziuk, V.; Scherbakov, N.; Murin, J.; et al. Intestinal congestion and right ventricular dysfunction: A link with appetite loss, inflammation, and cachexia in chronic heart failure. *Eur. Heart J.* **2016**, *37*, 1684–1691. [CrossRef] [PubMed]
27. Lennie, T.A.; Moser, D.K.; Heo, S.; Chung, M.L.; Zambroski, C.H. Factors influencing food intake in patients with heart failure: A comparison with healthy elders. *J. Cardiovasc. Nurs.* **2006**, *21*, 123–129. [CrossRef] [PubMed]
28. Colin-Ramirez, E.; McAlister, F.A.; Zheng, Y.; Sharma, S.; Ezekowitz, J.A. Changes in dietary intake and nutritional status associated with a significant reduction in sodium intake in patients with heart failure. A sub-analysis of the SODIUM-HF pilot study. *Clin. Nutr. ESPEN* **2016**, *11*, e26–e32. [CrossRef]

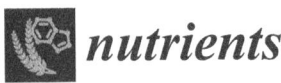

Article

Association between Vitamin D and Heart Failure Mortality in 10,974 Hospitalized Individuals

Kenya Kusunose [1,*], Yuichiro Okushi [1], Yoshihiro Okayama [2], Robert Zheng [1], Miho Abe [1], Michikazu Nakai [3], Yoko Sumita [3], Takayuki Ise [1], Takeshi Tobiume [1], Koji Yamaguchi [1], Shusuke Yagi [1], Daiju Fukuda [1], Hirotsugu Yamada [4], Takeshi Soeki [1], Tetsuzo Wakatsuki [1] and Masataka Sata [1]

[1] Department of Cardiovascular Medicine, Tokushima University Hospital, Tokushima 770-8503, Japan; yuuitirou_0110@yahoo.co.jp (Y.O.); pangtong2004@yahoo.ne.jp (R.Z.); myasan.abe@gmail.com (M.A.); isetaka@tokushima-u.ac.jp (T.I.); tobiume.takeshi@tokushima-u.ac.jp (T.T.); yamakoji3@tokushima-u.ac.jp (K.Y.); syagi@tokushima-u.ac.jp (S.Y.); daiju.fukuda@tokushima-u.ac.jp (D.F.); soeki@tokushima-u.ac.jp (T.S.); wakatsukitz@tokushima-u.ac.jp (T.W.); masataka.sata@tokushima-u.ac.jp (M.S.)

[2] Clinical Research Center for Developmental Therapeutics, Tokushima University Hospital, Tokushima 770-8503, Japan; y-okayama@tokushima-u.ac.jp

[3] Center for Cerebral and Cardiovascular Disease Information, National Cerebral and Cardiovascular Center, Osaka 564-8565, Japan; nakai.michikazu@ncvc.go.jp (M.N.); ysumi@ncvc.go.jp (Y.S.)

[4] Department of Community Medicine for Cardiology, Tokushima University Graduate School of Biomedical Sciences, Tokushima 770-8503, Japan; yamadah@tokushima-u.ac.jp

* Correspondence: kusunosek@tokushima-u.ac.jp; Tel.: +81-88-633-7851; Fax: +81-88-633-7894

Abstract: A broad range of chronic conditions, including heart failure (HF), have been associated with vitamin D deficiency. Existing clinical trials involving vitamin D supplementation in chronic HF patients have been inconclusive. We sought to evaluate the outcomes of patients with vitamin D supplementation, compared with a matched cohort using real-world big data of HF hospitalization. This study was based on the Diagnosis Procedure Combination database in the Japanese Registry of All Cardiac and Vascular Datasets (JROAD-DPC). After exclusion criteria, we identified 93,692 patients who were first hospitalized with HF between April 2012 and March 2017 (mean age was 79 ± 12 years, and 52.2% were male). Propensity score (PS) was estimated with logistic regression model, with vitamin D supplementation as the dependent variable and clinically relevant covariates. On PS-matched analysis with 10,974 patients, patients with vitamin D supplementation had lower total in-hospital mortality (6.5 vs. 9.4%, odds ratio: 0.67, $p < 0.001$) and in-hospital mortality within 7 days and 30 days (0.9 vs. 2.5%, OR, 0.34, and 3.8 vs. 6.5%, OR: 0.56, both $p < 0.001$). In the sub-group analysis, mortalities in patients with age < 75, diabetes, dyslipidemia, atrial arrhythmia, cancer, renin-angiotensin system blocker, and β-blocker were not affected by vitamin D supplementation. Patients with vitamin D supplementation had a lower in-hospital mortality for HF than patients without vitamin D supplementation in the propensity matched cohort. The identification of specific clinical characteristics in patients benefitting from vitamin D may be useful for determining targets of future randomized control trials.

Keywords: heart failure; vitamin D; mortality; big data

1. Introduction

The main treatment medications for heart failure (HF) remains to be β-blockers, angiotensin converting enzyme inhibitors, angiotensin receptor blockers, and aldosterone receptor antagonists in the guidelines [1]. Although it is well known that these medications can reduce the incidence of adverse cardiac events and improve cardiac function, HF is still a main cause of death worldwide [2]. Thus, supplementary treatment methods continue to be explored for improving the outcome of HF.

Vitamin D is a steroid hormone belonging to a group of lipid-soluble vitamins. Recently, many papers showed that a broad range of chronic conditions have been associated with vitamin D deficiency [3–5]. Around 90% of chronic HF patients have insufficient vitamin D levels, even in sunny climates [6,7]. Vitamin D has pleiotropic effects in the pathology of chronic HF [8]. Despite current evidence regarding the association of vitamin D with HF, there are many controversial results in previous clinical trials [9–11]. In these trials, lack of a large sample size and the small number of high-risk patients are major limitations. Our hypothesis was that vitamin D supplementation was associated with a decreased risk of in-hospital death in HF patients with specific clinical characteristics. Therefore, we sought to evaluate the outcomes of patients with vitamin D supplementation compared with a matched cohort using real-world big data based on HF hospitalizations.

2. Materials and Methods

2.1. Study Population

The study population was composed of hospitalized patients between April 2012 and March 2017 in The Japanese Registry of All Cardiac and Vascular Diseases and the Diagnosis Procedure Combination (JROAD-DPC) database. JROAD-DPC is a nationwide registry, a medical database with information of admission and discharge for cardiovascular diseases, clinical examinations and treatment status, patient status and hospital overview. JROAD-DPC database integrates the information composed by JROAD-DPC data, with analysis data sets covering 5.1 million cases in 1022 hospitals between April 2012 and March 2017. The identification of HF (I50.0, I50.1, I50.9) hospitalization was based on the International Classification of Diseases (ICD)-10 diagnosis codes. Data regarding patient age and sex, main diagnosis, comorbidity at admission, length of hospitalization and treatment content were extracted from the database. We recruited 654,737 patients hospitalized with HF. Diagnosis of HF was defined as the main diagnosis, admission-precipitating diagnosis or most resource-consuming diagnosis. We excluded patients of unknown age (n = 1073), readmission cases (n = 172,805), age < 20 years (n = 1477), death in 24 h after admission (n = 10,298), planned hospitalization (n = 54,713), and incomplete data (n = 320,679). As a result, total 93,692 (88,205 patients without vitamin D and 5487 patients with vitamin D) were recruited to assess hospital mortality (Figure 1). For vitamin D supplementation, oral 25(OH)D 3 (Calcifediol, Dedrogyl®) was prescribed at a daily dose of 0.5–1.0 µg/day based on the attending physician's discretion.

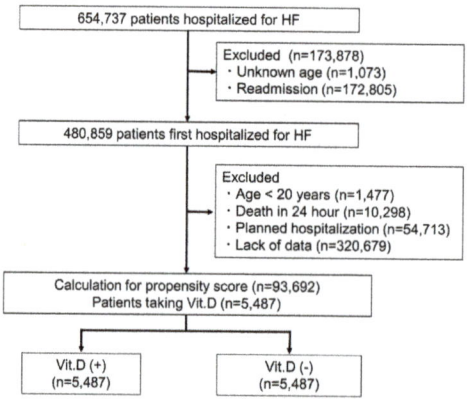

Figure 1. Flowchart of this study. HF, heart failure; Vit D, vitamin D supplementation.

2.2. Clinical Outcomes

The main outcome was in-hospital mortality (total number of deaths during hospitalization). Death $\leq$ 7 and 30 days after admission was assessed as secondary outcomes.

2.3. Sample Matching

Propensity score (PS) matching was used to reduce confounding effects related to differences in patient background. PS was estimated with a logistic regression model, with vitamin D supplementation as the dependent variable and the following clinically relevant covariates; age, sex, body mass index (BMI), smoking, New York Heart Association functional classification (NYHA), comorbidities (hypertension: HT, diabetes: DM, dyslipidemia: DL, osteoporosis, atrial fibrillation/atrial flutter: Af/AFL, stroke, myocardial infarction: MI, peripheral vascular disease: PVD, renal disease, liver failure, chronic obstructive pulmonary disease: COPD, rheumatoid arthritis: RA, dementia, cancer), treatment (catecholamine, intra-aortic balloon pumping: IABP, percutaneous cardiopulmonary support: PCPS, ventilation, hemodialysis: HD, percutaneous coronary intervention: PCI). These covariates were chosen for their potential association with reference to risk factor of heart failure and in-hospital mortality [12–14]. Matching was performed with greedy-matching algorithm (ratio = 1:1 without replacement), with a caliper of width 0.2 standard deviations of the logistic of the estimated propensity score. After matching, vitamin D and non-vitamin D groups of 5487 patients each were included in the final analysis. The area under the curve was 0.785 and the consistency of PS densities was matched after matching (Supplemental Figure S1). The balance of each covariate before and after matching between the 2 groups was evaluated by standardized differences. Absolute value of standardized differences less than 10% was considered to be a relatively small imbalance. Because the propensity score included cases in which vitamin D was used under the insurance of Japan (renal disease, osteoporosis, and dialysis), we believed the propensity score accounted for the factors that influence the prescription of vitamin D by general physicians in this analysis.

2.4. Statistical Analysis

Continuous variables are expressed as mean $\pm$ SD for parameters with normal distribution, as median (interquartile range; IQR) for parameters with skewed distribution, and categorical variables as proportion (%). We checked characteristics between groups with and without vitamin D supplementation using standardized difference. After matching, we estimated the OR for in-hospital mortality (total, within 7 days, 30 days) using mixed-effects logistic regression model with each institute as a random effect. We also analyzed subgroups in the PS-matched cohort. In-hospital mortality was assessed using Kaplan–Meier curves and log-rank test to compare the two groups. To clarify the beneficial group of vitamin D supplementation, odds ratios (ORs) and their 95% confidence interval (CI) for in-hospital mortality were calculated using multivariate models of multinomial logistic regression analysis in vitamin D (+) and vitamin D (−) groups. All statistical tests were 2-sided and p values less than 0.05 were considered statistically significant. Statistical analysis was performed using SAS version 9.4 and JMP version 14.0.

3. Results

3.1. Patient Characteristics

A total of 52.2% of patients in this study were male. Mean age was 79 ± 12 years, and half of all patients had hypertension (52.9%). Over 60% of the patients were NYHA class III or IV. Patients with vitamin D supplementation were more likely to have a history of chronic kidney disease, osteoporosis, hypoparathyroidism, or hemodialysis. There are differences for age, gender, BMI, smoking, hypertrophic cardiomyopathy, atrial fibrillation/atrial flutter, and rheumatoid arthritis between two groups. Around 19.7% took angiotensin converting enzyme inhibitors (ACE-I) or angiotensin-receptor blocker (ARB) and 9.1% took beta-blockers. About 19.4% of the patients took loop diuretic and 10.1% took K-sparing diuretics.

After propensity score matching, 10,974 patients were included in the survival analysis. In the matched cohort, there were no significant differences between groups for age, gender, comorbidities, and treatments (Table 1).

Table 1. Baseline characteristics before and after propensity score matching.

			Non Matching			Matching		
		All	Vit.D (+)	Vit.D (−)	std.diff (%)	Vit.D (+)	Vit.D (−)	std.diff (%)
Number		(n = 93,692)	(n = 5487)	(n = 88,205)		(n = 5487)	(n = 5487)	
Age average(years)		79 ± 12	80 ± 11	79 ± 13	10.6	80 ± 11	81 ± 11	8.4
Age(%)	20–30	0.2	0.1	0.2	−1.7	0.1	0.1	2.7
	30–40	0.8	0.4	0.8	−6.2	0.4	0.4	−0.2
	40–50	2.4	1.4	2.4	−7.8	1.4	1.1	2.5
	50–60	4.8	3.6	4.8	−6.3	3.6	3.1	2.6
	60–70	12.1	10.8	12.2	−4.4	10.8	9.8	3.3
	70–80	23.0	23.8	22.9	2.0	23.8	22.1	3.9
	80–90	39.8	42.4	39.7	5.5	42.4	44.2	−3.8
	>90	17.0	17.6	17.0	1.7	17.6	19.3	−4.2
Male (%)		52.2	33.9	53.4	−40.1	33.9	31.4	5.3
BMI		22.7 ± 5.0	21.8 ± 4.1	22.7 ± 5.0	−20.8	21.8 ± 4.1	21.7 ± 4.1	1.9
Smoking		30.2	21.1	30.8	−22.1	21.1	18.9	5.7
NYHA	1	12.2	12.8	12.2	1.9	12.8	13.2	−1.0
	2	24.4	24.5	24.3	0.3	24.5	25.0	−1.2
	3	32.2	32.1	32.2	−0.2	32.1	31.8	0.8
	4	31.2	30.5	31.2	−1.5	30.5	30.0	1.1
Comorbidities (%)								
Hypertension		52.9	48.8	53.2	−8.8	48.8	47.8	2.0
Diabetes mellitus		26.8	26.1	26.8	−1.7	26.1	25.1	2.2
Dyslipidemia		18.6	16.2	18.8	−6.7	16.2	14.9	3.7
Osteoporosis		3.0	24.5	1.7	72.1	24.5	21.2	7.1
Hypoparathyroidism		<0.1	0.2	<0.1	5.0	0.2	<0.1	4.5
HCM		3.4	1.4	3.5	−14.1	1.4	1.6	−2.0
DCM		1.2	1.0	1.3	−2.9	1.0	1.2	−2.8
Cardiac Amyloidosis		0.1	0.1	0.1	−0.8	0.1	0.1	<0.1
Cardiac Sarcoidosis		0.3	0.5	0.3	3.0	0.5	0.2	4.5
Af/AFL		35.5	27.5	36.0	−18.3	27.5	27.2	0.8
AT		0.9	0.6	0.9	−2.9	0.6	0.7	−0.9
Stroke		8.3	7.5	8.3	−3.3	7.5	7.2	1.1
MI		10.3	7.9	10.5	−9.1	7.9	7.2	2.6
PVD		3.8	4.8	3.7	5.1	4.8	3.9	4.3
CKD		14.1	38.6	12.6	62.5	38.6	35.3	6.9
Liver failure		0.1	0.1	0.1	−0.8	0.1	0.2	−2.7
COPD		7.4	6.1	7.5	−5.6	6.1	5.3	3.6
RA		1.3	4.2	1.2	19.0	4.2	4.9	−3.2
Dementia		6.2	6.9	6.2	3.1	6.9	7.0	−0.4
Cancer		11.0	11.0	11.0	0.1	11.0	10.6	1.3
Treatment (%)								
Catecholamine		12.4	11.3	12.5	−3.8	11.3	10.6	2.1
IABP		1.0	0.9	1.0	−1.1	0.9	1.1	−1.7
PCPS		0.1	0.0	0.2	−3.6	0.0	0.1	−0.5
Artificial Ventilation		21.3	21.1	21.3	−0.5	21.1	20.8	0.7
Hemodialysis		4.6	29.5	3.1	76.8	29.5	28.3	2.6
PCI		4.9	5.2	4.9	1.6	5.2	5.1	0.7
Drug (%)								
ACE-i/ARB		19.7	19.4	19.8	−0.8	19.4	21.0	−3.9
βblocker		9.1	8.0	9.2	−4.1	8.0	8.6	−1.9
Loop diuretic		19.4	18.4	19.4	−2.6	18.4	20.3	−4.8
K-sparing diuretic		10.1	7.4	10.3	−10.3	7.4	8.4	−3.7
Statin		13.1	13.5	13.0	1.2	13.5	13.7	−0.7
Hospital length (days)		18 (12–28)	19 (12–31)	17 (12–27)	13.1	19 (12–31)	18 (11–30)	14.9

Data are presented as percentage of patients or median (interquartile range). A standardized difference of < 10% suggests adequate balance. Abbreviations: Vit.D, vitamin D supplementation; std.diff, standardization difference; BMI, body mass index; NYHA, New York heart association functional class; HCM, hypertrophic cardiomyopathy; DCM, dilated cardiomyopathy; Af, atrial fibrillation; AFL, atrial flatter; AT, atrial tachycardia; MI, myocardial infarction; PVD, peripheral vascular disease; CKD, chronic kidney disease; COPD, chronic obstructive pulmonary disease; RA, rheumatoid arthritis; IABP, intra-aortic balloon pumping; PCPS, percutaneous cardiopulmonary system; PCI, percutaneous coronary intervention; ACE-I, angiotensin converting enzyme inhibitor; ARB, angiotensin II receptor blocker.

3.2. Outcomes

In-hospital mortality, mortality within 7 days and within 30 days of hospitalization are summarized in Table 2. Even after matching, patients with vitamin D supplementation had significantly lower in-hospital mortality (6.5 vs. 9.4%, $p < 0.001$; OR, 0.67, 95% CI: 0.58–0.77), mortality within 7 days of hospitalization (0.9 vs. 2.5%, $p < 0.001$; OR, 0.34, 95% CI: 0.25–0.48), and mortality within 30 days of hospitalization (3.8 vs. 6.5%, $p < 0.001$; OR, 0.56, 95% CI: 0.47–0.67).

Table 2. In-hospital mortality before and after propensity score matching.

In-Hospital Mortality	Non Matching				Matching			
	Vit.D (+)	Vit.D (−)	OR (95%CI)	p-Value	Vit.D (+)	Vit.D (−)	OR (95%CI)	p-Value
Total (%)	357 (6.5)	7256 (8.2)	0.79 (0.71–0.88)	<0.0001	357 (6.5)	515 (9.4)	0.67 (0.58–0.77)	<0.0001
7 days (%)	48 (0.9)	1761 (2.0)	0.44 (0.33–0.58)	<0.0001	48 (0.9)	138 (2.5)	0.34 (0.25–0.48)	<0.0001
30 days (%)	207 (3.8)	5171 (5.9)	0.64 (0.55–0.73)	<0.0001	207 (3.8)	358 (6.5)	0.56 (0.47–0.67)	<0.0001

Data given as proportion. Abbreviations: OR, odds ratio.

Kaplan–Meier curves of in-hospital mortality were shown in Figure 2. Vitamin D supplementation was strongly associated with survival rate ($p < 0.001$).

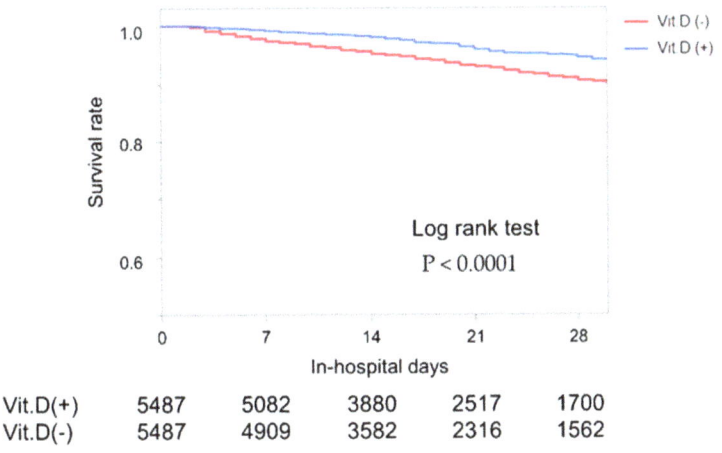

Figure 2. Kaplan Meier curves of in-hospital mortality and hospitalization days. Comparison between with and without vitamin D (Vit.D) supplementation.

Multivariate analysis was performed with covariates that were significant in the univariate analysis to assess the association with in-hospital mortality for all patients. Major contributors were age, BMI, NYHA, hypertension, peripheral vascular disease, chronic kidney disease, artificial ventilation, PCI, catecholamine, and atrial fibrillation/flutter in this cohort. After adjustment of clinical backgrounds, vitamin D supplementation was associated with low in-hospital mortality (OR, 0.63, 95% CI: 0.49–0.81, $p < 0.001$) (Table 3A).

Table 3. Multivariate analysis of covariates for in-hospital mortality.

A: In all patients. See abbreviations in Table 1.

	All			
	OR	Lower	Higher	*p*
Vit.D	0.63	0.49	0.81	0.0003
Age	1.06	1.05	1.08	<0.0001
BMI	0.93	0.90	0.96	<0.0001
NYHA	1.18	1.04	1.33	0.0070
Male	1.00	0.74	1.35	0.9884
Smoking	0.93	0.67	1.31	0.6867
HT	0.39	0.30	0.51	<0.0001
DM	0.80	0.60	1.07	0.1398
DL	0.83	0.57	1.22	0.3445
MI	1.17	0.76	1.80	0.4721
PVD	1.88	1.19	2.96	0.0064
Stroke	0.96	0.62	1.50	0.8659
Dementia	1.21	0.78	1.87	0.4000
COPD	0.95	0.56	1.59	0.8370
RA	1.10	0.65	1.89	0.7187
CKD	1.65	1.19	2.30	0.0030
Cancer	0.84	0.57	1.24	0.3764
Hemodialysis	0.84	0.58	1.22	0.3669
Artificial Ventilation	2.55	1.95	3.33	<0.0001
PCI	0.22	0.10	0.47	<0.0001
IABP	1.04	0.44	2.43	0.9355
Catecholamines	4.59	3.50	6.02	<0.0001
Osteoporosis	0.76	0.48	1.19	0.2331
HCM	0.61	0.18	2.09	0.4338
Sarcoidosis	2.60	0.55	12.18	0.2253
Af/AFL	0.68	0.51	0.92	0.0107

B: In patients with vitamin D supplementation. See abbreviations in Table 1.

	Vitamin D (+)			
	OR	Lower	Higher	*p*
Age	1.07	1.04	1.09	<0.0001
BMI	0.97	0.92	1.02	0.2186
NYHA	1.22	1.01	1.48	0.0379
Male	0.62	0.37	1.02	0.0589
Smoking	1.10	0.64	1.87	0.7396
HT	0.33	0.22	0.52	<0.0001
DM	0.70	0.44	1.11	0.1257
DL	1.11	0.64	1.90	0.7187
MI	1.36	0.71	2.59	0.3519
PVD	2.24	1.18	4.27	0.0138
Stroke	1.25	0.66	2.37	0.4844
Dementia	1.17	0.59	2.31	0.6536
COPD	0.86	0.38	1.94	0.7122
RA	0.80	0.30	2.12	0.6558
CKD	1.68	0.95	2.99	0.0746
Cancer	1.09	0.60	1.98	0.7663
Hemodialysis	0.98	0.52	1.85	0.9510
Artificial Ventilation	2.18	1.44	3.31	0.0003
PCI	0.19	0.06	0.64	0.0075
IABP	1.34	0.40	4.49	0.6352
Catecholamines	4.91	3.24	7.43	<0.0001
Osteoporosis	0.61	0.36	1.04	0.0707
HCM	1.57	0.34	7.23	0.5659
Sarcoidosis	2.14	0.26	17.31	0.4763
Af/AFL	0.66	0.41	1.06	0.0822

Table 3. Cont.

C: In patients without vitamin D supplementation. See abbreviations in Table 1.

		Vitamin D (−)		
	OR	Lower	Higher	p
Age	1.07	1.04	1.09	<0.0001
BMI	0.91	0.87	0.95	<0.0001
NYHA	1.14	0.97	1.33	0.1111
Male	1.36	0.93	2.01	0.1153
Smoking	0.83	0.54	1.30	0.4209
HT	0.43	0.30	0.60	<0.0001
DM	0.87	0.59	1.28	0.4857
DL	0.64	0.37	1.10	0.1087
MI	1.06	0.59	1.90	0.8573
PVD	1.53	0.79	2.95	0.2038
Stroke	0.77	0.40	1.45	0.4106
Dementia	1.20	0.67	2.15	0.5442
COPD	1.01	0.51	1.99	0.9816
RA	1.19	0.61	2.31	0.6059
CKD	1.55	1.02	2.36	0.0386
Cancer	0.75	0.45	1.26	0.2757
Hemodialysis	0.78	0.48	1.26	0.3036
Artificial Ventilation	3.03	2.12	4.32	<0.0001
PCI	0.25	0.09	0.65	0.0048
IABP	0.74	0.21	2.59	0.6374
Catecholamines	4.72	3.26	6.82	<0.0001
Osteoporosis	1.85	0.76	4.50	0.1746
HCM	0.24	0.03	2.05	0.1939
Sarcoidosis	3.58	0.35	36.60	0.2815
Af/AFL	0.70	0.48	1.02	0.0632

In multivariate analysis, there were many same risks (Table 3B,C: age, hypertension, artificial ventilator, PCI, catecholamine) for in-hospital mortality in vitamin D (+) and vitamin D (−). We have checked the difference of ORs between two groups for the risk distribution. Osteoporosis patients seemed to be protected in vitamin D (+) group, however, to be at increased risk in vitamin D (−) group. Based on this result, especially osteoporosis patients may have benefits from vitamin D supplementation during heart failure admissions. For hemodialysis and chronic kidney disease, there seemed to be small benefit in using vitamin D from ORs. BMI was associated with death in patients taking vitamin D (OR, 0.91, 95% CI: 0.87–0.95, $p < 0.001$), however, BMI was not associated with mortality in patients with vitamin D supplementation (OR, 0.97, 95% CI: 0.92–1.02, $p = 0.22$). The BMI may be an extra risk beyond the selection of patients with kidney disease or osteoporosis.

Predictive values using ROC analysis for in-hospital morality were good (Supplemental Figure S2: C-statistics: 0.85 for vitamin D (+) and 0.84 for vitamin D (−)) compared with the previous prediction models [15]. Thus, we thought that risk prediction performance was not different in both populations.

3.3. Subgroup-Analysis

Mortality in each sub-group, forest plots of OR are shown in Figure 3. Regardless of gender, BMI, NYHA, hypertension, and chronic kidney disease, patients with vitamin D supplementation had significantly lower in-hospital mortality than matched patients. Mortalities in patients with age < 75 (OR, 0.84, 95% CI: 0.59–1.24, $p = 0.54$), diabetes (OR, 0.75, 95% CI: 0.56–1.02, $p = 0.06$), dyslipidemia (OR, 0.67, 95% CI: 0.42–1.07, $p = 0.09$), Af/AFL (OR, 0.79, 95% CI: 0.58–1.07, $p = 0.13$), cancer (OR, 0.71, 95% CI: 0.47–1.07, $p = 0.10$), ACEi/ARB medication (OR, 0.72, 95% CI: 0.47–1.10, $p = 0.13$), and β-blocker usage (OR, 0.80, 95% CI: 0.41–1.57, $p = 0.51$) were not affected by vitamin D supplementation. Thus, this analysis suggested that there were specific clinical characteristics in patients benefitting from vitamin D supplementation.

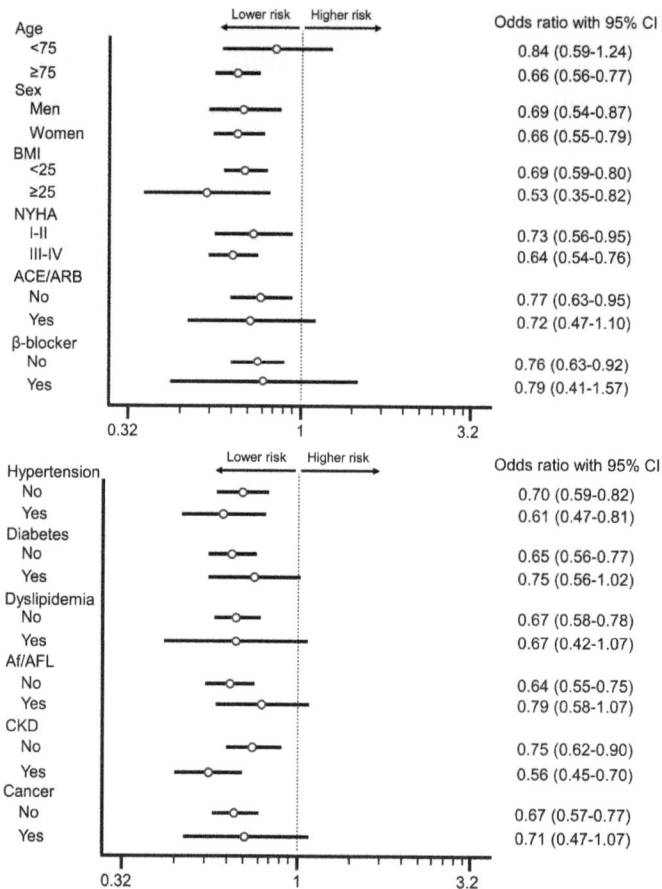

Figure 3. Odds ratio of in-hospital mortality. Patients with vitamin D compared with matched patients without vitamin D. Dots and lines mean OR and 95% CI, respectively.

4. Discussion

The main findings of the present study were (1) HF patients with vitamin D supplementation had significantly lower in-hospital mortality and mortality within 7 and 30 days of hospitalization in the propensity matched cohort; (2) mortalities in patients with age < 75, diabetes, dyslipidemia, atrial arrhythmia, cancer, renin-angiotensin system blocker medication, and β-blocker were not affected by vitamin D supplementation; (3) by multivariate analysis we identified that it was mainly osteoporosis patients that benefit from being treated with vitamin D supplementation when they were admitted for HF. Mortality was consistently low in patients with vitamin D supplementation at 7 days, 30 days, and during hospitalization. On the other hand, there are specific clinical characteristics in HF patients who do not benefit much from vitamin D. The identification of specific clinical characteristics in patients benefitting from vitamin D may be useful in determining targets of future studies.

4.1. Impact of Vitamin D on HF Mortality

Although there is much evidence showing that a lack of vitamin D could result in poor prognosis among patients with HF, different studies have reported controversial results about the benefit of vitamin D supplementation in patients with HF. In recent years, there were some randomized control trials for the effects of vitamin D on patients with HF. For example, the Vitamin D treating patients with chronic heart failure (VINDICATE) study showed that vitamin D supplementation has beneficial effect on left ventricular (LV) structure and function [11]. An individual participant data meta-analysis observed an association between low vitamin D level and increased risk of all-cause mortality [16]. On the other hand, another meta-analysis reported that vitamin D supplementation did not improve LV ejection fraction and 6-min walk distance in the treatment of chronic HF [17]. A recent updated meta-analysis also reported that vitamin D supplementation was not significantly associated with reduced major adverse cardiovascular events [18].

While randomized clinical trials (RCT) provide a foundation for clinical evidence, trials are often performed in highly controlled environments with narrow inclusion and exclusion criteria, which reduces their generalizability and external validity. Highly protocolled care in an RCT may differ substantially from interventions in routine settings [19]. The Mendelian Randomization study is a new concept of analysis, however, the genetic variants are unclear in the vitamin D3 levels [20]. A notably limitation of these trials is that none were focused on vitamin D supplementation in patients with high-risk cohort including NYHA 3 and 4. From our subgroup analysis, patients, the effect of vitamin D on in-hospital mortality was seemed to be greater in NYHA III-IV patients compared with NYHA I-II (NYHA III-IV: OR: 0.63, $p < 0.001$ and NYHA I-II: OR: 0.72, $p = 0.014$). We believe that the key to proving the worth of vitamin D supplementation is to create clinical studies that also involve a significant number of decompensated HF patients.

4.2. Mechanisms of Vitamin D for HF

There are some theories for the association between vitamin D and HF prognosis. In HF, cardiac contraction and relaxation are affected due to overload of Ca2+ ions in myocardial cells. Lack of vitamin D may intervene with the functions of Ca2+ in myocardial cells, resulting in cardiomyocyte hypertrophy, intra-organisational inflammatory reaction and fibrosis [21,22]. Low vitamin D levels may activate the renin–angiotensin system [23], give rise to inflammatory reactions [24] and result in endothelial dysfunction [25]. Interestingly, our subgroup analysis suggested that patients without ACEi/ARB had received more beneficial effects from vitamin D in regards to in-hospital mortality. The effect of vitamin D was more pronounced in patients without ACEi/ARB usage, hence suggesting an activated renin–angiotensin system in these patients.

The effects of vitamin D on the cardiovascular system are additionally mediated through elevated parathyroid hormone levels [26]. An age-related increase in parathyroid hormone levels has been demonstrated in several studies [27]. In our cohort, elderly patients (with suspected elevation of parathyroid hormone) with vitamin D supplementation were associated with lower in-hospital mortality (age < 75: OR: 0.84, $p = 0.40$ and age $\geq$ 75: OR: 0.66, $p < 0.001$). This result may suggest a link between vitamin D and elevated parathyroid hormone levels in the cardiovascular system. Based on the basic knowledge of these mechanisms, the link between vitamin D and prognosis in HF may be explained.

4.3. Clinical Implication

Even with the current wealth of guidelines and recommendations about HF and development of many new treatment methods, HF is associated with a high in-hospital mortality [1]. For patients with HF, vitamin D supplementation is a low-cost low-risk choice, and certain patients may benefit greatly from this therapy. According to our data from the large high-risk HF cohort, patients with vitamin D supplementation had lower mortality, and specific clinical characteristics were linked to better in-hospital mortality. The identified specific clinical characteristics that might be useful for future RCT studies.

4.4. Limitations

The study based on ICD codes has several limitations. First, we analyzed only patients with HF hospitalized in facilities contributing to the database, which may lead to selection bias. Second, the database has no information on echocardiography or laboratory data to assess the prognosis of HF. Third, the database lacked information on the specific doses of vitamin D supplementation in each patient. Dose dependency was unable to be examined. Forth, propensity score-matching reports the potential differences between groups, with only a certain degree of accuracy. Despite the application of propensity matching to the comparator group of patients, this non-randomized observational study could still be subject to hidden biases related to patient selection, because of unknown unadjusted differences. To overcome this issue, we used treatment devices and catecholamine medication as markers of HF severity. All-cause mortality was used as the primary end point in our patient population. The most likely cause of death in our patient population is HF, given the known high-risk nature of our patient population. The patients in this study are mostly Japanese. Results may differ due to racial or cultural differences in other countries. The JROAD-DPC dataset extracts only a record which contains all types of cardiovascular diseases in any categories of diagnosis based on the DPC dataset in Ministry of Health, Labor and Welfare in Japan. The DPC dataset has already been validated in past studies [28]. However, we were unable to check the undefined diseases by the coding system in our final dataset. This registry data does not include laboratory data. However, there would be no difference in background between the two groups as we corrected for many confounding factors. Finally, the results cannot be applied to all heart failure admissions. The results can be applied to the group of patients who should receive vitamin D supplementation but did not get it. The reason is that there were many osteoporosis and hemodialysis patients in both groups. Thus, the vitamin D group was suspected to have higher serum 25(OH)D compared with the non-vitamin D group. Considering these limitations, the present study should be considered as a hypothesis generating study for future RCT studies.

5. Conclusions

Patients with vitamin D supplementation had a lower in-hospital mortality for HF than patients without vitamin D supplementation in this propensity matched cohort. The causality should be tested in the future RCTs in specific population based on our study.

Supplementary Materials: The following are available online at https://www.mdpi.com/2072-6643/13/2/335/s1, Figure S1a: Receiver operating characteristic curve and concordance index. Figure S1b: comparison of the consistency of propensity score densities before and after matching. Figure S2: Predictive values for in-hospital mortality.

Author Contributions: K.K. conceived the idea for this study. Y.O. (Yuichiro Okushi) and Y.O. (Yoshihiro Okayama) conducted the data analyses. The initial draft of the manuscript was produced by K.K. and Y.O. (Yuichiro Okushi). All authors (K.K., Y.O. (Yuichiro Okushi), Y.O. (Yoshihiro Okayama), R.Z., M.A., M.N., Y.S., T.I., T.T., K.Y., S.Y., D.F., H.Y., T.S., T.W., and M.S.) were involved in interpreting the results and writing the manuscript. All authors have read and agreed to the published version of the manuscript.

Funding: This work was partially supported by Japan Society for the Promotion of Science Kakenhi Grants (Number 20K17084 to Y. Okushi, 19H03654 to M. Sata), the Takeda Science Foundation (to K. Kusunose), and Japan Agency for Medical Research and Development under Grant Number JP19lk1010035 (to K. Kusunose).

Institutional Review Board Statement: The study was conducted according to the guidelines of the Declaration of Helsinki, and approved by the Institutional Review Board of Tokushima University (protocol no. 3503).

Informed Consent Statement: Patient consent was waived because the analysis used anonymous clinical data.

Data Availability Statement: The datasets are available from the corresponding author on reasonable request.

Conflicts of Interest: The authors have no conflicts of interest to declare.

References

1. Tsutsui, H.; Isobe, M.; Ito, H.; Okumura, K.; Ono, M.; Kitakaze, M.; Kinugawa, K.; Kihara, Y.; Goto, Y.; Komuro, I.; et al. JCS 2017/JHFS 2017 Guideline on Diagnosis and Treatment of Acute and Chronic Heart Failure- Digest Version. *Circ. J.* **2019**, *83*, 2084–2184. [CrossRef] [PubMed]
2. Heidenreich, P.A.; Albert, N.M.; Allen, L.A.; Bluemke, D.A.; Butler, J.; Fonarow, G.C.; Ikonomidis, J.S.; Khavjou, O.; Konstam, M.A.; Maddox, T.M.; et al. Forecasting the impact of heart failure in the United States: A policy statement from the American Heart Association. *Circ. Heart Fail.* **2013**, *6*, 606–619. [CrossRef] [PubMed]
3. Wang, T.J. Vitamin D and Cardiovascular Disease. *Annu. Rev. Med.* **2016**, *67*, 261–272. [CrossRef] [PubMed]
4. Krul-Poel, Y.H.; Ter Wee, M.M.; Lips, P.; Simsek, S. Management of Endocrine Disease: The effect of vitamin D supplementation on glycaemic control in patients with type 2 diabetes mellitus: A systematic review and meta-analysis. *Eur. J. Endocrinol.* **2017**, *176*, R1–R14. [CrossRef] [PubMed]
5. Hewison, M. An update on vitamin D and human immunity. *Clin. Endocrinol.* **2012**, *76*, 315–325. [CrossRef] [PubMed]
6. Kim, D.H.; Sabour, S.; Sagar, U.N.; Adams, S.; Whellan, D.J. Prevalence of hypovitaminosis D in cardiovascular diseases (from the National Health and Nutrition Examination Survey 2001 to 2004). *Am. J. Cardiol.* **2008**, *102*, 1540–1544. [CrossRef] [PubMed]
7. Ameri, P.; Ronco, D.; Casu, M.; Denegri, A.; Bovio, M.; Menoni, S.; Ferone, D.; Murialdo, G. High prevalence of vitamin D deficiency and its association with left ventricular dilation: An echocardiography study in elderly patients with chronic heart failure. *Nutr. Metab. Cardiovasc. Dis.* **2010**, *20*, 633–640. [CrossRef]
8. Gardner, D.G.; Chen, S.; Glenn, D.J. Vitamin D and the heart. *Am. J. Physiol. Regul. Integr. Comp. Physiol.* **2013**, *305*, R969–R977. [CrossRef]
9. Schleithoff, S.S.; Zittermann, A.; Tenderich, G.; Berthold, H.K.; Stehle, P.; Koerfer, R. Vitamin D supplementation improves cytokine profiles in patients with congestive heart failure: A double-blind, randomized, placebo-controlled trial. *Am. J. Clin. Nutr.* **2006**, *83*, 754–759. [CrossRef]
10. Witham, M.D.; Crighton, L.J.; Gillespie, N.D.; Struthers, A.D.; McMurdo, M.E. The effects of vitamin D supplementation on physical function and quality of life in older patients with heart failure: A randomized controlled trial. *Circ. Heart Fail.* **2010**, *3*, 195–201. [CrossRef]
11. Witte, K.K.; Byrom, R.; Gierula, J.; Paton, M.F.; Jamil, H.A.; Lowry, J.E.; Gillott, R.G.; Barnes, S.A.; Chumun, H.; Kearney, L.C.; et al. Effects of Vitamin D on Cardiac Function in Patients With Chronic HF: The VINDICATE Study. *J. Am. Coll. Cardiol.* **2016**, *67*, 2593–2603. [CrossRef] [PubMed]
12. Win, S.; Hussain, I.; Hebl, V.B.; Dunlay, S.M.; Redfield, M.M. Inpatient Mortality Risk Scores and Postdischarge Events in Hospitalized Heart Failure Patients: A Community-Based Study. *Circ. Heart Fail.* **2017**, *10*. [CrossRef] [PubMed]
13. Peterson, P.N.; Rumsfeld, J.S.; Liang, L.; Albert, N.M.; Hernandez, A.F.; Peterson, E.D.; Fonarow, G.C.; Masoudi, F.A.; American Heart Association Get With the Guidelines-Heart Failure Program. A validated risk score for in-hospital mortality in patients with heart failure from the American Heart Association get with the guidelines program. *Circ. Cardiovasc. Qual. Outcomes* **2010**, *3*, 25–32. [CrossRef] [PubMed]
14. Hannan, E.L.; Wu, C.; Bennett, E.V.; Carlson, R.E.; Culliford, A.T.; Gold, J.P.; Higgins, R.S.; Smith, C.R.; Jones, R.H. Risk index for predicting in-hospital mortality for cardiac valve surgery. *Ann. Thorac. Surg.* **2007**, *83*, 921–929. [CrossRef]
15. Fonarow, G.C. Clinical risk prediction tools in patients hospitalized with heart failure. *Rev. Cardiovasc. Med.* **2012**, *13*, e14–e23.
16. Gaksch, M.; Jorde, R.; Grimnes, G.; Joakimsen, R.; Schirmer, H.; Wilsgaard, T.; Mathiesen, E.B.; Njolstad, I.; Lochen, M.L.; Marz, W.; et al. Vitamin D and mortality: Individual participant data meta-analysis of standardized 25-hydroxyvitamin D in 26916 individuals from a European consortium. *PLoS ONE* **2017**, *12*, e0170791. [CrossRef]
17. Jiang, W.L.; Gu, H.B.; Zhang, Y.F.; Xia, Q.Q.; Qi, J.; Chen, J.C. Vitamin D Supplementation in the Treatment of Chronic Heart Failure: A Meta-analysis of Randomized Controlled Trials. *Clin. Cardiol.* **2016**, *39*, 56–61. [CrossRef]
18. Barbarawi, M.; Kheiri, B.; Zayed, Y.; Barbarawi, O.; Dhillon, H.; Swaid, B.; Yelangi, A.; Sundus, S.; Bachuwa, G.; Alkotob, M.L. Vitamin D supplementation and cardiovascular disease risks in more than 83,000 individuals in 21 randomized clinical trials: A meta-analysis. *JAMA Cardiol.* **2019**, *4*, 765–775. [CrossRef]
19. Stuart, E.A.; Bradshaw, C.P.; Leaf, P.J. Assessing the generalizability of randomized trial results to target populations. *Prev. Sci.* **2015**, *16*, 475–485. [CrossRef]
20. Davies, N.M.; Holmes, M.V.; Davey Smith, G. Reading Mendelian randomisation studies: A guide, glossary, and checklist for clinicians. *BMJ* **2018**, *362*, k601. [CrossRef]
21. Weishaar, R.E.; Simpson, R.U. Involvement of vitamin D3 with cardiovascular function. II. Direct and indirect effects. *Am. J. Physiol.* **1987**, *253*, E675–E683. [CrossRef] [PubMed]
22. Chen, S.; Law, C.S.; Grigsby, C.L.; Olsen, K.; Hong, T.T.; Zhang, Y.; Yeghiazarians, Y.; Gardner, D.G. Cardiomyocyte-specific deletion of the vitamin D receptor gene results in cardiac hypertrophy. *Circulation* **2011**, *124*, 1838–1847. [CrossRef] [PubMed]
23. Vaidya, A.; Williams, J.S. The relationship between vitamin D and the renin-angiotensin system in the pathophysiology of hypertension, kidney disease, and diabetes. *Metabolism* **2012**, *61*, 450–458. [CrossRef]

24. Zhang, Y.; Leung, D.Y.; Richers, B.N.; Liu, Y.; Remigio, L.K.; Riches, D.W.; Goleva, E. Vitamin D inhibits monocyte/macrophage proinflammatory cytokine production by targeting MAPK phosphatase-1. *J. Immunol.* **2012**, *188*, 2127–2135. [CrossRef] [PubMed]
25. Caprio, M.; Mammi, C.; Rosano, G.M. Vitamin D: A novel player in endothelial function and dysfunction. *Arch. Med. Sci.* **2012**, *8*, 4–5. [CrossRef]
26. Schluter, K.D.; Piper, H.M. Left ventricular hypertrophy and parathyroid hormone: A causal connection? *Cardiovasc. Res.* **1998**, *39*, 523–524. [CrossRef]
27. Haden, S.T.; Brown, E.M.; Hurwitz, S.; Scott, J.; El-Hajj Fuleihan, G. The effects of age and gender on parathyroid hormone dynamics. *Clin. Endocrinol.* **2000**, *52*, 329–338. [CrossRef]
28. Yamana, H.; Moriwaki, M.; Horiguchi, H.; Kodan, M.; Fushimi, K.; Yasunaga, H. Validity of diagnoses, procedures, and laboratory data in Japanese administrative data. *J. Epidemiol.* **2017**, *27*, 476–482. [CrossRef]

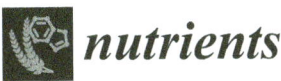

Article

Multidisciplinary Team-Based Palliative Care for Heart Failure and Food Intake at the End of Life

Tatsuhiro Shibata [1,2], Kazutoshi Mawatari [1], Naoko Nakashima [2,3], Koutatsu Shimozono [1], Kouko Ushijima [3], Yumiko Yamaji [3], Kumi Tetsuka [3], Miki Murakami [2,3], Kouta Okabe [1], Toshiyuki Yanai [1], Shoichiro Nohara [1], Jinya Takahashi [1], Hiroki Aoki [4], Hideo Yasukawa [1] and Yoshihiro Fukumoto [1,*]

[1] Division of Cardiovascular Medicine, Department of Internal Medicine, Kurume University School of Medicine, Kurume 830-0011, Japan; shibata_tatsuhiro@med.kurume-u.ac.jp (T.S.); mawatari_kazutoshi@kurume-u.ac.jp (K.M.); shimozono_koutatsu@med.kurume-u.ac.jp (K.S.); okabe_kouta@med.kurume-u.ac.jp (K.O.); yanai_toshiyuki@med.kurume-u.ac.jp (T.Y.); nohara_shoichiro@med.kurume-u.ac.jp (S.N.); takahashi_jinya@med.kurume-u.ac.jp (J.T.); yahideo@med.kurume-u.ac.jp (H.Y.)
[2] Kurume University Hospital Palliative Care Team, Kurume University, Kurume 830-0011, Japan; nakashima_naoko@med.kurume-u.ac.jp (N.N.); yoshigai_miki@med.kurume-u.ac.jp (M.M.)
[3] Department of Nursing, Kurume University Hospital, Kurume 830-0011, Japan; ushijima_kouko@kurume-u.ac.jp (K.U.); yumi0802minami@yahoo.co.jp (Y.Y.); tetsuka_kumi@kurume-u.ac.jp (K.T.)
[4] Cardiovascular Research Institute, Kurume University, Kurume 830-0011, Japan; haoki@med.kurume-u.ac.jp
* Correspondence: fukumoto_yoshihiro@med.kurume-u.ac.jp; Tel.: +81-942-31-7562

Abstract: Traditionally, patients with end-stage heart failure (HF) have rarely been involved in end-of-life care (EOLC) discussions in Japan. The purpose of this study was to examine the impact of HF-specific palliative care team (HF-PCT) activities on EOLC discussions with patients, HF therapy and care, and food intake at the end of life. We retrospectively analyzed 52 consecutive patients with HF (mean age, 70 ± 15 years; 42% female) who died at our hospital between May 2013 and July 2020 and divided them into two groups: before (Era 1, n = 19) and after (Era 2, n = 33) the initiation of HF-PCT activities in June 2015. Compared to Era 1, Era 2 showed a decrease in invasive procedures, an increase in opioid and non-intubating sedative use for symptom relief, improved quality of meals at the end of life, and an increase in participation in EOLC discussions. The administration of artificial nutrition in the final three days was associated with non-ischemic cardiomyopathy etiology, the number of previous hospitalizations for HF, and multidisciplinary EOLC discussion support. HF-PCT activities may provide an opportunity to discuss EOLC with patients, reduce the burden of physical and psychological symptoms, and shift the goals of end-of-life nutritional intake to ensure comfort and quality of life.

Keywords: heart failure; palliative care; end-of-life care discussion; advance care planning; food intake; artificial nutrition

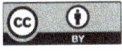

1. Introduction

Recent developments in new drugs, monitoring systems, and device therapies have evolved heart failure (HF) therapy; however, these developments may stabilize HF but rarely cure it. Furthermore, these advances are often only available for a limited number of patients. During HF progression, patients experience a high symptom burden and poor quality of life similar to that reported by patients with cancer [1,2]. HF often follows an unpredictable illness trajectory, with stable periods interrupted by exacerbations and sometimes resulting in sudden cardiac death, leading to difficulties in estimating survival [3]. When focusing on end-of-life decision making, such prognostic uncertainty complicates the patients' plans concerning their end-of-life wishes and sometimes leads to an overestimation of survival [4]. Furthermore, traditionally in Japan, patients rarely participate in discussions about their own goals and preferences for end-of-life care (EOLC), because their families may hesitate to bring bad news. As patients tend to lose their decision-making ability toward the end of life [5], they sometimes have no opportunity to express their wishes and preferences regarding their EOLC. Until recently in Japan, these situations often led to providing life-prolonging treatment to critically ill patients, regardless of the medical futility [6]. In addition, at the end-stage of HF, associated symptoms such as anorexia, nausea, vomiting, and dyspnea are observed, and food intake decreases [7]. In patients with end-stage HF, the goal of nutritional care is to optimize quality of life and comfort. Even though patients eventually lose their appetite spontaneously, artificial nutrition has often been attempted in the past.

Palliative care comprises a multidisciplinary team approach for patients and their families facing serious illnesses that focuses on improving quality of life and death. Recently, palliative care has been recommended by the Japanese Circulation Society (JCS)/Japanese Heart Failure Society (JHFS) and American College of Cardiology (ACC)/American Heart Association (AHA) HF guidelines [8,9]. The core elements of a multidisciplinary palliative care team (PCT) include not only expert assessment of physical and psychosocial distress but also the establishment of care goals and support for advance care planning (ACP) and complex decision-making, including EOLC discussion. In Japan, a multidisciplinary PCT is available in most of the regional cancer centers; however, it is only available in 9% of JCS-authorized cardiology training hospitals [10]. One of the major reasons is that PCT intervention had not been reimbursed for patients with HF by April 2018. Given that these services are not yet widely available, there has been insufficient clinical data regarding PCTs in patients with HF in Japan. Moreover, even in Western countries, only limited evidence is available regarding the patient-centered EOLC discussions of inpatient PCTs with patients with HF [11,12].

Therefore, the main purpose of this study was to compare changes in HF therapies in terms of palliative care and EOLC discussions, with a focus on food intake at the end of life in HF, before and after the initiation of HF-specific PCT (HF-PCT) activities at our institute.

2. Materials and Methods

2.1. Study Design and Population

The study was performed at Kurume University Hospital, a 1000-bed tertiary medical center located in the southern part of Fukuoka Prefecture, Japan. We retrospectively analyzed the medical records of 215 consecutive patients who died at the Division of Cardiology of our hospital between May 2013 and July 2020. Among these, we excluded 163 cases of non-HF deaths, including acute myocardial infarction, and patients treated only in the intensive care unit. HF was diagnosed by at least two specialist cardiologists based on the Framingham criteria [13]. Thus, we conducted a final analysis of 52 patients with HF who died in our department. These patients were divided into two groups according to their time of death before (Era 1; May 2013 to May 2015) and after (Era 2; June 2015 to July 2020) the HF-PCT activity started in June 2015. In this study, a multidisciplinary palliative approach for patients and their families was provided by an HF-PCT, which consisted of cardiologists, palliative care physicians, nurses (inpatient, outpatient, and a certified palliative care nurse), pharmacists, a psychologist, a medical social worker, and a managerial dietitian. The HF-PCT was available for all HF patients and assisted the treatment of patients with HF through refractory symptom relief, the establishment of care goals, psychosocial support, support of ACP and EOLC discussions, and provision of nutritional support for EOLC.

The demographic and clinical information of each patient was extracted from the electronic medical records of Kurume University Hospital. We obtained data on the patients' background, etiology of HF, duration of HF, comorbidities, echocardiographic findings, HF treatments, sedative medications, laboratory data, location of death, invasive procedures undergone before death (cardiopulmonary resuscitation, intubation, direct current shocks, and mechanical circulatory support) and length of hospital stay. We also assessed differences in the palliative care intervention, such as the use of opioids and sedative medications for refractory symptoms, psychiatric support, and multidisciplinary support for EOLC discussions, between the patients who died in Era 1 and those who died in Era 2. To assess the nutritional status of patients with end-stage HF, we examined the method of receiving nutrition three days prior to death and nutritional interventions (discontinuation of salt reduction, allowing non-hospital meals, and use of oral nutritional supplements) for patients who were maintaining oral intake at the time. We also examined factors associated with the use of artificial nutrition (total parenteral nutrition and tube feeding) three days prior to death.

2.2. Statistical Analysis

Continuous variables are presented as mean ± standard deviation (SD) or median (interquartile range (IQR)), as appropriate; they were compared using Student's t-test. Categorical baseline variables are presented as numbers (percentage) and compared using the chi-square or Fisher's exact test. Univariate associations between baseline characteristics and multidisciplinary support for end-of-life discussions were performed using univariate logistic regression. Variables relevant to the model were selected based on a univariate threshold p-value (≤ 0.05) and included in a multivariate logistic model to predict the odds of receiving artificial nutrition in the final three days prior to death. Adjusted odds ratios (ORs) and 95% confidence intervals (CIs) were calculated. Statistical significance was set at $p < 0.05$. All statistical analyses were performed using EZR (Saitama Medical Center, Jichi Medical University, Saitama, Japan), which is a graphical user interface for R (The R Foundation for Statistical Computing, Vienna, Austria). More precisely, it is a modified version of R Commander designed to add statistical functions that are frequently used in biostatistics.

3. Results

3.1. Patient Characteristics

Patient characteristics are shown in Table 1. Among the 52 patients, 22 (42%) were female, with an age of 70.0 ± 15.1 years. The median number of HF hospitalizations prior to death was 3 (IQR 1–5, and 42% of patients had non-ischemic cardiomyopathy (NICM) etiology. The median left ventricular ejection fraction was 35% (IQR 20–56%), and the median N-terminal B-type natriuretic peptide (NT-proBNP) was 12,683 pg/mL (IQR 5181–31,264 pg/mL). Nineteen patients who died during Era 1 and 33 patients who died during Era 2 were included in the analyses. There were no significant differences in demographics or clinical characteristics between the two groups, except for the etiology of "Others".

Table 1. Baseline characteristics of patients.

	Total (n = 52)	Era 1 (n = 19)	Era 2 (n = 33)	p Value
Age, year	70.0 ± 15.1	69.5 ± 18.1	70.3 ± 13.4	0.861
Female, n (%)	22 (42)	8 (42)	14 (42)	0.982
Duration of HF, months	58.4 (10.9–173.2)	80.7 (2.0–207.8)	56.5 (11.8–158.4)	0.643
No. of previous HF hospitalization, n	3 (1–5)	3.0 (1.0–5.0)	3.0 (1.0–4.5)	0.992
Left ventricular ejection fraction, %	35 (20–56)	30 (16–52)	37 (20–63)	0.666
Intensive care unit hospitalization, n (%)	6 (12)	1 (5)	5 (15)	0.283
Etiology				
Ischemic, n (%)	7 (13)	4 (21)	3 (9)	0.223
Valvular, n (%)	12 (23)	5 (26)	7 (21)	0.674
Non-ischemic cardiomyopathy, n (%)	22 (42)	6 (32)	16 (48)	0.235
Pulmonary arterial hypertension, n (%)	8 (15)	1 (5)	7 (21)	0.125
Others, n (%)	3 (6)	3 (14)	0 (0)	0.019 *

Table 1. Cont.

	Total (n = 52)	Era 1 (n = 19)	Era 2 (n = 33)	p Value
Comorbidities				
Cerebrovascular disease, n (%)	9 (17)	5 (26)	4 (12)	0.193
Hypertension, n (%)	12 (23)	6 (32)	6 (18)	0.270
Diabetes, n (%)	21 (40)	7 (37)	14 (42)	0.693
Atrial fibrilation, n (%)	27 (52)	9 (47)	18 (55)	0.618
Malignancies, n (%)	5 (10)	1 (5)	4 (12)	0.419
Cardiac resynchronization therapy, n (%)	19 (37)	8 (42)	11 (33)	0.527
Implantable cardioverter defibrillator, n (%)	19 (37)	7 (37)	12 (36)	0.973
Systolic blood pressure, mmHg	104.0 ± 26.5	113.2 ± 29.0	98.7 ± 23.7	0.056
NYHA class III or IV, n (%)	43 (83)	15 (79)	28 (85)	0.592
Medication on admission				
ACE-I/ARB, n (%)	29 (56)	13 (68)	16 (48)	0.163
β-blocker, n (%)	31 (60)	11 (58)	20 (61)	0.848
Mineralocorticoid receptor antagonist, n (%)	25 (48)	7 (37)	18 (55)	0.219
Loop diuretic, n (%)	44 (85)	15 (79)	29 (88)	0.390
Laboratory data				
NT-proBNP, pg/mL	12,683 (5181–31,264)	12,684 (4512–38,571)	13,728 (5526–31,109)	0.770
Blood urea nitrogen, mg/dL	46.0 ± 24.9	52.1 ± 25.6	42.5 ± 24.2	0.180
Creatinine, mg/dL	1.8 ± 1.2	2.1 ± 1.4	1.6 ± 1.0	0.148
Sodium, mEq/L	135.0 ± 7.4	133.6 ± 8.1	135.8 ± 7.0	0.310

Data are presented as mean ± SD, median (IQR) and n (%); HF = heart failure; HFrEF = HF with reduced ejection fraction; NYHA = New York Heart Association functional classification; ACE-I = angiotensin-converting-enzyme inhibitor; ARB = angiotensin II receptor blocker; NT-proBNP = n-terminal b-type natriuretic peptide. * $p < 0.05$.

3.2. Palliative and End-of-Life Care

Table 2 presents an overview of the palliative care and EOLC provided prior to death. In patients who died during Era 2, the rates of attempted cardiopulmonary resuscitation, intubation, and direct current shock at the end of life were significantly lower than in those who died in Era 1 (53% vs. 6%; $p < 0.001$, 47% vs. 0%; $p < 0.001$, 37% vs. 6%; $p = 0.005$, respectively). Compared to Era 1, a greater proportion of patients who died in Era 2 received opioids (11% vs. 70%). All the patients who received opioids were non-intubated and the administration was indicated to relieve dyspnea resistant to hemodynamic interventions (afterload reduction, diuretics, and inotropes). Sedative medications were significantly more commonly used in intubated patients who died in Era 1 and non-intubated patients who died in Era 2 ($p < 0.05$). Sedative medications without intubation were used for refractory symptoms, such as dyspnea, malaise, and delirium. Patients who died in Era 2 received more psychiatric consultations, although the difference was not significant. In Era 2, 70% of patients received multidisciplinary EOLC discussion support, a significant increase from 5% in Era 1 ($p < 0.001$).

Table 2. Palliative and end-of-life care.

	Era 1 (n = 19)	Era 2 (n = 33)	p Value
Length of hospital stay until death, days	20 (9–59)	24 (14–91)	0.448
Transfer to intensive care unit prior to death, n (%)	2 (11)	0 (0)	0.057
Invasive treatment at the time of death			
Cardiopulmonary resuscitation, n (%)	10 (53)	2 (6)	<0.001 *
Intubation, n (%)	9 (47)	0 (0)	<0.001 *
Direct current shocks, n (%)	7 (37)	2 (6)	0.005 *
Mechanical circulatory support, n (%)	1 (5)	0 (0)	0.183
Palliative care intervention			
Use of opioid, n (%)	2 (11)	23 (70)	<0.001 *
Use of sedative medication, n (%)	6 (32)	13 (39)	0.573

Table 2. Cont.

	Era 1 (n = 19)	Era 2 (n = 33)	p Value
For intubated patients, n (%)	5 (26)	1 (3)	0.020 *
For non-intubated patients, n (%)	1 (5)	12 (36)	0.018 *
Specialized psychiatric care, n (%)	4 (21)	15 (45)	0.078
Multidisciplinary support for EOLC discussions, n (%)	1 (5)	23 (70)	<0.001 *

Data are presented as median (IQR) and n (%); EOLC = end-of-life care. * $p < 0.05$.

3.3. Nutrition in the Three Days Prior to Death

Among the patients who died in Era 1 and Era 2, total parenteral nutrition was provided to 7 (37%) and 11 (33%), tube feeding to 1 (5%) and 5 (15%), and 9 (47%) and 12 (36%) patients fasted, respectively. There were no significant differences in nutrition administration methods between the two groups. Food intake three days before death was maintained in 9 out of 19 patients (47%) in Era 1 and 16 out of 33 patients (48%) in Era 2. The characteristics of the patients who maintained food intake three days prior to death are summarized in Table 3. Compared to the patients who died in Era 1 (n = 9), significantly more patients who died in Era 2 (n = 16) maintained food intake during opioid administration (11% vs. 63%, respectively, $p = 0.013$). In addition, food intake during sedation was not observed in Era 1 but was observed in 19% of patients who died in Era 2 ($p = 0.166$). Nutritional counseling was more frequently provided to patients who died in Era 2 than to those who died in Era 1 (33% vs. 81%, respectively, $p = 0.017$), and the change from a low-sodium diet to a regular-sodium diet was also significantly more frequent (59% vs. 22%, respectively, $p = 0.025$). Permission for non-hospital foods, such as bringing a patient's favorite meal cooked by their family, also tended to be more frequently granted to patients who died in Era 2 as compared to those who died in Era 1 ($p = 0.053$).

Table 3. Characteristics of patients who maintained oral intake in the three days prior to death.

	Era 1 (n = 9)	Era 2 (n = 16)	p Value
Use of artificial nutrition, n (%)	0 (0)	3 (19)	0.166
Food intake under opioid administration, n (%)	1 (11)	10 (63)	0.013 *
Food intake under sedative medication administration, n (%)	0 (0)	3 (19)	0.166
Nutritional Counselling, n (%)	3 (33)	13 (81)	0.017 *
Change from low-sodium to regular-sodium diets, n (%)	2 (22)	11 (59)	0.025 *
Permission for non-hospital meals, n (%)	2 (22)	10 (63)	0.053
Use of oral nutritional supplements, n (%)	3 (33)	10 (63)	0.161

Data are presented as n (%). * $p < 0.05$.

Logistic regression analysis of factors associated with the administration of artificial nutrition three days prior to death was performed (Table 4). In the univariate regression analysis, the number of previous hospitalizations for HF (OR 0.69; 95% CI 0.51–0.93; $p = 0.014$) and HF due to NICM (OR 3.30; 95% CI 1.03–10.60; $p = 0.045$) were significantly associated with the administration of artificial nutrition in the final three days of life. Multivariate analysis demonstrated that the number of previous HF hospitalizations (OR 0.63; 95% CI 0.44–0.91; $p = 0.014$), NICM-caused HF (OR 15.8; 95% CI 2.42–103.00; $p = 0.004$), and multidisciplinary support for EOLC discussions (OR 0.15; 95% CI 0.03–0.91; $p = 0.039$) were independent factors related to the administration of artificial nutrition three days prior to death.

Table 4. Results of univariate and multivariate analysis associated with the administration of artificial nutrition three days prior to death.

	Univariate Analysis			Multivariate Analysis		
	OR	95% CI	*p* Value	OR	95% CI	*p* Value
Age	1.01	0.97–1.05	0.74	1.00	0.95–1.06	0.86
Female	1.20	0.39–3.70	0.76	1.22	0.27–5.58	0.80
ICM	0.60	0.11–3.44	0.57			
NICM	3.30	1.03–10.60	0.045 *	15.80	2.42–103.00	0.004 *
VHD	0.75	0.19–2.91	0.68			
NYHA class III or IV on admission	0.43	0.10–1.84	0.25			
Number of previous hospitalizations for HF	0.69	0.51–0.93	0.014 *	0.63	0.44–0.91	0.014 *
Multidisciplinary support for EOLC discussions	0.29	0.09–1.00	0.05	0.15	0.03–0.91	0.039 *

OR = odds ratio; CI = confidence interval; ICM = ischemic cardiomyopathy; NICM = non-ischemic cardio myopathy; VHD = valvular heart disease; HF = heart failure; EOLC = end-of-life care. * $p < 0.05$.

4. Discussion

In this study, we compared the changes in HF therapies in terms of palliative care and EOLC discussions before and after the initiation of HF-PCT activities at our institute, with a focus on food intake at the end of life. The major findings were that after HF-PCT activities, (a) fewer invasive procedures were performed, (b) the use of opioids and non-intubated sedatives for symptom relief increased, (c) support from the multidisciplinary team in EOLC discussions increased, and (d) quality of meals was improved at the end of life in patients (from low-sodium diet to regular diet, adequate symptom relief with opioids, provision of non-hospital meals such as patients' favorite meals mainly by family members). Furthermore, the administration of artificial nutrition in the final three days prior to death was associated with NICM etiology, number of previous hospitalizations for HF, and multidisciplinary EOLC discussion support. To the best of our knowledge, this is the first report on changes in HF palliative care and end-of-life food intake after the initiation of HF-PCT activities.

4.1. End-of-Life Discussion with Patients with HF

Considering the plateau in diagnostic capacity and treatment efficacy for HF, new problems have arisen related to difficult EOLC decision-making under uncertain disease trajectories [14]. In addition, physicians often discuss EOLC with the families rather than the patients in Far East Asian countries such as China, South Korea, and Japan [15–17], where physicians and patients' families traditionally tend to avoid giving unfavorable information to patients. However, Matsushima et al. showed that 85% of English-speaking Japanese Americans desired to make treatment decisions on their own, as compared to only 36% of Japanese individuals living in Japan [18]. Another Japanese study had shown that only 4.7% of patients with end-stage HF participated in EOLC discussions [19]. In the present study, EOLC discussions were more frequent in patients who died in Era 2. Moreover, the number of patients who underwent invasive procedures prior to death was significantly lower among patients who died in Era 2. Our findings suggest that HF-PCT activities might facilitate EOLC discussions based on patient values and preferences and could avoid unnecessary invasive treatment prior to death.

The current study did not confirm the existence of the ACP process. However, EOLC discussions with patients are an extension of the ACP process. The latest survey, conducted by the Japanese Ministry of Health, Labour and Welfare in 2017, indicated that 64.9% of Japanese individuals approved ACP and that 66% of them agreed to make an advance directive [20]. Furthermore, the newly revised Japanese Guidelines on the Diagnosis and Treatment of Acute and Chronic Heart Failure consider ACP as a class I recommendation for the management of HF [9]. Reflecting such situations, ACP and patient-centered decision-making processes have become an increased focus in Japan.

4.2. Symptom Management

In this study, many patients who died in Era 2 received opioids for refractory dyspnea. Kuragaichi et al. reported in a nationwide survey that dyspnea is the most common symptom requiring palliative care in patients with HF [10]. Some small studies have shown that low-dose opioids, especially morphine, relieve breathlessness in these patients [21,22], although another study does not support this finding [23]. Further studies are required to investigate appropriate opioid use in patients with HF and refractory dyspnea. Furthermore, there has been little evidence for palliative sedation in non-cancer patients, including HF [24]; however, in this study, 36% of non-intubated patients with HF who died in Era 2 received palliative sedation. Palliative sedation is only performed to relieve intractable distress at the end of life, but not to hasten death [25]. Clinicians should discuss the indication of palliative sedation with a multidisciplinary team such as an HF-PCT in terms of the patients' benefits, goals, and risks, as well as the limited prognosis and presence of treatable factors. Psychological issues are also important problems in patients with HF. In particular, depression has an independent impact on morbidity and mortality in HF [26,27]. It is important to recognize psychological problems that may occur in the complex disease trajectory of HF. In this study, specialized psychiatric care was more often performed in patients with HF who died in Era 2; therefore, the HF-PCT may promote psychological support.

4.3. Diet in Palliative Care of Patients with HF

Food intake is extremely important in human life. Clinical evidence on the administration of artificial nutrition at the end of life is limited, even in oncology, and even more in HF. However, the goal of nutritional care at the end of life may be the same in both cancer and HF, in which it needs to change from maintaining nutritional status and function to ensure the patient's well-being and quality of life [7]. In addition, the enjoyment of food may increase when restrictions are lifted. In Era 2 of this study, patients with HF, who had maintained food intake until three days prior to death, were provided symptomatic relief using opioids and dietary modification—providing a normal diet, not a low-sodium diet. Extensive communication and psychosocial support between the healthcare team and patients and/or families are important to alleviate distress related to food intake and weight loss, eliminate false expectations about nutrition, and set goals for nutritional care [28]. In this study, discussing EOLC with multidisciplinary support was associated with a decrease in the use of artificial nutrition in the last three days of life. If HF-PCT activities provide more opportunities to discuss EOLC in the future, the administration of unnecessary artificial nutrition may be avoided, and patients may be able to enjoy their meals at the end of life.

4.4. Limitations

The present study has several limitations. First, the retrospective and single-center nature of this study, including the small number of study patients, might have resulted in a certain extent of bias. Second, patients who die at a university hospital may be a selected group, incorporating bias. Thus, future studies should include a larger population and more hospitals. Third, although palliative care should be provided at the early stage of a life-threatening illness, only patients with HF who died at our hospital were included in this study. Further research is required to confirm whether palliative care would benefit patients from an earlier stage of HF. Fourth, since this study focuses on correlations between eras, reverse causality and hidden causal relationships may exist. Fifth, Era 1 and Era 2 differ not only in the existence of HF-PCT but also in the time background of HF palliative care awareness. The time background may be responsible for the differences found between the two eras. Sixth, because of the retrospective nature of the study, we could not evaluate objective health-related quality of life indicators in determining the effectiveness of HF-PCT consultation. Seventh, we will examine a longer period before death in the next study in near future. Finally, further research is required to examine how to provide HF palliative care that is adapted to the healthcare system in Japan.

5. Conclusions

Despite increasing attention on palliative care in HF, providing optimal palliative care at the end of life presents many challenges and complexities. The present study indicated that HF-PCT activities provide an opportunity to discuss EOLC with patients, reduce the burden of physical and mental symptoms, and may shift the goals of end-of-life nutritional care to ensuring comfort and quality of life.

Author Contributions: Conceptualization, T.S., K.M., K.S. and N.N.; methodology, H.A. and Y.F.; formal analysis, T.S.; investigation, K.U., Y.Y., K.T., M.M., K.O. and T.Y.; data curation, T.S.; writing—original draft preparation, T.S.; supervision, S.N., J.T. and H.Y.; project administration, Y.F. All authors have read and agreed to the published version of the manuscript.

Funding: This research received no external funding.

Institutional Review Board Statement: The study was conducted in accordance with the guidelines of the Declaration of Helsinki and approved by the Institutional Review Board of Kurume University (No. 18066).

Informed Consent Statement: The release of research information in this study allowed us to collect and analyze data without obtaining written informed consent from each patient.

Data Availability Statement: Data supporting the results obtained in this study are available from the corresponding author upon reasonable request. All data were obtained from the subjects and are not available to the public for ethical reasons.

Acknowledgments: The authors thank the great contribution of the Heart Failure Support Team of Kurume University Hospital (Tomomi Sano, Toyoharu Oba, Takanobu Nagata, Naoki Horikawa, Hiroshi Eguchi, Koji Akasu, Kyoko Nuruki, Michiko Mukae, Moe Tokunaga, Mika Sumiyoshi, Masae Aoki, Yuki Umeno, Ryoko Fukumori, Tomoko Ishikawa, Miki Sakaguchi, Natsumi Maruyama, Yuki Kamori, Hideki Kojima, and Keiko Nishie) and all medical staff involved in this study.

Conflicts of Interest: The authors declare no conflict of interest.

References

1. Moens, K.; Higginson, I.J.; Harding, R.; Brearley, S.; Caraceni, A.; Cohen, J.; Costantini, M.; Deliens, L.; Francke, A.L.; Kaasa, S.; et al. Are There Differences in the Prevalence of Palliative Care-Related Problems in People Living with Advanced Cancer and Eight Non-Cancer Conditions? A Systematic Review. *J. Pain Symptom Manag.* **2014**, *48*, 660–677. [CrossRef]
2. Bekelman, D.B.; Havranek, E.P.; Becker, D.M.; Kutner, J.S.; Peterson, P.N.; Wittstein, I.S.; Gottlieb, S.H.; Yamashita, T.E.; Fairclough, D.L.; Dy, S.M. Symptoms, Depression, and Quality of Life in Patients with Heart Failure. *J. Card. Fail.* **2007**, *13*, 643–648. [CrossRef]
3. Allen, L.A.; Stevenson, L.W.; Grady, K.L.; Goldstein, N.E.; Matlock, D.D.; Arnold, R.M.; Cook, N.R.; Felker, G.M.; Francis, G.S.; Hauptman, P.J.; et al. Decision making in advanced heart failure: A scientific statement from the Amer-ican Heart Association. *Circulation* **2012**, *125*, 1928–1952. [CrossRef] [PubMed]
4. Allen, L.A.; Yager, J.E.; Funk, M.J.; Levy, W.C.; Tulsky, J.A.; Bowers, M.T.; Dodson, G.C.; O'Connor, C.M.; Felker, G.M. Discordance between patient-predicted and model-predicted life expectancy among am-bulatory patients with heart failure. *JAMA* **2008**, *299*, 2533–2542. [CrossRef]
5. Silveira, M.J.; Kim, S.Y.; Langa, K. Advance Directives and Outcomes of Surrogate Decision Making before Death. *N. Engl. J. Med.* **2010**, *362*, 1211–1218. [CrossRef]
6. Makino, J.; Fujitani, S.; Twohig, B.; Krasnica, S.; Oropello, J. End-of-life considerations in the ICU in Japan: Ethical and legal per-spectives. *J. Intensive Care* **2014**, *2*, 9. [CrossRef]
7. Yamamoto, K.; Tsuchihashi-Makaya, M.; Kinugasa, Y.; Iida, Y.; Kamiya, K.; Kihara, Y.; Kono, Y.; Sato, Y.; Suzuki, N.; Takeuchi, H.; et al. Japanese Heart Failure Society 2018 Scientific Statement on Nutri-tional Assessment and Management in Heart Failure Patients. *Circ. J.* **2020**, *84*, 1408–1444. [CrossRef]
8. Yancy, C.W.; Jessup, M.; Bozkurt, B.; Butler, J.; Casey, D.E., Jr.; Drazner, M.H.; Fonarow, G.C.; Geraci, S.A.; Horwich, T.; Januzzi, J.L.; et al. 2013 ACCF/AHA Guideline for the Management of Heart FailureA Report of the American College of Cardiology Foundation/American Heart Association Task Force on Practice Guidelines. *J. Am. Coll. Cardiol.* **2013**, *62*, e147–e239. [CrossRef]
9. Tsutsui, H.; Isobe, M.; Ito, H.; Okumura, K.; Ono, M.; Kitakaze, M.; Kinugawa, K.; Kihara, Y.; Goto, Y.; Komuro, I.; et al. JCS 2017/JHFS 2017 Guideline on Diagnosis and Treatment of Acute and Chronic Heart Failure—Digest Version. *Circ. J.* **2019**, *83*, 2084–2184. [CrossRef] [PubMed]

10. Kuragaichi, T.; Kurozumi, Y.; Ohishi, S.; Sugano, Y.; Sakashita, A.; Kotooka, N.; Suzuki, M.; Higo, T.; Yumino, D.; Takada, Y.; et al. Nationwide Survey of Palliative Care for Patients with Heart Failure in Japan. *Circ. J.* **2018**, *82*, 1336–1343. [CrossRef]
11. Hopp, F.P.; Zalenski, R.J.; Waselewsky, D.; Burn, J.; Camp, J.; Welch, R.D.; Levy, P. Results of a Hospital-Based Palliative Care Intervention for Patients with an Acute Exacerbation of Chronic Heart Failure. *J. Card. Fail.* **2016**, *22*, 1033–1036. [CrossRef]
12. Sidebottom, A.C.; Jorgenson, A.; Richards, H.; Kirven, J.; Sillah, A. Inpatient palliative care for patients with acute heart failure: Outcomes from a randomized trial. *J. Palliat. Med.* **2015**, *18*, 134–142. [CrossRef]
13. McKee, P.A.; Castelli, W.P.; McNamara, P.M.; Kannel, W.B. The Natural History of Congestive Heart Failure: The Framingham Study. *N. Engl. J. Med.* **1971**, *285*, 1441–1446. [CrossRef]
14. Mizuno, A.; Shibata, T.; Oishi, S. The Essence of Palliative Care Is Best Viewed as the "Problematization". *J. Palliat. Med.* **2019**, *22*, 6. [CrossRef] [PubMed]
15. Weng, L.; Joynt, G.M.; Lee, A.; Du, B.; Leung, P.; Peng, J.; Gomersall, C.D.; Hu, X.; Yap, H.Y.; Chinese Critical Care Ethics Group. Attitudes towards ethical problems in critical care medicine: The Chinese perspective. *Intensiv. Care Med.* **2011**, *37*, 655–664. [CrossRef] [PubMed]
16. Shin, D.W.; Lee, J.E.; Cho, B.; Yoo, S.H.; Kim, S.; Yoo, J.-H. End-of-life communication in Korean older adults: With focus on advance care planning and advance directives. *Geriatr. Gerontol. Int.* **2015**, *16*, 407–415. [CrossRef] [PubMed]
17. Akabayashi, A.; Slingsby, B.T.; Kai, I. Perspectives on advance directives in Japanese society: A population-based questionnaire survey. *BMC Med. Ethic.* **2003**, *4*, 5. [CrossRef] [PubMed]
18. Matsumura, S.; Bito, S.; Liu, H.; Kahn, K.; Fukuhara, S.; Kagawa-Singer, M.; Wenger, N. Acculturation of attitudes toward end-of-life care: A cross-cultural survey of Japanese Americans and Japanese. *J. Gen. Intern. Med.* **2002**, *17*, 531–539. [CrossRef] [PubMed]
19. Nakamura, K.; Kinugasa, Y.; Sugihara, S.; Hirai, M.; Yanagihara, K.; Haruki, N.; Matsubara, K.; Kato, M.; Yamamoto, K. Sex differences in surrogate decision-maker preferences for life-sustaining treatments of Japanese patients with heart failure. *ESC Heart Fail.* **2018**, *5*, 1165–1172. [CrossRef]
20. Ministry of Health, Labour and Welfare. Survey on Attitudes toward Medical Care in the End Stages of Life. Available online: https://www.mhlw.go.jp/toukei/list/dl/saisyuiryo_a_h29.pdf (accessed on 20 June 2021).
21. Johnson, M.; McDonagh, T.; Harkness, A.; McKay, S.; Dargie, H. Morphine for the relief of breathlessness in patients with chronic heart failure-a pilot study. *Eur. J. Heart Fail.* **2002**, *4*, 753–756. [CrossRef]
22. Williams, S.G.; Wright, D.J.; Marshall, P.; Reese, A.; Tzeng, B.H.; Coats, A.J.; Tan, L.B. Safety and potential benefits of low dose diamorphine during exercise in patients with chronic heart failure. *Heart* **2003**, *89*, 1085–1086. [CrossRef]
23. Oxberry, S.G.; Torgerson, D.; Bland, J.M.; Clark, A.L.; Cleland, J.G.; Johnson, M. Short-term opioids for breathlessness in stable chronic heart failure: A randomized controlled trial. *Eur. J. Heart Fail.* **2011**, *13*, 1006–1012. [CrossRef] [PubMed]
24. Swart, S.J.; Rietjens, J.A.; van Zuylen, L.; Zuurmond, W.W.; Perez, R.S.; Van Der Maas, P.J.; Van Delden, J.J.; Van Der Heide, A. Continuous Palliative Sedation for Cancer and Noncancer Patients. *J. Pain Symptom Manag.* **2012**, *43*, 172–181. [CrossRef] [PubMed]
25. Romano, M. The Role of Palliative Care in the Cardiac Intensive Care Unit. *Healthcare* **2019**, *7*, 30. [CrossRef] [PubMed]
26. Gathright, E.C.; Goldstein, C.M.; Josephson, R.A.; Hughes, J.W. Depression increases the risk of mortality in patients with heart failure: A meta-analysis. *J. Psychosom. Res.* **2017**, *94*, 82–89. [CrossRef]
27. Rutledge, T.; Reis, V.A.; Linke, S.E.; Greenberg, B.H.; Mills, P.J. Depression in Heart Failure: A Meta-Analytic Review of Prevalence, Intervention Effects, and Associations with Clinical Outcomes. *J. Am. Coll. Cardiol.* **2006**, *48*, 1527–1537. [CrossRef]
28. Orrevall, Y. Nutritional support at the end of life. *Nutrition* **2015**, *31*, 615–616. [CrossRef]

MDPI
St. Alban-Anlage 66
4052 Basel
Switzerland
Tel. +41 61 683 77 34
Fax +41 61 302 89 18
www.mdpi.com

Nutrients Editorial Office
E-mail: nutrients@mdpi.com
www.mdpi.com/journal/nutrients

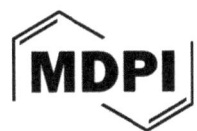

www.ingramcontent.com/pod-product-compliance
Lightning Source LLC
LaVergne TN
LVHW070715100526
838202LV00013B/1098